THE ENCYCLOPEDIA OF
HEALING
PLANTS

Also by Chrissie Wildwood

The Complete Guide to Reducing Stress

Create Your Own Aromatherapy Perfumes

The Bloomsbury Encyclopedia of Aromatherapy

Sensual Aromatherapy

The Aromatherapy and Massage Book

Aromatherapy Massage with Essential Oils

Flower Remedies For Women

Flower Remedies, Natural Healing with Flower Essences

The Book of Aromatherapy Blends

Aromatherapy Made Easy

THE ENCYCLOPEDIA OF HEALING PLANTS

A Complete Guide to Aromatherapy, Flower Essences & Herbal Remedies

CHRISSIE WILDWOOD

PIATKUS

First published in 1998 by
Judy Piatkus (Publishers) Ltd
5 Windmill Street, London W1P 1HF

This paperback edition published in 1999

The moral right of the author has been asserted

A catalogue record for this book is available from the British Library

ISBN 0-7499-1710-5 hbk
ISBN 0-7499-1875-6 pbk

Edited by ESTHER JAGGER
Designed by PAUL SAUNDERS
Plant watercolours by LYNN CHADWICK/ILLUSTRATION
Massage illustrations by BIZ HULL/ARTISTS PARTNERS
Decorative illustrations by MADELEINE DAVID

Data capture and manipulation by
Create Publishing Services, Bath
Printed in Great Britain by
Bath Press Colourbooks, Blantyre, Scotland
Bound at The Bath Press, Bath

CONTENTS

ACKNOWLEDGEMENTS

Many thanks to everyone who contributed in some way towards the birth of this book. First, Peter Lemesurier (historian) for his invaluable comments and advice and for dispelling a few myths about the life and work of Paracelsus; Sue Minter (Curator of the Chelsea Physic Garden) and Dr Peter Houghton (Department of Pharmacology, King's College Hospital) for their help in exploring the herbal uses of certain plants employed in the Bach flower system of healing; Moira Gardiner (Assistant Librarian at the Glasgow Homoeopathic Hospital) for allowing me to make use of some interesting research material concerning agents which have been found to antidote homoeopathic medicines; Dr Peter Wilde for explaining the Phytonics process of extraction and for sending me some intriguing aromatic samples; and to members of staff at Weleda (UK) Ltd, Amyris Essential Oils, Simmonds Herbal Suppliers and Higher Nature for their informed opinions and advice. I am also indebted to the research team at *What Doctors Don't Tell You* for responding so generously to my numerous queries and for producing a highly informative periodical. A big thank you to Lynn Chadwick (illustrator of the remedy plants) for all her hard work and artistic talent, also to Biz Hull for the massage pictures and Madeleine David for the fillers. Finally, I would like to thank everyone at Piatkus for believing in this project, especially Anne Lawrance for her unflustered competence and empathetic nature.

INTRODUCTION

WITH THE CURRENT DELUGE of books on the various aspects of botanic medicine, what makes this one different? It is the first in-depth guide to the combined use of aromatherapy, herbal remedies and flower essences for healing body, mind and soul. Although aimed at people wishing to employ plant remedies to promote health and vitality in themselves and their families, this book will interest students and practitioners of any of the three branches of botanic medicine. It will also prove useful to proponents of other therapeutic approaches (including orthodox medicine) who feel drawn to the idea of incorporating at least one aspect of green healing as an adjunct to their work.

THE BENEFITS OF THE COMBINED APPROACH

It is common for the newly-qualified health practitioner to adopt a kind of missionary zeal about the virtues of their chosen therapeutic tool. With experience comes the realisation that no single therapy is effective, by itself, for *every* health problem, nor for *every* individual, nor in *every* circumstance. It must often be used in conjunction with other supportive measures. For example, while herbal remedies work slowly towards easing the pain and stiffness of arthritis, an aromatherapy massage can bring immediate relief. As the herbs (which are usually combined with dietary reform, salt baths and gentle exercise)

begin to take effect, the frequency of massage treatments can be gradually reduced. Eventually, pain and stiffness can be greatly relieved by means of a sensible diet and lifestyle, perhaps supported by an occasional aromatherapy massage.

Flower therapy is perhaps the most versatile of the three healing tools because it works solely on the psycho-spiritual level and will not interfere with any other therapeutic measure – in fact, it enhances other forms of treatment. Unlike most systems of healing, however, the flower remedies' mode of action is impossible to describe in ordinary materialistic terms. While some people regard the flower remedies (also known as flower essences) as a form of spiritual healing from the plant kingdom – a merging of human intent with the spiritual essence of flowers – others of a more pragmatic nature categorise them as a form of energy medicine. Flower therapy is also commonly described as vibrational medicine.

The best known system of vibrational medicine is homeopathy, which flower therapy mimics to a degree. While both systems employ minute amounts of medicinal agents, the effects of homeopathic medicines, however, are quite different from those of flower remedies (see pages 158–9). Although the basic principles of homeopathy are explored, and a few homeopathic remedies are profiled, such information should not be regarded as prescriptive. Homeopathic references are included solely to round out the picture, to enable you to glimpse the multi-dimensional potential of healing plants.

Above all, since homeopathy also encompasses medicines of animal and mineral origin, it cannot be regarded as a branch of botanic medicine.

ACTIVATING THE VITAL FORCE

As this book sets out to prove, whatever the therapeutic tool (including conventional drug therapy), successful treatment involves something over and above the material element. While orthodox medicine denigrates this unknown quantity by referring to it as the placebo effect, complementary therapists welcome the phenomenon, but recognise it as the self-healing process. Without doubt, the restoration of health and a sense of wellbeing is dependent upon the activation of this latent force.

Conventional drug treatment, on the other hand, aims to suppress symptoms as quickly as possible. Side-effects (unfortunately, sometimes long-term problems) are regarded as the inevitable price we must pay for a quick fix, no matter how temporary. From an ecological perspective, the over-use of antibiotics (especially over the last thirty years) has created highly resistant strains of bacteria so that problems become even more unyielding to treatment. Yet by taking steps to strengthen the body's immune defences, which may have become weakened through suppressive treatments and an unbalanced way of living, we become more receptive to the gentle healing actions of plant-based therapies.

Aromatherapy, herbalism and flower therapy, in common with all *holistic* systems of healing, aim to strengthen the *mind/body's* self-healing capacity. This approach requires more time and effort and may even demand a complete overview of one's conditioned attitudes, dietary habits and way of living.

The holistic therapist also recognises that the key to good health and a sense of wellbeing lies in the realisation that we need not become victims of our own distress. In a world permeated with mechanical noise, electromagnetic radiation, exhaust fumes, industrial pollutants, cigarette smoke, devitalised food, deadlines, job insecurity and much else besides, little wonder that psycho-physical stress is at the root of almost all illness. Even in cases of hereditary illness, it is widely recognised that emotional disharmony can exacerbate existing symptoms.

However, almost everyone can take steps to buffer the adverse effects of stress. This can be achieved through simple measures such as eating a varied wholefood diet, taking a brisk half-hour walk every day and allowing time in your daily routine for some form of nurturing, creative or frivolous activity – something that enables you to completely unwind. This can be anything from sitting with your feet up with a nice cup of tea, listening to the birds, playing with the children, flying a kite, dancing to music on the radio, singing at the top of your voice whilst doing the dishes, having a long soak in the bath, putting on some uplifting music – or having a good belly laugh with friends! Indeed, one of the basic tenets of holistic philosophy is to rediscover the simple joys of life.

The ability to surrender to joy enables us to connect with the spiritual aspect of self. The spiritual aspect is our guiding impulse, the part we call 'I', the part which is aware of our true purpose in life. When we lose sight of our own sense of purpose, perhaps as a result of following the dictates of others, we become depressed or apathetic; life then appears bleak and meaningless. Even when we do not follow a conscious spiritual path in terms of a religious faith, we may in fact be realising our purpose in some other way. It could be through painting, writing, gardening, or some other creative outlet no matter how humble, or simply through our work, family, relationships, a love of animals or nature – or more actively perhaps by working towards the realisation of a humanitarian ideal.

THE VISION OF HOLISM

The vision of the holistic healer, and indeed all those within the green movement, is that the expression of such qualities as compassion, intuition, and nurturing will raise the consciousness of humanity as a whole. In so doing, we will once again honour the living earth, as did the green healers and farmers of antiquity, realising that we are an interrelated part of nature and the cosmos. Of course, putting intuition back into medicine does not mean we have to go completely overboard into the realms of earth magic at the total expense of rational thought. There needs to be a marriage between the two seemingly opposing principles – between the archetypal Feminine and Masculine. In other words, we need to integrate science with mysticism, and the best of orthodox medicine with the best of the gentler approaches. For as day cannot exist without night, nor the sun without the moon, the high-tech approach to medicine is dehumanised without the balance of intuition and feeling.

THE PATTERN OF THIS BOOK

The book is divided into three parts and offers a complete overview of green medicine. Although certain conclusions have been drawn from ancient healing philosophies, the modified approach advocated is entirely compatible with current modes of living and thinking.

Part 1 begins with a history of botanic medicine, revealing how ancient peoples displayed a profound understanding of the interrelatedness of mankind, nature and the cosmos. With the growing interest in the esoteric and in traditional medicine, this approach is once again highly topical. This section of the book includes an overview of plant chemistry explained in simple terms, followed by an intriguing diversion into realms of vibrational healing. Undoubtedly, the material things health practitioners do for their patients are not the sum total of the medicine they practise. This chapter is followed by a comprehensive section on working with herbal remedies, essential oils and flower essences. It includes a clearly illustrated, step-by-step guide to massage with aromatic oils, and offers detailed advice on harvesting and preparing herbal medicines, blending essential oils, and potentising flower essences.

Part 2 is concerned with the practice of green healing. It begins with an introductory chapter on the philosophy of holism, including advice on promoting health and vitality through good nutrition, movement, correct breathing, deep relaxation, guided imagery and meditation. The rest of this section comprises clearly presented charts outlining holistic treatment strategies for many common ailments, ranging from anxiety, depression and stress, through to chronic conditions such as arthritis, eczema and asthma. Special attention is given to women's health, including advice on safe and effective hormone-free treatments for PMS and menopausal distress.

Part 3 is a comprehensive directory providing details of over 80 healing plants, listing their properties and their main uses in herbalism, aromatherapy, homeopathy and flower therapy. The majority of the plants are illustrated in beautiful watercolour – just looking at the paintings can be a healing experience in itself!

To help you choose the correct flower essences for yourself and others there is a comprehensive repertory of emotional and psychological states in the Appendices. This is followed by a repertory of common health problems, along with suggested herbal remedies and essential oils. Here you will also find glossaries of botanical, medical and general terms used throughout the book, plus a useful addresses section and suggested reading list.

TAKING IT FURTHER

If you would like to train in any of the therapies explored in this book, contact the appropriate umbrella organisation given in the Useful Addresses section (see page 264). Although the majority of accredited training courses are primarily aimed at those intending to gain professional qualifications, most schools also conduct short introductory workshops for those wishing to learn how to use herbal medicines, essential oils, homoeopathic remedies and flower essences at home.

At the time of writing, I am discussing with colleagues the possibility of founding a new school of healing incorporating aromatherapy, flower therapy and herbal medicine. To find out more, readers can write to me c/o Piatkus Books.

Chrissie Wildwood
Midsummer, 1997

PART ONE

THE
FOUNDATIONS

There is life on earth – one life, which embraces every animal and plant on the planet. Time has divided it up into several million parts, but each is an integral part of the whole. A rose is a rose, but it is also a robin and a rabbit. We are all of one flesh, drawn from the same crucible.

LYALL WATSON, SUPERNATURE, 1973

CHAPTER ONE

A POTTED HISTORY
OF BOTANIC MEDICINE

BOTANIC MEDICINE has been practised by all peoples and cultures since the beginning of time. Even without prior knowledge of the pharmacological properties of the remedies employed, it is remarkable how often the same plants are administered for the same purposes in primitive cultures all over the world. Moreover, biochemical analysis of traditional plant remedies usually verifies their specific curative properties. But how did our forebears discover the healing plants in the first place?

IN THE BEGINNING

In the wild, animals instinctively eat the kind of food that nourishes them, ignoring whatever is poisonous. And when feeling unwell most creatures (even carnivores like dogs and cats) will nibble on certain medicinal plants to make them feel better. Likewise, our early ancestors were endowed with finely attuned senses which are today seen only in the few remaining native tribes. We in the industrialised world perceive our environment through comparatively dulled senses, presumably because we no longer rely on our animal instincts for sheer survival.

Not only did our early ancestors find edible and medicinal plants, they discovered those which they believed were endowed with magical powers: for example, narcotic or hallucinogenic plants like cannabis resin, the opium poppy and henbane. Such plants were deemed sacred and were used only by the shaman, the tribal medicine man or woman. When taken as a drug – with the help of ritualistic drumming, dancing and chanting – they facilitated entry into the trance state. This enabled the shaman to intercommunicate with the ancestral Great Ones and with nature spirits.

Since illness was generally attributed to loss of soul power (the sick person's soul having been abstracted by spirits), the shaman's function was to go in pursuit of that soul and arrange for its return. The ritual would almost always involve 'smoking' the patient with smouldering incense to facilitate the healing process. Echoes of this practice remain in our modern word 'perfume', derived from Latin *per fumen*, which means 'through the smoke'.

By the time European explorers and missionaries started to involve themselves with tribal peoples in Africa and elsewhere, diagnosis and treatment had become what observers regarded as rational. The shaman performed consciously, administering herbal drugs and dealing with fractures and dislocations. Nevertheless, the psychic element survived. Herbs were often found by dowsing, either by using a pendulum or by holding the hands above the plant in order to sense the healing vibrations, and administered with the assistance of a spell or incantation.

ANCIENT EGYPT AND MESOPOTAMIA

For centuries, the vast repository of herbal lore was passed down by way of the oral tradition. However, with the development of the early civilisations came the first drug inventories. The oldest of these are the cuneiform clay tablets of Mesopotamia (modern Iraq) and the medical papyri of Egypt. From such records we learn that magic was still included in many prescriptions, which often featured exorcism to drive out evil spirits responsible for disease.

Interestingly, archaeological evidence suggests that many Egyptians produced 'sheep' faeces, which are caused by intestinal cramps and tend to be associated with stress and agitation. This tells us that a pressurised lifestyle lay behind many of their health problems. Some of the remedies employed for 'freeing and provoking' obstinate stools included castor oil and sycamore seed. In addition, they used enemas of water, beer or milk.

The Ancient Egyptians are generally regarded as the true founders of aromatherapy; indeed, their knowledge of aromatic plants was considerable. Aromatics were employed in a variety of ways for religious, cosmetic and medicinal purposes (including body massage with perfumed oils), and plant essences were integral to the process of embalming. The survival of Egyptian mummies over thousands of years is a tribute not just to the skills of the embalmers, but also to the amazing preservative powers of aromatic oils and resins. When in recent times forensic scientists unwrapped a three-thousand-year-old mummy, myrrh and cedarwood could still be smelt on the inner bandages.

Among further uses, aromatics were employed as fumigants and as mood-altering incense. Some of the most potent psycho-active blends are known to us today because their formulae were carved on the stone walls of special chambers within temples where the priest-healers made up their fragrant prescriptions. Unfortunately, however, some of the plants are referred to only by their local names which cannot now be deciphered. But if pollen samples and other residues of these mystery aromatics are found and analysed in modern laboratories it is possible that the compounds can be re-created.

One of these concoctions, Kyphi, is known to have included at least sixteen ingredients: a mixture of calamus (which contains a narcotic and hallucinogenic substance called asarone), saffron, cassia, spikenard, cinnamon and juniper, were worked into a paste with honey, raisins and wine. The result was burned as soporific incense, taken as medicine, or applied to wounds and skin disorders. However, Egyptians' aromatic compounds were not all plant-based and sometimes contained substances of mineral and animal origin such as lead, alabaster, saltpetre, serpent skin, crocodile dung and spittle!

For many years archaeologists believed that the Ancient Egyptians had no knowledge of distillation, a skill attributed to the Arabs and Persians of the eleventh century AD. The majority of the Egyptian healing oils and unguents involved blending aromatic plant material into a base of vegetable oil or animal fat, then leaving it for some weeks to infuse in the heat of the sun. Interestingly, distillation pots have been found at Tepe Gawra, near ancient Nineveh. They are thought to date back to 3500 BC, which suggests that the technological achievements of the Mesopotamians have been underrated. Moreover, the drug inventories of Egypt, Mesopotamia and India show such remarkable similarities that there was obviously continual exchange of ideas and practices.

Unlike the Ancient Egyptian prescriptions, those of the Mesopotamians gave neither weights nor measures. It would seem that there was a tacit understanding among physicians regarding the matter of dosage. We know that the time of day when the medicine was prepared and administered was seen as important. Medicinal brews were usually prepared in the evening and taken by the patient in the morning before eating, with a second dose being taken at sundown. A 'tea' for stimulating the flow of bile, for example, contained pine resin, galbanum (a bitter gum resin), mustard and glasswort (*Salicornia* spp.) Modern herbalists would confirm that the effect of this herbal compound would be the same as that suggested by the ancients.

THE MEDICINE OF CHINA AND INDIA

A parallel development in plant medicine took place in China. Ancient Chinese knowledge of the effects of drugs on living organisms was incredibly advanced, and indeed continues to impress and amaze researchers. The compendium entitled *Pen-Ts'ao Kang-Mu*, reputed to be the work of the

Emperor Shen-nung (3737–2697 BC), records in its final published version of AD 1597 a vast array of medicinal substances used as drugs. These include ginseng root, star anise, camphor, pomegranate root, and the minerals arsenic, iron, mercury and sulphur. Legend has it that the Emperor deliberately poisoned himself many times over, but always managed to find an antidote! Remarkably, even though the bubonic plague bacillus was not discovered until the late nineteenth century, the Chinese had long understood that there was a connection between fleas and rats in propagating the disease.

Meanwhile in India, the Ayurvedic system of healing had developed to an advanced degree. The name comes from two Sanskrit words, *ayus* or 'life' and *veda*, meaning 'knowledge'. Its principal aim is the prolongation of life. The roots of this complex system of healing are believed to date back more than five thousand years. Just like traditional Chinese herbal medicine (and acupuncture), Ayurveda has enjoyed an unbroken tradition of practice for thousands of years. As well as plant medicines, it incorporates dietetics, hydrotherapy (water cure), aromatherapy massage, yoga and meditation. Ayurveda continues to evolve, and now embraces more recently developed therapies such as homeopathy and flower therapy.

Ancient Indian philosophy and medicinal formulae have been preserved in priestly collections such as the *Rig Veda*. The botanical medicines of India became known throughout Asia, finding their way into the pharmacopoeias of Middle Eastern countries and eventually into Europe. The best-known Indian botanicals are spices like black pepper, cloves, cardamom, ginger, cinnamon and nutmeg. Other indispensable plant remedies include aloe vera, sandalwood (the essential oil), sesame oil and castor oil.

THE GREEKS AND ROMANS

The medicinal knowledge of the Egyptians and Mesopotamians was absorbed by Greek physicians. Hippocrates (c.460–377 BC), known as the 'father of medicine', was one of the Asclepiadae, a group of physicians named after Aesculapius, a deified healer whose name means 'always gentle'.

Hippocrates' approach to medicine was pragmatic yet holistic, relying on observation rather than magic. He taught his students to treat the whole person, not just the symptoms of disease; to examine not just the individual on the sickbed, but also the life and habits of that person; and to nurture the latent capacity of the human body to heal itself. This recommended treatment therefore included dietetics, 'Let food be your medicine and medicine your food'; hydrotherapy; fresh air and sunlight; adequate exercise; and aromatherapy massage. So effective were these, especially massage with aromatic oils, that the philosopher Plato is said to have reproached Herodicus, one of Hippocrates' teachers, for protracting the miserable existence of the aged!

According to Hippocrates, disease is the consequence of some imbalance in the body's 'humours' (a similar theory is expounded in the healing philosophies of China and India). He held that there were four vital principles: Earth, Water, Fire and Air. The representatives of these four principles in the human organism are the four body fluids or cardinal humours: blood, phlegm, yellow bile and black bile. When these are in harmony, a person is healthy; when one of these elements is deficient or excessive, a person becomes ill.

An excess of phlegm (Water), for example, gives rise to 'cold' problems like lethargy, catarrh, respiratory infections and fluid retention. Therefore, warming and drying plant remedies like thyme, cinnamon, and ginger would be prescribed to correct the imbalance. An excess of yellow bile (Fire), on the other hand, results in 'hot' symptoms such as angry outbursts, and liver and digestive problems. In such cases, cooling and moistening herbs like dandelion and violet were perceived as restoring equilibrium.

The Greeks also liked to decorate their heads with chaplets and garlands of sweet-smelling flowers, in order to harness the psychotherapeutic properties of scent. The physician Marestheus wrote a treatise on the subject, dividing plants into those which depressed the spirits and caused fatigue, and those which had an exhilarating effect. The rose, the hyacinth and most fruity or spicy scents were found to invigorate a tired mind; the lily and narcissus, on the other hand, were deemed oppressive and said to create feelings of tiredness.

In the first century AD the Greek physician Dioscorides, who served under the Roman Emperor Nero, completed his impressive herbal *De Materia Medica*. Building on the work of Hippocrates, it contained monographs of over five hundred medicinal plants and set the pattern for professional herbals in the succeeding centuries.

Claudius Galenus or Galen, who was born around AD 130, began his career as a physician in the school for gladiators in Alexandria and later became the personal physician to the Emperor and philosopher Marcus Aurelius in Rome. His teachings were based on the findings of Hippocrates, but he also pursued his own studies, recording the results in eleven books, notably *De Simplicibus*, a tome which was to become a major source for Arabian physicians.

However, many of Galen's prescriptions were unnecessarily elaborate and costly. For example Galene, based on an older Egyptian formula called Theriac, contained dozens of plant extracts mixed with honey and wine, along with scraps of viper's flesh and a little bitumen for good measure! Galene (which was popular right up until the nineteenth century) was said to be a sovereign remedy for all imaginable poisons and ills, even bubonic plague!

Since the Romans adopted the ways of the Greeks in most matters, they contributed little of their own to the development of medicine. However, they certainly led the way in hygiene, and in particular to the provision of abundant supplies of pure water. As well as extolling the virtues of naturally warm spa waters to ease rheumatic pain and alleviate skin diseases, they were particularly fond of aromatherapy massage. The wealthy would while away their days at the baths, being rubbed with perfumed oils by slaves skilled in the art of pummelling and kneading.

According to historical records, the educated classes in Imperial Rome were highly susceptible to nervous complaints and mental illness. This tells us something about the exacting demands of the Roman educational system and indeed about the competitive and insecure nature of life in general. Add to this the whims of the various mentally unbalanced Emperors, and it is little wonder that stress was a major cause of illness.

THE PHYSICIANS OF PERSIA AND ARABIA

With the decline of the Roman Empire from about the third century AD, and the subsequent period of apparent stagnation known as the Dark Ages, came the rise of the Arabian Empire. Seats of learning were established and encouraged at Baghdad, Cordova and Toledo. The Middle Eastern physicians were able to draw not only on Greek and Egyptian teaching, but also on the Ayurvedic and Persian traditions.

Prominent among them was the Persian physician, philosopher and mathematician Avicenna (AD 980–1037). He is credited with having perfected the art of distillation for capturing the essential oils of aromatic plants and producing alcohol. So advanced was his method that the apparatus for distillation has barely altered in nine hundred years. He chose for his first experiments the favourite flower of the Middle East, the rose, from which he succeeded in extracting attar of roses (a semi-sold perfume) and rosewater, a by-product of the distillation process. For centuries afterwards, 'perfumes of Arabia' were the most precious in the world.

During his seven years as court physician in Isfahan (1014–21), Avicenna completed his monumental *Canon Medicinae* in which he describes 811 medicinal substances. Many of the plant medicines are of Indian, Tibetan and Chinese origin, though not all have been identified. As well as aromatic remedies like camphor, chamomile, lavender and rose, he was not averse to administering poisonous minerals like mercury and lead. Avicenna's treatments also encompassed dietetics, massage therapy and traction (for fractured and dislocated limbs).

THE HEALING TRADITIONS OF BRITAIN

Even before the Romans introduced many of their own plants to the British Isles, knowledge of the native herbal lore was extensive. The traditions of the Druid priest-healers, for instance, dated back to thousands of years before Christ. They were highly skilled in the use of medicinal plants, which included their seven sacred herbs: clover, henbane, monks-hood, pasque flower, primrose, vervain and mistle-toe. Julius Caesar's Druid friend Divitiacus the Aeduan told him about the remarkable properties of the mistletoe, also known as all-heal, which was deemed the most magical of all plants.

As a point of interest, biochemical analysis of the leaves shows that mistletoe is primarily sedative, tonic and diuretic (in common with many other plants) and therefore hardly a panacea. But since tra-ditional plant lore has so often proved to have solid foundations, homeopathic doctors in Switzerland carried out extensive research on the whole plant (leaves, stems, berries and flowers). The remarkable results were published in the *British Homoeopathic Journal* in 1969. The remedy appears to have anti-tumour activity, and is reported to be beneficial in the treatment of certain forms of cancer. None the less, conventional medical science dismisses the claim as unproven.

The oldest remaining Saxon herbal is *The Leech Book of Bald*, 'leech' being the old name for a healer or doctor. The book was written in the tenth century AD by a herbalist named Bald, who was closely asso-ciated with the court of King Alfred. The Saxons thought that many diseases were the work of mali-cious elves which could only be kept under control by the use of magic spells, charms and herbal remedies. One typical remedy from *The Leech Book* is a salve to ward off the dark elves responsible for causing nightmares and nocturnal visions. It contained fourteen herbs, including wormwood, henbane, viper's bugloss, garlic and fennel, which were boiled together with butter and mutton fat. The salve was then applied to the patient's feet, head and eyelids, accompanied by incantations.

Alongside the Druid priest-healers and Anglo-Saxon leeches was an independent school of healers in Wales, known as the physicians of Myddfai. This tradition was well established by the time the first emissaries of Christianity arrived in the sixth century, and continued into the eighteenth century. It was Hippocratic in its emphasis and therefore holistic in its approach, looking for the causes of a disease as well as attempting to alleviate its symptoms.

Unlike Galen, the Myddfai healers preferred to use herbs singly, though occasionally combined with a few others, when making their infusions, oint-ments and poultices. Their favourite plant remedies included garlic for troublesome coughs; elecampane for suspected consumption; lily roots pounded with egg white to dress burns; and white horehound for pneumonia.

Most of the Myddfai prescriptions (recorded in a manuscript now housed in the British Museum) are for eye complaints, skin disorders, broken bones, wounds, chest diseases and intestinal worms. There are few prescriptions for nervous conditions, heart problems, rheumatism and arthritis, disorders which are common today. This suggests that a great deal of illness stemmed from poor living conditions. For ex-ample, smoky fires affecting the eyes; worms affecting the gut; and damp, unhygienic housing contributing to lung disease.

THE MONASTIC INFLUENCE

During the Dark Ages, when much of European culture was suppressed or destroyed, the task of keeping alive official herbal knowledge fell to the monasteries, where monks copied out texts, practised healing and tended their vegetable and herb gardens. Under the Holy Roman Empire, which was subse-quently established by Charlemagne in the late eighth century and covered a large part of western Europe, monks (and convent nuns) were ordered to devote their lives to caring for sick people – their own, the poor and passing strangers.

Until the first universities were established, in the eleventh and twelfth centuries, the monks were also responsible for training physicians. However, neither the Church nor the physicians approved of unautho-rised healers like illiterate herbalists and village midwives. This attitude led to an horrific persecution of alleged witches in the late fifteenth century.

Yet the monastic healers drew on herbals like *The Leech Book of Bald*, whose prescriptions are often accompanied by magical incantations. They also had partial access to classical texts which came back with Crusaders from the Middle East. The Crusaders also brought exotic spices and complex herbal com-pounds – the legendary 'perfumes of Arabia' – together with the knowledge of distillation.

Since the Church had condemned bathing as a sin, people smothered their unwashed bodies and clothes with perfume and carried little bouquets of aromatic herbs (tussie mussies) to mask the stench of the filthy streets. It was also the custom in Medieval Europe to strew sweet-smelling herbs like lavender, thyme and rosemary on the floor, which released their aromas when crushed underfoot. Most aromatic plants have insecticidal and bactericidal properties, so they must have played an important role in helping to ward off infectious illness.

Nevertheless, plant remedies proved powerless against the greatest scourge of all – bubonic plague. Alas, in its slow journey westwards the Black Death spread to Europe in 1348, killing off an estimated third of its population. The physicians tried every therapy known to contemporary medicine, including blood-letting and fumigation with aromatic plant material to destroy 'the corruption of the air': flight or seclusion proved more effective.

At the close of the Middle Ages, treatment for the sick – for those who could afford it – was largely in the hands of physicians dedicated to Galen. The poor continued to rely on self-medication reinforced by the ministrations of the village wise-woman, cunning man or bonesetter, a person with a natural talent for healing fractures and correcting dislocations.

Orthodox treatment involved prescribing increasingly complex apothecary compounds, alongside brutal practices such as cauterising, purging and blood-letting to 'evacuate excess humours'. This was all quite different from Hippocrates' approach, which aimed to balance the humours using plant remedies, dietetics and other reasonable measures. The concept of holism – that the body will heal itself if given the right conditions – had sunk almost out of sight.

It should be mentioned, however, that blood-letting was developed with a degree of wisdom, even though it was then commonly misapplied. A recent survey has revealed that cardiovascular disease is very low among blood donors. Apparently, people (usually men) who are prone to heart attacks and strokes have an extremely high blood viscosity and red corpuscle count. Regular donation of blood makes the blood more fluid and lowers the red corpuscle count, thus lessening the danger of thrombosis and stroke.

PARACELSUS THE REVOLUTIONARY

After the invention of printing at the end of the fifteenth century, herbals were among the first and most popular books to be published and widely circulated. However, many errors were perpetuated by European scholars who sometimes misinterpreted the classical texts which formed the mainstay of medicinal knowledge. With the spread of such information (and misinformation) came the opportunity to re-examine the treatises of Avicenna and Galen. The most vociferous of the nonconformists was the Swiss German physician and alchemist Phillipus Aureolus Theophrastus Bombastus von Hohenheim, popularly known as Paracelsus (1493–1541).

In 1515 Paracelsus received his doctorate in medical science at the famous school for physicians at Ferrara in Italy. He also studied at many of the leading European universities, published numerous books and exchanged ideas with the most learned men of his time. But he never assumed that the learned knew everything, and neither did he imagine that the unschooled were ignorant. Much of his life was spent travelling through Europe and Russia, learning the ways of gypsies, wise-women and other folk-healers.

Paracelsus came to reject contemporary medicine's over-reliance on classical texts, abstract reason, complex compounds and cathartic treatments. Far from being curative, such methods, he considered, were downright harmful. He also criticised the apothecaries' preference for costly foreign medicines, when an abundance of medicinal herbs could be found growing locally.

In a theatrical display of defiance he publicly burned the works of Avicenna and Galen, provoking the wrath of established authorities everywhere. In 1529 he humiliated the medical establishment further by offering to cure any patient deemed incurable – and promptly succeeded with nine out of fifteen lepers! But despite his incredible healing skills, many of his contemporaries refused to recognise his genius, preferring instead to remain entrenched in ancient dogma.

Paracelsus believed it was his mission to found a new medical science based on experiment, observation and a philosophy of correspondences between the macrocosm and the microcosm – a philosophy which acknowledged the evidence of the senses and the interrelatedness of mankind, nature and the universe. Although he rejected Galenism, he accepted the wisdom of the Hippocratic school's reliance upon nature's healing force. However, he took the theory a stage further, believing that the genuine physician was a magus capable of channelling cosmic energy into medicinal substances and thus increasing their effectiveness.

His belief in cosmic correspondences made him a proponent of the Doctrine of Signatures, an understanding which was also shared by Hippocrates. According to the Doctrine, plants have been signed by their Creator with visible clues to their usefulness. For example, yellow-flowered plants such as dandelion and celandine are effective against jaundice. The perforations in the leaves of St John's wort infer its usefulness in the treatment of wounds. The skullcap flower resembles the shape of the human skull, which suggests its ability to alleviate headaches and insomnia. In fact, the biochemical constituents of the aforementioned plants confirm their efficacy in the conditions for which they have been used for centuries.

So Paracelsus denounced the humoral theory and its dependence on the healing power of contraries: for instance, a 'hot' remedy would cure a 'cold' ailment. Instead, he subscribed to the axiom which three centuries later became the basis of homeopathy: that like is cured by like. For example, he treated kidney stones with powdered lapis lazuli (a gemstone) and scorpion poisoning with highly diluted scorpion venom. He also employed chemical remedies like mercury (for syphilis) and arsenic (for tumours) – but in minute, carefully calculated doses, and in chemically treated formulations.

Unfortunately, the physicians and quacks who followed Paracelsus' lead gave metallic medicine a bad press. They administered infinitely larger doses of poisonous substances, often with devastating results. The use of mercury for treating syphilis, for example, produced some horrific side-effects such as

excessive salivation (several pints a day), terrible grimacing, loss of teeth, disintegration of the jaw, tremors and sometimes total paralysis. Although the disease might be eradicated, the treatment killed many sufferers. In fact, dying of syphilis was a rather better option than the so-called cure.

Even though Paracelsus is popularly perceived as being the founder of pharmaceutical chemistry, he never abandoned the use of herbal remedies. He also employed the essential oils of aromatic plants which he distilled in his laboratory. The fragrances of plant essences, he believed, were of a similar nature to the human spirit and therefore capable of healing psychic distress.

Contrary to popular belief, Paracelsus' lifelong search for the essential virtue of substances was somewhat different from the modern preoccupation with isolating from a medicinal plant its biochemical 'active principle'. Paracelsus was seeking a soul-like force which he believed determined the nature of a substance rather than its (visible) chemical components. He regarded substances as merely crystallised deposits of an underlying vibrational force which he called *Archeus*. Hippocrates called it *vis medicatrix naturae*. In India it has always been called *prana*; in China it is known as *ch'i*.

ENGLISH HERBALS AND HERBALISTS

The best-known of the English herbals are those of John Gerard (1545–1607) and Nicholas Culpeper (1616–54). Gerard, the Elizabethan physician who superintended the gardens of Elizabeth I's great statesman Lord Burghley, combined his delight in flowers and plants with a practical knowledge and philosophy. In 1597 he published his *Historie of Plants*, which was also an intriguing compendium of plant folklore. It was in 1653 that Culpeper, a London astrologer and physician, published *The English Physician, or Herball*. His interest in astrology lends additional fascination to the work, despite the fact that he is much criticised by modern herbalists for combining occultism with the serious practice of herbalism.

HOMEOPATHY

In the eighteenth century the German physician Samuel Christian Hahnemann (1755–1843) became disillusioned with medicine as it was then being practised. Like Paracelsus, he was appalled by the constant use of purging and blood-letting, and by the highly complex, exorbitantly priced (and often ineffective) apothecary brews. And so he began to cast around for an alternative.

In 1790 he decided to research the effects of *Cinchona*, a South American bark from which quinine is derived, and which was the primary treatment for malaria. Experimenting on himself, Hahnemann found that decoctions of the bark produced in his own body the same kind of feverish symptoms as were experienced by people who had malaria. When he stopped taking the drug, all the symptoms gradually disappeared.

Over several years he continued experimenting, both on himself and on healthy volunteers, with other drugs then in current use. He had similar results, and concluded that a remedy can cure a disease if it produces in a healthy person symptoms similar to those of the disease. He had, in fact, stumbled upon the Law of Similars – that like will be cured by like. The system of healing which developed from these initial experiments Hahnemann called 'homeopathy', from the Greek *homoios* (similar) and *pathos* (suffering). He called conventional medicine 'allopathy', meaning 'opposite suffering', because it employs contrary remedies such as the treatment of constipation with laxatives.

Hahnemann was then inspired to seek the smallest possible dose needed for medicines to remain effective. He discovered that if he were to succuss (shake vigorously) his remedies each time he diluted them, this would dramatically increase their potency. Although the material substance (the actual quantity of the drug) became less and less during the process of dilution and succussion, amazingly the potency continued to increase. He believed that shaking released the energy of the substance (involving some kind of imprinting on the water/alcohol solvent), with none of its toxic effects remaining.

Hahnemann numbered the potentised remedies according to the number of times they had been diluted and succussed: a remedy diluted to one part in ten is termed 1× or first decimal potency. When a drop of the 1× solution is similarly diluted and succussed it becomes a 2×, and so on. The most commonly used potency is 6×, which means that the drug is present in the dilution as one part per million. However, once a substance like sea salt has been diluted to the 30th potency, not a single molecule of the material is left in the test solution – and yet the remedy remains effective.

Today, homeopaths may prescribe infinitely higher potencies, for example, 1M (diluted one thousand times), 10M (ten thousand times) and CM (one hundred thousand times). It is believed that higher potencies act predominantly on the mind and spirit, whereas low potencies, being more material, act predominantly on the body. Indeed, homeopathy recognises the paramount importance of the mind and its interplay with the body, and so remedies are selected for their psychological influence as much as for anything else.

Hahnemann set down his findings in *The Organon of Rational Medicine*, published in 1810. In this treatise he asserts that the healing power of homeopathic remedies can only be explained by the acceptance of a dynamic energy or vital force animating the body, and a similar vibrational principle embodied in every medicinal substance. The method of potentisation imparts a vibration on the diluted substance which releases the vital force – even from substances such as certain metals, charcoal and sand, which appear to be therapeutically inactive.

In 1812, when an epidemic of typhoid fever swept through Napoleon's army, Hahnemann treated 180 cases; only one soldier died. From this point his fame spread throughout Europe. Similarly, in 1831 when cholera raged through central Europe, he at once set about finding a remedy. Camphor proved to be the most efficacious at the onset of the disease, while other remedies were helpful during the later stages. However, even though Hahnemann's new system of medicine had spread far and wide, with practitioners in other countries reporting good results, the orthodox medical establishment refused to accept the validity of homeopathy.

THE RISE OF PHARMACEUTICAL DRUGS

The eighteenth and nineteenth centuries saw the development of organic chemistry. A pattern was established that continues today: chemists set out to purify drugs in order to isolate their 'active principles' and eventually to synthesise them. However, certain drugs like morphine (an alkaloid derived from the opium poppy) cannot be successfully synthesised, so pharmacists continue to rely on the biochemical isolate. As a point of interest, morphine was isolated for the first time in 1803 by a twenty-year-old German apothecary's apprentice called Friedrich Serturner.

However, the so-called impurities of a plant medicine are often a necessary part of the whole because they work in harmony with the active principle, quenching the activity of what would otherwise be a powerful drug with unpleasant side-effects (see Chapter 2). For example, the alkaloid ephedrine (isolated from the Chinese herb ma huang, *Ephedra sinica*) was once marketed as a drug for asthma. But in isolation the chemical raises blood pressure to dangerous levels, which is why today the drug is rarely ever used. Yet the crude medicinal plant has been widely used in China for thousands of years, with no harmful side-effects.

In a pharmacological breakthrough, salicylic acid crystals (derived from salicin, a substance extracted from willow bark) were produced synthetically in 1852. By the time acetylsalicylic acid – a less irritant version of salicylic acid – was synthesised in 1899 by the German company Bayer, and given the name of aspirin, there was already a steady demand for this popular drug.

Unfortunately, however, orthodox medicine in the nineteenth century was still biased towards drugs based on antimony, arsenic and other toxic substances. Since these and other chemical drugs could be patented, resulting in higher profits for the manufacturer, there was little incentive to promote botanic medicines (a situation which unfortunately still prevails). Only country people were left, in the main, relying on herbal remedies, as were the enthusiasts of botanic medicine who crossed over from the USA to lecture in Britain and other parts of Europe.

In Britain professional herbal medicine survived only through the establishment in 1864 of the National Association of Medical Herbalists, which thrives today under the name of the National Institute of Medical Herbalists.

THE DEVELOPMENT OF FLOWER THERAPY

Dr Edward Bach (pronounced 'batch') was born at Moseley, near Birmingham, in 1886 and trained as a pathologist and bacteriologist in London shortly before the First World War. Even though Bach attained eminence as a consultant physician, he became disenchanted with orthodox medicine, which focused on relieving the symptoms of disease rather than its true causes. For a while he worked with vaccine therapy, and later with homeopathic principles. Despite a great deal of success in both areas of research, he became convinced that poisonous substances of animal, plant or mineral origin should play no part in healing – even when used in minute doses as in homeopathy.

Equally important to Bach was the realisation that prolonged emotional disharmony lowered a person's resistance to disease. He also observed that people suffering from the same disease and with similar personalities responded well to a particular remedy, but that those of differing temperament needed other treatment. Thus Bach's axiom became: take no notice of the disease, think only of the personality of the one in distress. According to Bach, 'disease is a consolidation of a mental state', a message from our inner being calling for a change in our way of living and our mental outlook.

Building on these newly formed ideas, Bach started to focus more on his intuitive faculties. He strongly believed that the key to true healing lay not in the laboratory but within the plant kingdom, and that these special plants would be found growing wild. During a visit to rural Wales, his sensitivity began to blossom fully. He felt that certain flowers (rather than other parts of the plant or tree) emanated a special kind of healing vibration, an energy which resonated in harmony with the soul and was capable of transmuting negative emotions like fear, anger and sadness into courage, optimism and joy. In this manner, he felt, they addressed the origin of disease.

Even though his researches were entirely intuitive, his conclusions were grounded in a certain kind of logic. Rather like the ancient herbalists who ascribed to the Doctrine of Signatures, Bach believed that a plant's outward mode of being signified its subtle healing virtues. For example, when the ripe seed pods of the Himalayan balsam (*Impatiens glandulifera*) are touched, they burst open and with alarming force the seeds are shot out in all directions – a perfect demonstration of the explosive irritation of the person for whom this flower remedy is best suited!

To take another example, the Bach remedy Aspen is prepared from the flowers of a tree whose leaves are always trembling, even on calm days when the breeze is barely perceptible. So the flower remedy is for fear, but of a specific kind. Bach describes it as a fear of 'vague unaccountable things which cannot be explained. As if something dreadful is going to happen, without any idea as to what it might be.'

Originally, the first few remedies discovered were prepared from tinctures potentised by the homeopathic method of successive dilution and succussion. Later, Bach felt it would be better to devise an easier method which could be followed by lay people.

In 1930 he decided to give up his lucrative London practice; for the next six years he travelled around southern England and Wales, seeking flowers for his developing system of healing. Through his heightened senses, Bach discovered that the dew which collected on the petals encompassed the healing energy of the plant upon which it rested. Moreover, dew exposed to sunlight was far more potent than that found on flowers growing in the shade. But collecting dew proved to be too time-consuming. After much experiment, he eventually devised two methods of extraction or 'potentisation', as he preferred to call it – the Sun Method and the Boiling Method (see pages 102–4). They were simple methods which anyone could employ, and which would not damage the parent plant or tree.

The resulting flower remedies or essences (there are thirty-eight altogether) are similar to homeopathic remedies in that they are diluted almost infin-

itesimally. They are employed not for their chemical constituents, but for the healing energy harnessed within the water-based carrier.

Bach came to believe that the homeopathic Law of Similars (that 'like cures like') is born of an incomplete understanding of the nature of the whole: for disease itself is like curing like. The purpose of disease, he asserted, is to teach us to correct our ways and harmonise our lives with the dictates of our soul. True healing occurs not by repelling disease with the darkness of substances of a similarly low vibration (for example, the use of homeopathic 'nosodes' which are prepared from substances of pathological origin, rather like conventional vaccines), but as a result of flooding our being with the light of a higher vibration – in the presence of which 'disease melts away like snow in the sunshine'.

Whatever the arguments for or against this view, in Bach's own hands the flower remedies undoubtedly proved most efficacious – indeed, on occasions miraculous. However, we need to consider how much of this can be attributed to Bach's own extraordinary gift of healing (there are a number of recorded instances of Bach having healed patients through the laying-on of hands), and how much to the flower remedies themselves. In my own experience, which is mirrored by other therapists of my acquaintance, flower remedies cannot totally obviate the need for homeopathy – or any other form of treatment for that matter – especially in serious or chronic illness. Nevertheless the remedies are extremely supportive and, on occasions, can be sufficient in themselves.

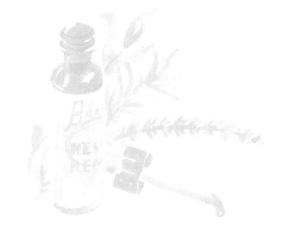

Not surprisingly, the conventional medical establishment repudiated Bach's theories and regarded him as the victim of some kind of mental aberration – as did most herbalists, in the fear that he would bring herbal medicine into disrepute. The General Medical Council even threatened to remove his name from the medical register, though in the end they never carried out the threat. But Bach was so convinced of the benefit of his remedies that he would not be distracted from his purpose.

Shortly before he died in 1936 Bach declared his work complete. For many years his remedies stood alone. Then in the mid-1970s interest in flower therapy was revived. American psychologist Richard Katz began to develop essences from organically grown flowers, employing his intuitive faculties (enhanced by meditation) and Bach's Sun Method of potentisation. In 1979 he founded the non-profit-making Flower Essence Society in California. FES is now a worldwide organisation of professional health practitioners and interested lay people who are devoted to the development and application of flower therapy.

As well as embracing the mental states recognised by Bach, some of the new flower essences address psycho-spiritual states which Bach himself apparently overlooked. Examples are problems relating to sexuality, communication and creativity. Unlike the Bach remedies, many of the new flower essences are also prescribed for certain physical symptoms; for example muscular aches and pains (Dandelion), catarrh (Jasmine), headaches (Feverfew) and digestive problems (Chamomile).

Since the 1970s flower essences have continued to be developed by a number of individuals, not only in Britain and the mainland of the USA, but also in Hawaii, New Zealand, Australia, Canada, the Amazonian rain forests, the Himalayas and other wild and beautiful places throughout the world.

THE REBIRTH OF AROMATHERAPY

Although the origin of healing body and soul using aromatic oils can be traced back to the earliest civilisations, the healing oils of antiquity were very different from the vast array of highly refined essences captured by modern methods of distillation. So in this sense, unlike herbal medicine, massage combined with essential oils does not have an unbroken tradition of practice spanning many centuries. The word 'aromatherapy' was first used in 1937 when the French chemist and perfumier René Gattefossé published a book entitled *Aromatherapie*. Gattefossé was not the first scientist to recognise the healing properties of essential oils – the volatile extracts of aromatic plants captured by steam distillation – but his ideas helped form the basis of aromatherapy as it is practised today.

Gattefossé was not a part of the natural health movement, but as a perfumier he recognised the potential of fragrance to uplift the human spirit. He was also interested in the remarkable antiseptic, painkilling and regenerative powers of plant essences. This was demonstrated to him in 1910 when he badly burned his hand in a laboratory explosion and treated the injury with undiluted lavender essence, which straightaway eased the pain. Moreover, the skin healed extremely well, with no trace of infection and no scar.

He also found out that when essential oils are rubbed into the skin they can pass into the bloodstream. From here they interact with the chemistry of the body, exerting a therapeutic effect similar to that resulting from oral doses of the same substance (see page 39).

Considerable interest in aromatherapy arose in France as a result of Gattefossé's experiments. A former army surgeon, Dr Jean Valnet, is felt to have made the greatest contribution to the medical assessment and acceptance of aromatherapy. Inspired by Gattefossé, in the Second World War Valnet used essential oils for treating wounded soldiers. Not only did the fragrances of the essential oils mask the putrid smell of gangrene, but they actually retarded putrefaction.

In his first book, entitled *Aromatherapie*, and published in 1964 (the English translation is called *The Practice of Aromatherapy*), Valnet describes how he successfully treated several long-term psychiatric patients with essential oils, dietetics and herbal remedies. These people also had physical symptoms caused by the side-effects of the drugs they had been given to control their depression and hallucinations. They were gradually weaned off the drugs and treated with essential oils both externally, with aromatic baths and liniment rubs, and internally, by mouth or interdermal injections (through the upper layers of the skin rather than into a vein). Both physical and mental symptoms were relieved, sometimes within days of discontinuing the drugs.

Other researchers, such as the Italian doctors Gatti and Cajola in the 1920s, were primarily interested in the psychotherapeutic value of smelling essential oils. They wrote: 'The sense of smell has, by reflex action, an enormous influence on the function of the cental nervous system.'

In the early 1970s another Italian, Professor Rovesti of Milan University, used citrus essences like bergamot, orange and lemon to raise the spirits of people suffering from depression. He held wads of cotton wool soaked in essential oils under the noses of his patients, and said that the aromas helped to bring out and release suppressed memories and emotions which were having harmful effects on the psyche of these people. Among other anxiety-relieving essences which were listed by Professor Rovesti are marjoram, cypress, rose and lavender.

Another prominent figure in the aromatherapy world was the Austrian-born cosmetologist Marguerite Maury, who in the 1950s suggested combining essential oils with massage. She disliked the idea of administering essential oils internally (the favoured method of French aromatherapy doctors) and preferred to dilute them in vegetable oil and then massage them into the skin. Drawing on traditional Tibetan medicine, she developed a technique of massaging the oils into the skin along the nerve centres of the spinal column. She also came up with the concept of the 'individual prescription' – essences selected to suit the physical and emotional needs of the recipient. As the mental and physical pattern altered, so did the aromatic prescription.

Marguerite Maury worked closely with her husband, the French homeopathic physician Dr E. A. Maury. They concluded that aromatherapy massage was an excellent prerequisite to homeopathic treatment, for it created a state of heightened receptivity to the remedies. None the less, massage with essential oils was also seen as a marvellous therapy in itself. Many of Marguerite Maury's clients (mostly wealthy women seeking rejuvenation) reported a whole range of benefits, including deeper sleep, relief from rheumatic pain, increased sexual pleasure and a generally improved mental state. In 1962 and 1967 she was awarded two international prizes for her research into essential oils and cosmetology.

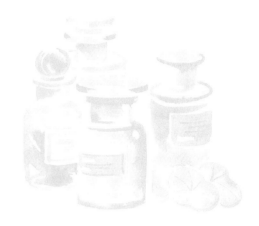

In the introduction to the English edition of her book, entitled *Marguerite Maury's Guide to Aromatherapy*, Danielle Ryman – an ex-pupil of Maury who has continued her work for over twenty-five years – writes, 'Marguerite Maury possessed some of the eccentricities of genius . . . she was a veritable whirlwind of energy and enthusiasm, working ceaselessly until, quite literally, she died of sheer overwork [aged seventy-three] of a stroke during the night of 25 September, 1969.'

In the late 1970s British researcher Robert Tisserand published one of the first books in English on this therapy, which had been hitherto elusive except in France. It would be fair to say that this work, *The Healing Art of Aromatherapy*, has perhaps generated more worldwide interest in the therapeutic use of essential oils than any other book.

AROMATHERAPY TODAY

Since the 1980s, the practice of aromatherapy has spread to many countries throughout the world. In France a number of medical schools now include the study of essential oils as part of their curriculum. However, since few European aromatherapy doctors hold certificates in massage therapy, the majority employ essential oils in the treatment of infectious illness, and oral dosage is the principal method of administration. In this instance the word 'aromatherapy' is something of a misnomer, since the oils are chosen for their pharmacological action rather than for the subtle effect of the aroma upon mood.

To ascertain the most efficacious oils for a particular person, French aromatherapy doctors employ the *aromatogram*. This involves taking a swab from an infected area of the patient, culturing it in the laboratory and then testing several different essences to find out which blend of oils would be most effective for that person's infection. The most potent oils are then encapsulated and administered by mouth, or sometimes in the form of a suppository. Surprisingly, a different patient suffering from the same named

bacterial invasion will need a different blend of oils in order to combat the infection. From this we may conclude that even our germs carry the essence of our individuality!

In Britain, Japan, the USA, Australia, Canada and Norway, the art of massage is the mainstay of aromatherapy. It combines the physical and emotional effects of nurturing touch with the medicinal and psychotherapeutic properties of plant essences.

Unlike more clinical therapies such as homeopathy and herbal medicine, aromatherapy's healing potential stems from its ability to engender joy or tranquillity in the recipient. Indeed, the more wonderful the experience, the more healing the effect!

CHAPTER TWO

THE CHEMISTRY OF MEDICINAL PLANTS

THERE IS A WHOLE branch of science known as pharmacognosy, which is devoted to investigating the active principles of plants used traditionally in folk medicine. Most typically, a pharacognosist is interested in isolating and describing these biochemicals. This might lead to attempts to synthesise them, or to experiment with changing them slightly, to achieve certain desired effects such as increased activity and greater stability. Around 50 per cent of pharmaceutical drugs are either derived from natural sources or synthesised from natural models.

While it is interesting to take a closer look at the individual components of herbs and essential oils, it is important not to lose sight of the whole. Assigning actions to an essential oil or herbal remedy based upon examination of isolated components can be misleading. The therapeutic properties of a plant remedy are the result of synergism – an interaction of all its chemical constituents working harmoniously together, so that the effect of the whole becomes greater than the sum of its parts.

The compounds and substances which the drug manufacturers seek to eliminate work in concert with the 'actives', making them more easily utilised in the body. They also buffer the action of what are otherwise powerful chemicals, thus protecting the body from side-effects. Some even help to protect us from taking too much of a particular active principle by causing nausea if the body's safety level of tolerance is exceeded.

Moreover, as every chemist knows, it is impossible to replicate a natural chemical. Indeed, 'nature identical' drugs (a euphemism for synthetic) always carry with them a small percentage of undesirable substances which are not found in nature. What effect some of the new synthetic drugs will have on people in the long term is little understood. Most herbal medicines, on the other hand, have been on trial for thousands of years, which means their effects upon the mind/body complex are well documented.

Medicinal and culinary plants have a natural affinity with the human organism, for all living things are composed of related organic compounds. For example, sex hormones akin to those found in the human body have been found in frankincense resin, hops, yeast, certain fungi and soya beans. Many plants also contain compounds similar to the endorphins and encephalins (brain hormones) which control human pain response.

Of course, not all medicinal plants are safe for home use. Despite their natural synergy, plants like foxglove, larkspur and aconite can be lethal unless administered with extreme caution in carefully controlled doses. (Incidentally, when taken in homeopathic form these same remedies do not cause toxicity problems, yet they retain a certain level of potency.)

Foxglove leaves have, at times, been mistaken for those of the comparatively benign comfrey – with devastating consequences. There are also a few reported cases of deliberate misuse of essential oils (for example, taken internally to induce abortion). All in all, however, the safety record of both herbal medicine and aromatherapy, when used correctly with a proper understanding of their effects, is impressive.

None the less, potentially dangerous drugs do have a role to play in the holistic scheme of things. Examples of these are the heart drug digoxin (derived from the foxglove), the painkiller morphine (from the opium poppy), and vincristine sulphate (from the Madagascar periwinkle), which can be vital in the treatment of childhood leukaemia.

MAIN GROUPS OF CONSTITUENTS IN MEDICINAL PLANTS

ALKALOIDS

These are a diverse group of compounds with nitrogen comprising a major part of their structure. Generally, they exert a marked effect on the nervous and circulatory systems. Isolated alkaloids usually have a more potent action than the plant material from which they are derived. Several thousand alkaloids are known, the most familiar being morphine, nicotine and caffeine.

GLYCOSIDES

All glycosides (there are several main groups) have sugar as part of their chemical structure. Among the most important are the cardiac glycosides, which have the capacity to support a weakened or failing heart. Plants containing cardiac glycosides include foxglove and lily of the valley. Herbalists favour the latter because the active principles are released more slowly; they are also easily excreted, thus avoiding toxic accumulation. Many plants containing anthraquinone glycocides are pigmented and have been used as dyes – for example, madder. If taken as medicine, most exert a laxative effect: rhubarb and senna are well-known examples.

SAPONINS

This group has a chemical nature very similar to that of the glycosides, but the saponins are distinguished by the fact that they produce a soapy lather when shaken with water. The most interesting of these are the tri-terpenoid saponins, which act as precursors to steroid (sex) hormones – oestrogens, progesterone and androgens. This means they provide the raw materials out of which the body can make whatever hormones are needed to enhance health. Examples of such plants are ginseng, wild yam and chaste tree.

BITTER PRINCIPLES OR COMPOUNDS

As their name implies, these substances have a bitter taste. They irritate the taste buds, and in so doing stimulate the appetite and the flow of digestive juices. Bitter tastes also stimulate the liver, further improving digestion. Examples of plants which contain bitters are dandelion, hops, centaury and gentian.

TANNINS

These are complex compounds with the ability to coagulate proteins, heavy metals and alkaloids. They are used to cure or tan leather – a process in which the proteins in animal hides are broken down, rendering them impervious to putrefaction. Tannins have astringent and antiseptic properties; plants containing them are helpful for such problems as diarrhoea, slow-healing wounds, mouth infections and haemorrhoids. The substance is usually concentrated in the bark and leaves. Examples are rose, willow, witch-hazel and oak.

FATTY OR FIXED OILS

Plant-derived fatty oils are mixtures of triglycerides, which are insoluble in water. Unlike essential oils, they are not volatile, hence the term 'fixed'. Many of these oils are liquid at room temperature but congeal and become cloudy in cooler temperatures. They contain fat-soluble nutrients such as vitamins A and E. A few, like evening primrose and borage, contain essential fatty acids (EFAs). As their name implies, EFAs are essential to health. As well as helping to maintain the tone and elasticity of the skin, they have important functions in the activity of brain cells and other physiological processes.

Other examples of fatty oils with nutritional and medicinal applications are almond, olive, sunflower seed and corn.

FLAVONOIDS

These often appear in the plant as glycosides, but may be present in their free state too. They are widely distributed as water-soluble pigments in the cell sap of certain plants. Flavonoids and their derivatives have been used as dyes and give many flowers such as cowslip their yellow colour (the Latin word *flavus* means yellow). Flavonoids exert a range of physiological actions. For example, those found in liquorice and parsley are antispasmodic, while those in broom are diuretic. Certain flavonoids are known as bioflavonoids (formerly called vitamin P). They act to strengthen the capillary walls and increase the body's ability to make use of vitamin C. They also have antibacterial and antiviral properties. Plants rich in bioflavonoids include buckwheat and rue.

MUCILAGES AND PECTINS

These are polysaccharides (sugars) which dissolve and swell in water to form a soothing gel. When they pass through the digestive tract they form a protective coat over the mucous membranes and prevent irritants from reaching inflamed surfaces. Medicinal plants high in mucilages are used to treat infections of the chest, throat and intestinal tract. Good examples are marshmallow, comfrey and Iceland moss.

Pectins are classed as plant mucilages because they are also polysaccharides and form gels in the same way. They are found in many fruits, especially blackberry, blackcurrant, apple and quince.

ORGANIC ACIDS

There are many different types of organic acids. The best-known is ascorbic acid or vitamin C. Others, like citric and tartaric acid, are most concentrated in unripe fruits – though they give even ripe fruit its refreshing quality. Their action is generally laxative and diuretic. However, oxalic acid, which is found in rhubarb and wood sorrel, is potentially lethal if taken in quantity.

VITAMINS AND TRACE ELEMENTS

Many herbs are good sources of vitamins and trace elements and make excellent additions to the diet. For example, nettles (taken as an infusion or cooked like spinach) and kelp (a seaweed) are a good source of iron and other important trace elements. Dandelion is rich in potassium, which makes it an excellent diuretic because, unlike its pharmaceutical counterparts, it does not leach potassium from the body. Nasturtium leaves, borage leaves and rosehips are excellent sources of vitamin C. Another health-giving plant is garlic, which contains numerous constituents (including essential oil) and high levels of potassium and phosphorus, together with vitamin C and some B vitamins.

ESSENTIAL OILS, RESINS AND BALSAMS

Essential oils are odoriferous, volatile substances which accumulate in certain tissues, specialised cells or intercellular spaces in aromatic plants. Chemically their principal constituents are complex mixtures of terpenoid substances with diverse properties. Most are antiseptic, and a great many exert a beneficial action on the digestive system. They have numerous other properties, including the capacity to uplift mood through their pleasing aromas. While steam-distilled essences form the basis of aromatherapy, the oils' properties can be employed in their crude form – for example, as culinary herbs and spices or as herbal infusions. Some of the most useful essential oil-yielding plants are lavender, rosemary, garlic, peppermint, sage and chamomile.

Other substances associated with essential oils in many trees and shrubs are resins and balsams. Resins occur as viscous aromatic exudations. They usually harden on exposure to the air, but soften and melt when heated (for example, frankincense resin). Balsams are very similar to resins in that they usually occur dissolved with essential oils. However, they are characterised by their high content of benzoic acid, benzoates, cinnamic acid or cinnamates (for example, balsam of Peru). Like essential oils, resins and balsams are produced by specialised plant cells and are secreted into cavities or, in conifers (for example pines), into resin ducts. When heated, the vapours of resins and balsams exert a marked effect on the respiratory system, acting as expectorants and disinfectants.

ARE ESSENTIAL OILS WHOLE?

Some herbalists shun the use of essential oils in the belief that they are not 'whole'. Separating the essential oil from the plant cells, they would argue, is akin to using a bioactive isolate as employed in conventional medicine. Moreover, the chemistry of a captured essential oil is different from that which is retained within the living plant cells.

It is true that essential oils do not contain certain chemical constituents found in the living plant material, for example water-soluble constituents such as tannins, bitter compounds, sugars, mucilages and pectins, all of which play an important role in the medicinal action of the plant. Nevertheless, essential oils are incredibly complex substances – so complex that they cannot be replicated in the laboratory. A 'nature identical' oil is not the same as the oil which is locked within the plant fibres, neither is it exactly like a steam-distilled essence; for it is impossible to isolate (and therefore replicate) the numerous trace elements and compounds which make up the whole substance. As we have seen, the broad spectrum of properties attributed to a single essential oil (or herbal remedy) is the result of biochemical synergism.

Admittedly, once plant material is collected its chemical composition starts to alter, resulting in eventual reduction of potency. But in the case of certain plants and essential oils, chemical change of this kind is actually desirable. The laxative effect of the herbal remedy cascara (*Rhamnus purshiana*), for example, is the result of enzymic changes that take place during the drying process. The essential oil of German chamomile contains the valuable anti-inflammatory agent chamazulene, which is not present in fresh plant material but occurs as a direct result of distillation.

Heat, of course, brings about further chemical changes to herbal medicines; but fibrous material such as barks and roots need to be simmered in water for some time in order to extract the medicinal compounds and make them readily available for absorp-

tion. If carried out with care, the remedy remains effective.

These natural forms of chemical change are very different from the changes which occur to a chemical drug in the making. Synthetic drugs contain 'shadow' chemicals which are not found in nature, rendering them incompatible with the human organism. As we have seen, unpleasant side-effects are the inevitable outcome of employing such substances in medicine. Despite the pitfalls of separating the parts that make up the whole, this chapter now concludes with a simplistic survey of the chemistry of essential oils.

THE MAIN CHEMICAL COMPONENTS OF ESSENTIAL OILS

TERPENES

These are a diverse group of chemicals with widely varying properties, so it is difficult to generalise about their therapeutic actions. However, common terpenes include limonene, an antiviral agent found in high concentration in pine and turpentine oils, while others, such as chamazulene and farnesol (found in chamomile oil), have anti-inflammatory and bactericidal properties.

ESTERS

Found in many essential oils, esters include linalyl acetate (in clary sage and lavender), and geranyl acetate (sweet marjoram). Esters are fungicidal and sedative and usually possess a fruity aroma.

ALDEHYDES

These substances are found mainly in lemon-scented essences like lemongrass and citronella. Aldehydes generally have a sedative, though uplifting, effect.

KETONES

Certain essential oils contain appreciable quantities of toxic ketones, so should be avoided by the home user. For example, mugwort, tansy, wormwood and common sage contain thujone, while pennyroyal contains pulegone. Non-toxic ketones include jasmone (found in jasmine) and fenchone (found in sweet fennel). Ketones ease congestion and aid the flow of mucus, so plants and essences with a relatively high concentration of these substances are usually helpful in dealing with conditions of the upper respiratory system.

ALCOHOLS

Among the commonest alcohols are linalol (found in lavender), citronellol (rose, lemon, eucalyptus and geranium) and geraniol (geranium and palmarosa). These substances often have good antiseptic and antiviral properties and are uplifting.

PHENOLS

These bactericidal substances have a very strong, stimulating effect on the central nervous system. But essential oils which contain relatively large amounts of certain phenols are potentially irritant to skin and mucous membranes. Among common caustic phenols are eugenol (found in clove oil), thymol (thyme) and carvacrol (oregano). Those that have no caustic properties include anethole (found in sweet fennel) and estragole (tarragon).

OXIDES

Found in a wide range of essences, especially those of a camphoraceous nature, such as rosemary, eucalyptus, tea tree and cajuput. Oxides tend to have an expectorant effect, a well-known example is eucalyptol (found in eucalyptus).

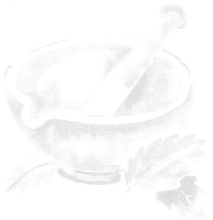

CHAPTER THREE

THE HEALING POWER
OF VIBRATION

SINCE THE LATE 1970s there has been a flurry of books which detail with authority the connections between Eastern mysticism, the philosophy of holism and recent developments in quantum (subatomic) physics. Although the various schools of thought differ in many details, they all emphasise the basic unity of all things. The cosmos is seen as one inseparable reality – forever in motion, alive, organic; spiritual and material at the same time.

The quantum physicist recognises a realm beyond the atom, proton, electron and quark, all of which can be broken down into smaller particles and therefore take up space. Whatever it is that shapes the universe and bestows it with life is non-material and takes up no space. In the subatomic realm there is no distinction between animate and inanimate, between mind and matter. Everything in the universe is a reflection of an underlying vibration. The only difference between the myriad manifestations of nature is the frequency at which they vibrate. Mind energy (like electricity), for example, vibrates so fast that it is apparently invisible; whereas stone (or any other 'solid' object) vibrates so slowly that we are unaware of its essential dynamism. Vibration is also another word for energy. Life is essentially energy – so we return to the ancient realisation that All is One.

ENERGY FIELDS

According to Dr Richard Gerber, author of *Vibrational Medicine*, flower essences (and indeed other forms of 'energy medicine' such as homeopathy and crystal healing) emanate high-frequency subtle energies. These resonate with the vital force – the energy which permeates every aspect of our being.

Many practitioners of vibrational medicine believe that the healing effect is triggered within the subtle body or 'aura' which surrounds and interpenetrates the physical form. From this field, which is essentially a thought form, the remedies' effect filters 'inwards', as it were, to the physical level. In contrast, pharmacologically active medicines move 'outwards' from the physical level, eventually affecting the auric field.

Although healers describe the auric field differently (according to their own level of psychic perception), it is generally agreed that it is a rainbow-coloured emanation radiating half a metre or more around the physical form. It is said to be composed of at least three, and possibly seven, bands of energy, each band vibrating at a different frequency.

Before we go any further, the idea that all living things emanate energy fields follows a law of physics – that the movement of any electrical charge creates a magnetic field. The biochemical reactions which regulate the metabolic processes in the human organism follow this law. That the body emits light (mainly in the invisible ultra-violet and infra-red range) has been verified by a research team headed by John Zimmerman, an ex-professor of Colorado Medical School in the USA.

The part of the electromagnetic field closest to the physical form, emanating about 2.5 centimetres from the body, is known as the *etheric* or *vital* body. Its function is to receive and transmit vital energy from the air we breathe (the Sanskrit term *prana* is commonly used to describe this energy). Interestingly, the etheric body vibrates at a frequency which can be detected by a high-voltage technique called Kirlian photography. The information captured by this process shows a kind of luminescence and streams of energy flowing from the hands or feet. To the trained eye, these patterns reflect the emotional and physical state of the individual and can be used as a diagnostic tool.

British scientist Harry Oldfield, the world's leading authority on Kirlian photography, has developed a much more advanced diagnostic (and healing) technique known as electrocrystal therapy. In this system quartz crystals, mechanically stimulated by high-energy, high-frequency radio signals (reputedly harmless), are beamed into the body. The nature and frequency of the body's returning signals – which are displayed on a VDU screen in technicolour detail – indicate whether the energies emitted from the body tissues being scanned are healthy or otherwise. The equipment can then be used as a healing tool by beaming beneficial electromagnetic waves into the body.

Changes in the energetic body occur well before they manifest on the physical level. Subtle scanning devices can therefore be used as an early warning sign of impending illness. The energy system can then be balanced using various measures such as plant remedies, improved nutrition and relaxation techniques. In this way it is possible to nip the disease process in the bud, before it takes root in the physical body.

What is particularly revealing about the electrocrystal instrument is that it works better with another person standing close by (especially a person with marked healing ability). The human element acts to increase the crystals' therapeutic effect. As Oldfield puts it: 'It's as if the crystals are picking up the nearby human signals and amplifying them for the benefit of the aberrant cells of the patient.'

Similarly, I have seen Kirlian photographs of the energy field of a piece of wholemeal bread, before and after being touched by a healer. The photographs showed the ability of the healer to influence positively the energy field of the bread, the radiance of which was significantly increased. It is therefore also highly likely that an aromatherapist, flower remedy practitioner or herbalist with a genuine desire to heal has the ability to increase the potency of any remedy they may prepare for the recipient. Conversely, of course, the energies of certain individuals may act to diminish the vibratory quality of substances.

In the 1950s a pioneering professor of biochemistry, Dr Bernard Grad of McGill University in Canada, carried out some remarkable experiments with a then famous healer, Colonel Esterbany. Esterbany was requested to transfer healing thoughts to some water with 1 per cent salt added, which was then used to water plants (normally, land plants cannot tolerate such high levels of salt). The growth rates were compared with those of plants treated with non-energised salt-water. The results confirmed that the plants on the energised water grew more quickly. Dr Grad asked sceptical medical students to energise unsalted water in the same manner as the healer had done. However, plants watered in this way suffered even more than those treated with salt-water in the control. Apparently the negative thought waves of the students exerted a growth-depressing effect!

The results of Grad's tests lend credence to the age-old belief that some people have 'green fingers', and others certainly do not. The implications of this may well extend into the field of personal relationships and their co-effects.

THE BENVENISTE HERESY

In 1987, the French immunobiologist Jacques Benveniste demonstrated that certain highly diluted substances could be as potent as vastly greater quantities of the same substance – that is to say, provided the test tube holding the triggering agent was vibrated vigorously between each dilution. In laboratory tests, he demonstrated that living cells could be influenced by Immunoglobulin E in dilutions so high that it was unlikely that a single molecule remained in the water solvent. Only the energy pattern or 'memory' of the original material could have triggered the effect.

Even though Benveniste's findings were published in the June 1988 edition of the prestigious British scientific journal *Nature*, the editors frankly declared their disbelief. For he was lending credence to homeopathy, which employs minute amounts of antagonistic substances to heal the body. Still in the throes of belief system shock, shortly after publishing the results of the trials *Nature* sent a team of experts to France to view Benveniste's findings. To add insult to injury, one member of the visiting team was a magician with an interest in exposing how allegedly paranormal phenomena can be duplicated by sleight of hand.

Unfortunately, Benveniste was unable to duplicate his results consistently: some trials worked, but others did not. So *Nature* condemned Benveniste's work, calling his results a 'delusion' and ignoring the fact that the original paper had been signed by twelve other researchers in four countries. Strangely, they failed to comment on the experiments which did work. In view of what we have learned about the power of mind over matter, is it possible that the negative vibrations emanating from the sceptical observers actually hampered the trials?

The medical establishment is most reluctant to enter into the realms of quantum reality. For it is believed that the laws of ordinary Newtonian physics work perfectly satisfactorily. When dealing with cells, tissues, organs and the pharmacological effects of drugs, this may well be true. However, the same laws break down when dealing with phenomena which are galactically huge, subatomically small or travelling at high speed. The mode of action of the Benveniste experiments operates beyond the laws of materialism, which means that it can only be understood in terms of quantum theory. Moreover, the assertion that quantum physics is a separate branch of science, and therefore totally out of touch with ordinary physics, is akin to believing in the separateness of mind (quantum reality) and body (Newtonian reality): an outmoded and non-holistic concept.

AROMATIC SIGNATURES

Believe it or not, no two people can create an identical aromatherapy blend, even though they may use exactly the same quantities from the same bottles. The oil will always take on an aspect of the blender's personality. Taking the two extremes of personality as an example, the introverted person's blend is likely to emit a dulcet tone, while the extrovert's formula will broadcast its presence loud and clear!

Moreover, an oil blended while you are feeling depressed or angry will not smell right, no matter how beautiful the ingredients. It may smell flat, murky or harsh. On the other hand, a blend mixed while you are feeling relaxed and optimistic will be much more vibrant.

Nevertheless, even when a blend for self-use is composed while you are feeling downhearted, this does not necessarily mean that the oil has lost its healing potential. By the homeopathic Law of Similars ('like cures like'), this kind of self-blended aromatic formula may still have the power to uplift the spirits and restore a sense of harmony. In truth, the mysterious law of paradox permeates the universe – something we must learn to accept with an open heart.

Incidentally, many schools of holistic therapy recognise that devitalisation can occur to either person in the therapeutic partnership. Therefore, it is usual to recommend practitioners to engender in themselves a state of inner calm and stability (a 'grounded' feeling) before offering any form of treatment or counselling. This can be achieved through various breathing and visualisation techniques, or by taking certain flower essences such as Rosemary, St John's wort or a composite of Rescue Remedy/Walnut.

Just for interest, you might like to participate in the following experiment. Get together with a group of three or four people, preferably of widely differing personalities. Then prepare an identical aromatherapy blend, say 5 drops of lavender, 2 drops of bergamot and 2 drops of cedarwood, in a 30ml bottle of vegetable oil such as almond or sunflower seed. Each person should label their own blend with their name, then keep the bottle on their person for at least fifteen minutes for the oil to become imbued with their personal 'vibes'. Once everyone has completed the task, compare aromas. This little experiment never fails to amuse and intrigue!

THE UBIQUITOUS PLACEBO EFFECT

Give a sick person a dummy pill and, as long as he or she believes in its healing potential, there is likely to be some improvement – even more so if the recipient has great confidence in the doctor. However, instead of setting out to explore the amazing potential of the self-healing phenomenon, orthodox practitioners disregard it and refer to it dismissively as the 'placebo effect'. And as far as medical researchers are concerned it is a tiresome distraction, serving only to mask the genuine pharmacological effects of test drugs.

For obvious reasons holistic practitioners are reluctant to acknowledge the role of the placebo effect in therapy, yet they constantly put it to good use. For example, most recognise the importance of empathy in the healing partnership. They are also quick to point out that people cannot be healed if at one level (often unconscious) they do not wish to be healed, or if they cannot trust, or cannot let go of any fears that may be blocking the healing process. Indeed every health practitioner, orthodox or otherwise, has come across the person who just does not get better – despite their doing everything 'right'.

As we have seen, although a therapeutic substance has healing potential in its own right, its efficacy can be enhanced (or decreased) by the persona or vibrational influence of the practitioner. And this is where things move on from the placebo effect as defined by orthodox medicine. Moreover, faith in the treatment is not always necessary – which is why even babies and animals can respond to such methods as flower therapy, homeopathy and spiritual healing. Rather, the efficacy (or otherwise) of the treatment is affected by the psycho-spiritual state of the recipient. If the person is open and receptive to the treatment primarily on the *unconscious* level of

their being, healing can occur through an exchange of energies, as it were, between the practitioner and the recipient, facilitated by the chosen therapeutic tool. In other words, the health practitioner is merely a catalyst in the recipient's *self-healing* process.

If only medical science would divert part of its research into harnessing the placebo effect, rather than seeking to over-ride its influence! But since the word 'placebo' has negative implications, it is little wonder that health practitioners from both camps would prefer to ignore it. A step in the right direction, of course, would be to broaden the meaning of the term and to embrace its presence as an essential part of the healing process. Without doubt, the material things that health practitioners do for their patients are not the sum total of the medicine they practise.

THE ESSENCE OF TRUE HEALING

In the past, doctors were inclined to think that, having done everything they could to save a patient's life, but failed, they had discharged their responsibility. The advent of the hospice movement in Britain, with its emphasis on the quality rather than the quantity of life, has helped to change matters.

Hospice workers are well aware of the fact that, when people feel depressed, unloved or fearful, even the painkilling effect of morphine is significantly inhibited. However, following successful counselling and a great deal of tender loving care and support from loved ones and professional carers – sometimes including gentle aromatherapy massage – the body's own natural opiates are released, and the need for morphine is often markedly reduced.

Indeed, even when the pathological condition has progressed beyond all hope of healing on the physical level, it is still possible to become healed in a spiritual sense. In the words of Nora Weeks (a close friend and colleague of Dr Edward Bach), talking of those who took flower remedies before passing on, 'Well, they at least died happy!'

Without doubt, whatever the therapeutic tool – be it aromatherapy, herbal medicine, flower essences, even conventional medicine – the vibration of Love is the greatest healer of all.

CHAPTER FOUR

AROMATHERAPY

AROMATHERAPY IS THE therapeutic use of essential oils to promote health of body and serenity of mind. The most popular approach is to combine the physical and emotional effects of massage with the medicinal and psychotherapeutic properties of plant essences. As well as being an enjoyable way to maintain health and a sense of wellbeing, aromatherapy reigns supreme as a treatment for stress-related ailments, including anxiety, moderate depression, insomnia, fatigue, emotionally induced sexual difficulties, muscular aches and pains, headaches and digestive disturbances. The therapy is also helpful for premenstrual syndrome (PMS) and menopausal distress.

Aromatherapy is beneficial in more serious conditions, though an aromatherapist (or home user of essential oils) should always seek the cooperation of a doctor before treating people with long-term health problems. But what exactly are essential oils, and how do they exert their beneficial effects?

ABOUT ESSENTIAL OILS

Essential oils (also known as essences, aromatic oils or volatile oils) are the odoriferous liquid components of aromatic plants and trees. They accumulate in specialised tissues in different parts of the plant, for example in the petals (rose), leaves (eucalyptus), roots of grass (palmarosa), heartwood (sandalwood), rind (lemon), seeds (angelica), rhizomes or roots (ginger), gum resin (frankincense) and sometimes in more than one part of the plant. The orange tree, for instance, yields three different-smelling oils with differing therapeutic properties: petitgrain (leaves), orange (rind of the fruit) and neroli (flowers).

To the sensitive nose every plant has an odour of some kind, though not every plant produces an essential oil. This means that scent is not vital to the life of plants as a whole. When plants do secrete an essential oil, there are two main reasons for its presence: fragrance in flowers attracts pollinating insects, and the aromas of leaves are protective. During hot weather, the essential oil forms a protective veil of oil vapour around the plant to prevent the desiccating effects of heat. Besides helping to keep the plant moist, essential oils also function as repellents to harmful insects and other creatures that might attempt to feed on leaves and stems. It is also thought that these oils help protect plants from fungal and bacterial disease.

Plant essences are soluble in oil and alcohol, but only partially soluble in water. Even though they are technically classified as oils, they are quite different from 'fixed' or fatty oils such as olive, corn or soya. They are highly volatile and will evaporate when left in the open air. Most have the consistency of water or alcohol, though others, such as myrrh and vetiver, are viscous (thick and sticky). Rose otto is unique because it is semi-solid in cool temperatures but becomes liquid with the slightest warmth. While many essences are virtually colourless, others may be greenish (bergamot), yellowish (lavender) or amber (patchouli). A few are endowed with an idiosyncratic hue. Tagetes, for example, is orange-yellow, whereas German chamomile is deep blue.

The more oil glands present in the plant, the less costly the oil, and vice versa. One of the most expensive essences is rose, for it takes 100 kilos of petals to produce half a litre of essential oil; whereas the same quantity of lavender yields almost 3 litres of oil, hence its relatively low price.

CAPTURING AROMATIC ESSENCES

Technically, the term 'essential oil' denotes an aromatic oil captured by steam distillation. However, the term is often stretched to include aromatic extractions of other origins, including those captured by volatile solvents. There is also the costly carbon dioxide method, which employs the gas at extremely high pressure in order to dissolve the essential oils from the plant material. The latest innovation is the Phytonics process developed by British microbiologist Dr Peter Wilde. Let us take a closer look at the most popular methods of extraction.

DISTILLATION

The process of distillation involves placing plant material in a metal still (usually stainless steel, though older models are made of copper or iron) and subjecting it to concentrated steam, which releases the aromatic molecules from the plant cells. The aromatic vapour moves along a series of glass tubes, covered in a cold water 'jacket', which serve as a condenser. The essence is then separated from the water by siphoning it off through a narrow-necked container called a florentine. The remaining aromatic water is a useful by-product: rosewater, orange flower water and lavender water are well-known examples.

It has to be said that the heat and water employed in distillation are to some degree harmful to certain fragile constituents of the essential oil, as reflected in the aroma. It is never identical to that which emanates from the living plant.

EXPRESSION

Most citrus essences are extracted from the rind of the fruit by means of expression. Although this was once done by hand, by squeezing the rind and collecting the oil in a sponge, machines using the principle of centrifugal force are now used. The process involves no heat, so the aroma and chemical structure of the oils is almost identical to those of the oil when still in the skin of the fruit. Unfortunately, however, expressed oils have only a relatively short shelf-life. Although distilled citrus essences with a longer shelf-life are also produced, the quality of aroma is comparatively poor.

SOLVENT EXTRACTION

Volatile solvents such as petroleum ether or hexane are employed to capture the fragrances of flowers like jasmine, hyacinth, narcissus and tuberose. Such fragile scents would be completely ruined by the intense heat of distillation. After being treated with the solvent the plant material produces a waxy substance called a concrete, which then undergoes repeated evaporation under a gentle vacuum. The aromatic viscous 'oil' that results is known as an absolute. If a similar process is applied to resinous material such as benzoin or myrrh, the extract is known as a resinoid.

The fragrance of a solvent-extracted aromatic is closer to that of the living plant, but in a concentrated form. Unlike essential oils, which are composed entirely of volatile substances, absolutes and resinoids also contain non-volatile components such as waxes and fatty acids.

It has to be mentioned that solvent-extracted aromatics may not be suitable for aromatherapy. While many essential oils are produced in the knowledge that they will be used for therapy, the same cannot be said for floral absolutes. These costly substances are produced mainly for the perfume industry, which means they are extremely vulnerable to adulteration with synthetic perfume compounds (see page 88). For this reason, French aromatherapy doctors never employ absolutes for medicinal purposes.

Certainly, the use of benzoin resinoid for aromatherapy purposes should be questioned. It is captured by means of the potentially carcinogenic substance benzene. The same volatile agent is employed in the manufacture of polystyrene and insecticides. While there are those who would argue that the use of benzene is acceptable because barely a trace of it remains in the resulting aromatic liquid, this is short-sighted. Quite apart from the outrageous fact that a known carcinogenic solvent is being employed for extracting a medicinal product, there is also the problem of air pollution in and around the distilleries – hardly in keeping with the holistic principle.

Admittedly, it is difficult not to concede to the occasional use of exquisite-smelling floral absolutes (captured by hexane or petroleum ether rather than benzene) in the making of mood-enhancing room scents and personal perfumes. However, the new Phytol extracts are preferable because the process is reputedly kind to the environment.

THE PHYTONIC PROCESS

This process has been developed around a family of solvents collectively known as phytosols, whose unique character ensures that the plant essences can be captured at or below room temperature. This means that the exceptionally fragile, heat-sensitive components of the aromatic oil are not lost, or radically altered, in the extraction process.

The odour intensity of these extracts is generally stronger than that of distilled essences, which means smaller quantities can be employed for most aromatherapy applications. Chemical analysis reveals Phytol extracts to be somewhat different from essential oils. For example, English Rose Phytol (produced from several varieties of rose) contains over 290 separate identifiable components (including the water-soluble phenylethyl alcohol), whereas the best available rose absolutes contain around 210 components.

Proponents of the Phytonics process assert that the method is non-polluting, for the small amount of solvent employed is constantly recycled. Since the extraction equipment is small and portable it can be taken out into the field, ensuring that the flowers are gathered at the peak of perfection. Moreover, the flowers and herbs (though not necessarily the spices and other exotics) chosen for the process are cultivated without the use of poisonous sprays and artificial fertilisers.

A word of warning: at the time of writing, Phytol extracts have not been extensively tested for possible adverse reactions on human skin. Therefore, it may be wise to use them solely as mood-enhancing room scents, or perhaps as handkerchief perfumes.

THE PROPERTIES OF ESSENTIAL OILS

Most essential oils are antiseptic to some degree: good examples are eucalyptus, thyme and tea tree. A number also have antiviral properties: garlic (available in capsule form) and tea tree are two of the most powerful. Other oils, such as lavender and patchouli, are antifungal and therefore helpful for conditions such as athlete's foot, ringworm and candida. Many essences, in particular rosemary and juniper, are antirheumatic. After being rubbed into the skin they will stimulate the circulation and increase the supply of oxygen to problem areas, which in turn assists in eliminating tissue wastes such as uric and lactic acids which contribute to the pain experienced by arthritis and rheumatism sufferers.

A great many essential oils also have cytophylactic properties, which means they trigger the release of white blood cells (leucocytes) in the body's fight against infection. Examples of such essences are chamomile (Roman and German) and thyme. Then there are those oils which have a cicatrising effect: they stimulate the growth of healthy skin cells and promote the formation of scar tissue. Among the most remarkable is marigold oil (Calendula officinalis). Sadly, the plant produces too little essential oil to make distillation commercially viable; however, infused oil of calendula can be used instead (see page 96). Other renowned cicatrisant essential oils include frankincense, geranium and lavender.

Another major area of influence is the effect of essential oils (and indeed their herbal remedy counterparts) upon the female reproductive system. A number of essential oils, for example chamomile, rose and clary sage, help to regulate the menstrual cycle. Others, such as fennel, dill and caraway, are known to promote the flow of breast milk. If, for some reason, the milk supply needs to be stopped,

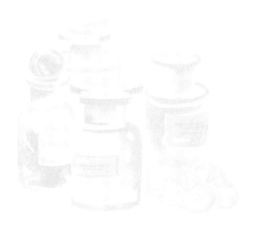

peppermint will have the desired effect. Indeed, British aromatherapy midwives successfully employ peppermint compresses for that purpose.

HOW ESSENTIAL OILS ENTER THE BLOODSTREAM

For many people, however, the influence of scent upon the mind and the emotions is the most fascinating aspect of aromatherapy. But before beginning to explore the art of aromatic mood enhancement, it is important to have a basic understanding of the two main routes by which external applications of essential oils reach the bloodstream – by skin absorption and by diffusion across the tiny air sacs in the lungs. We shall also look at the function of smell.

THROUGH THE SKIN

The skin is capable of both absorption and excretion. When we eat spicy or garlicky food, for example, the odour will be noticeable on our breath; the odoriferous molecules will also be secreted through the pores of the skin with our sweat. Although water cannot be absorbed into the bloodstream through the skin, certain other substances can be conveyed in this way to the systemic circulation, provided that their molecular structure is small enough.

When essential oils are applied to the skin – for example, diluted in a vegetable base oil for massage, or a few drops added to the bathwater – the tiny aromatic molecules pass through the hair follicles.

These contain an oily liquid called sebum, with which essential oils have an affinity. From here, the oils diffuse into the bloodstream or are taken up by the lymph and interstitial fluid (a liquid surrounding all body cells) and carried to other parts of the body.

Evidence accumulated by herbalists would suggest that the skin can also absorb the medicinal properties of herbs when applied externally. For example, when a strong decoction of herbs is added to the bathwater the passage of the medicinal molecules through the skin is facilitated by warmth and moisture (a process known as osmosis).

External applications of therapeutic agents are increasingly employed by drug companies. For example, oestrogen and trinitrin can be administered by means of a patch applied to the skin. The advantage of these so-called transdermal applications of drugs over oral dosage is that much smaller quantities may be administered. This is because nothing is lost through digestion, nor is the substance immediately broken down by the liver. The external method also avoids irritating the gastrointestinal tract, which is a frequent side-effect of many drugs.

Similarly, smaller quantities of essential oils applied externally may be just as efficacious as larger quantities taken orally. (A word of warning: although essential oils are commonly prescribed by European aromatherapy doctors to be taken by mouth, the method should be avoided by lay people and aromatherapists who do not have formal medical qualifications.)

THROUGH THE LUNGS

Once breathed in, the aromatic molecules of essential oils arrive in the lungs, from where they diffuse across tiny air sacs (called alveoli) into the surrounding blood capillaries. Soon they find their way into the systemic circulation from where they exert their therapeutic effect.

THE PHARMACOLOGICAL ELEMENT

As already explained, essential oils are composed of numerous biochemical compounds including terpenes, esters, aldehydes, ketones, alcohols and oxides. Whether absorbed through the skin or inhaled, once in the bloodstream and body fluids the essences are believed to exert a pharmacological effect – even though the amount absorbed is very small. According to Gattefossé, essential oils diluted to a degree at which they have no effect on living cultures in the laboratory still have a clear, rapid and beneficial action on the body.

Essential oils are sometimes described as bio-catalysts. Having triggered their healing effect, the aromatic molecules are rapidly excreted from the body – via the skin, sweat, urine, faeces, or, in the case of certain essences such as eucalyptus and garlic, mainly through exhalation – and yet the aromatic molecules remain almost unchanged in themselves.

THE ENIGMATIC SENSE OF SMELL

If you were asked to describe the fragrance of some exotic flower, chances are that you would be lost for the exact word or phrase. At best, its qualities can be transposed to the other senses through simile and metaphor. The flower may smell like 'cooked cherries', 'maple syrup' or 'vanilla fudge'. Or it may smell 'fruity', 'sharp', 'rounded', or perhaps 'sweet and cloying'. Or, more imaginatively, 'airy and ethereal like a bluebell wood'. Encounter another fragrance and it may elicit the frustrated response, 'It reminds me of something, but I can't think what.' Indeed, the silent language of smell is indefinable, evocative and unforgettable. But why does scent have such a profound influence on memory, mood and imagination?

The olfactory cells in the upper part of the nose are specialised neurones (technically they are brain cells), each of which connects with the brain by means of a single long nerve fibre. Smell is unique among the senses in not having connections through the thalamus (the brain's relay system) to the neo-cortex, the part of the brain which gives rise to our intellect. Instead, smell impulses go directly to the brain area formerly called the rhinencephalon (from the Greek, meaning literally 'smell brain') and now known as the limbic system (from the Latin *limbus*, meaning 'border'). The various structures which comprise the limbic system form a border around the neo-cortex.

Although the limbic system is still largely uncharted territory, we do know that it is concerned with our instincts: emotion, intuition, memory, creativity, hunger, thirst, sleep patterns, sex drive and probably much else besides. Scent, as a result, can evoke memories, feelings and images, or move us to actions without our even realising it.

THE BLOOD–BRAIN BARRIER

The tiny capillaries which carry blood through the brain are protected by a lipid (fatty) membrane known as the blood–brain barrier. Its purpose is to pass certain molecules to the brain cells whilst inhibiting the passage of others. Blood and most prescription drugs cannot pass through the protective sheath. Those substances which can reach the brain cells have a tiny molecular structure and are soluble in lipids; examples include oxygen molecules, nutrients from food, nicotine, alcohol, heroin, benzodiazepene and possibly essential oils.

Receptors for drugs like benzodiazepene and cocaine are located throughout the brain. They include the olfactory bulb, a part of the brain which actually extends into the nose. Without the appropriate receptor with which to bind, such drugs could not work. As Professor Susan Schiffmann of Duke University in the USA points out: 'Now, they did not evolve over millions of years so they could be around to bind Valium when it was invented, so why *are* they there in our noses? My guess is that they might be there to bind things that we smell, natural substances that have a similar effect.'

AROMATHERAPY AND EPILEPSY

British consultant psychiatrist Dr Tim Betts at the Queen Elizabeth Psychiatric Hospital in Birmingham has been researching into the uses of essential oils in the treatment of epilepsy, and with a good deal of success. Some patients have been able to withdraw from medication.

Initially, patients are taught to develop a conditioned response to their chosen essential oil (aroma preference is very important). This is achieved by encouraging the recipient to inhale the essence whilst in a state of deep relaxation. Those patients who are chronically tense – they have no concept of what being relaxed is like – respond best if the treatment involves massage. Others are taught to relax using an auto-hypnotic technique. Patients also carry the essential oil around with them (dropped on to a handkerchief or in a small bottle), enabling them to inhale the scent at the first sign of an oncoming seizure. (Many people with epilepsy experience certain premonitory sensations such as the epileptic 'aura', a current of cold air rising from some part of the body to the head.)

Those patients who have been able to use this technique to control their seizures are the ones who experience premonitory sensations; those who do not experience such warnings respond less well. A few have even reached a point at which they merely have to recall the memory of the scent in order for it to exert the same seizure-stopping effect!

None the less, there is evidence to suggest that the beneficial effect may be over and above that of mere odour association. Intriguingly, 36 out of 50 patients chose ylang ylang essential oil. Dr Betts believes that the oil may contain a pharmacological agent, as yet unidentified, which reduces seizure activity.

As a point of interest, Dr Betts's approach is not entirely new. In former times physicians encouraged their epileptic patients to inhale the vapours of certain odoriferous substances of animal origin. For example, ambergris (a sweet-smelling substance excreted by the male sperm-whale), musk (from the scent glands of the male musk-deer) and civet (from the scent glands of the male civet cat). It should also be mentioned that strong synthetic perfumes have been known to *provoke* seizures in susceptible subjects.

ODOUR ADAPTATION

A unique and as yet unexplained phenomenon of smell is that of adaptation. After a few minutes' exposure to a certain scent, we become unaware of or 'blind' to it. Moreover, prior exposure to one scent will decrease the ability to detect another. A higher concentration of the second odorant is therefore required in order for it to be perceived fully.

When odour researchers record the electrical activity that smelling an odour triggers in the brain (see below), they find that, even though the subjects can no longer detect the test scent – say, of jasmine – the electrical signals continue unabated. This means

that the mind/body effects of scent do not depend upon conscious recognition of the odour molecules. Moreover, odour researchers at Warwick University in the UK discovered that humans can respond to subtle levels of fragrance – that is to say, so highly diluted that it is imperceptible to the conscious mind. This suggests that even those who have lost their sense of smell (a condition known as anosmia) may still benefit from the healing power of fragrance, albeit on a subliminal level.

MONITORING THE EFFECT OF ESSENTIAL OILS

Research into the mind/body effects of odorants, employing EEG (electroencephalogram) scanning equipment, is being carried out by scientists all over the world, notably at Warwick University, Toho University in Tokyo and Yale University in the USA.

It has been found that essences like sandalwood, chamomile and clary sage tend to produce alpha, theta and delta brainwave patterns. This translates into feelings of relaxation and inner ease. Other essences such as black pepper, rosemary and coriander produce beta brainwaves, indicating a state of alertness and wellbeing. Then there are those oils which have an adaptogenic effect – they gently stimulate those who feel lethargic, and lower anxiety levels in those who feel tense and nervy. Bergamot, lavender and geranium have been cited as especially helpful. If an aroma is disliked, however, its effect on the central nervous system is effectively blocked – hence the importance of personal preference when choosing oils for healing the emotions.

Despite the undoubted psychotherapeutic properties of natural aromatics, it should be mentioned that the people who fund research into mood-scents are almost entirely concerned with developing synthetic products. Why? It is the same old story – natural healing agents cannot be patented. Since patented products are potential money-spinners, clearly there is no incentive to extol the virtues of unmodified essential oils.

A growing number of companies and retail outlets have taken to pumping synthetic mood-scents through commercial diffuser systems to improve productivity in their workers and to lure customers to buy their products. But even though synthetic odorants seem to elicit the desired behavioural responses, we need to consider the safety aspects as well as the ethical issue.

SOMETHING IN THE AIR

Dr Richard Lawson, quoted in the British journal *What Doctors Don't Tell You* (September 1996), recounts over fifty cases of emotional illness triggered by synthetic perfumes found in commercial air fresheners. Symptoms include palpitations, insomnia, black moods and tiredness. Even more disturbing, one patient described what would have gone on record as a textbook case of 'nervous breakdown' – anxiety, tremor, weepiness and feelings of unreality. She had even been given to wandering around outside late at night. Another women patient suffering from emotional imbalance found that she was reacting to the aroma chemicals in a 'feminine hygiene' product. Needless to say, once the offending odorants were removed every one of Dr Lawson's patients made a speedy recovery.

But what about the health of people who may be exposed to environmental fragrance in the workplace? Sadly, this is a problem that over-enthusiastic odour researchers have yet to acknowledge. While the overuse of natural essential oils can also be deleterious to wellbeing, symptoms are infinitely less severe than those just described. Idiosyncratic allergies apart, the early warning signs of essential oil 'overload' (and presumably also with synthetic odorants) are usually headache or a sudden aversion to the aroma.

Yet for those subjected to 'Big Brother' fragrance, such warnings cannot always be heeded. Without doubt the concept should be reconsidered, preferably before the art of gentle persuasion develops into a science of subtle manipulation.

AROMA PREFERENCE

Generally, a scent which is perceived as unpleasant is likely to trigger discomfiting thoughts and mood states, whereas a pleasant fragrance is likely to evoke happy memories or feelings and may also enhance creativity and inspiration. However, the perception of 'pleasant' and 'unpleasant' is highly subjective. For example, while some people enjoy the aroma of farmyard manure, others (particularly those who have always lived in the urban environment) may perceive it as disgusting! Moreover, a certain scent may make us fell uneasy if we have learned to associate it with some unpleasant experience. According to the hill walker who twisted his ankle whilst rambling among the heather, the honey-like scent is 'nothing to write home about'!

Aroma preference, however, is not solely governed by odour association. Scents are multi-faceted; a single odoriferous material may be composed of a myriad overtones and undertones. For this reason you may perceive a particular scent quite differently from someone else, perhaps detecting a mere nuance of the whole. Or you may lack conscious awareness of the entire odour. For instance, it is common to be anosmic (odour blind) to some musks or to sandalwood essence, which has a musky undertone. Some people, while not being totally insensitive to sandalwood oil, may have a partial anosmia to the scent. One person may focus on the soft woody-balsamic notes, whereas another may be repulsed by the musky note lingering beneath the surface. Various other 'animal' notes (collectively known as pheromones) may be perceived as 'sweaty', 'urinous' or 'faecal', such as those emitted by heavily-scented flowers like azalea, freezia, lilac, jasmine, orange blossom and narcissus.

HUMAN PHEROMONES

Just like plants, insects and animals, people secrete subtly fragrant pheromones. The word pheromone derives from the Greek *pherin* to transfer, and *hormone* to excite. While hormones are broadly classified as internal messengers, secreted into the bloodstream to influence the activity of target cells, the closely-related pheromones are external messengers. They are secreted by the apocrine glands in the skin (found mainly in the armpits, pubic area, face and nipples) to evoke a response in other people. The musky androstenone, which is produced in the bodies of both men and women, is reputedly the raw fuel of the libido.

However, it is important to emphasise that human androstenone acts merely to entice, rather than compel. Unlike animals, whose sexual cycles are governed by the release of pheromones, we can maintain a measure of control over our basic instincts. Indeed, we relate to one another in a variety of sophisticated, emotionally complex and imaginative ways. Yet in the light of what we have learned about flower pheromones, whose biochemical make-up is akin to that of our own essences of desire, there may well be some truth in the age-old belief that putting plant secretions (perfumes) on the skin can help capture an erotic allure!

Not all human pheromones, however, are erogenic; some contribute to our characteristic body scent. While no two people smell exactly alike, there are similarities within races. Moreover, along with the 'fingerprint' odour there is the person's essential 'male' or 'female' scent, which can be recognised within any ethnic group. Body scent is also influenced by the type of food eaten, the odours of which appear in the body fluids, most noticeably in sweat.

Moreover, emotion, illness, the pill, HRT (and other drugs), as well as hormonal changes such as puberty, pregnancy, menstruation and menopause, all influence body odour and our aroma preferences. This explains why the same perfume or essential oil smells different on each person and why we tend to go off certain scents and flavours from time to time and begin to enjoy ones previously distasteful to us. As we grow older our bodies secrete different pheromones, and consequently a favourite perfume of our youth may no longer appeal to us in maturity.

AROMATIC MOOD ENHANCEMENT

The aromatic oils included in the chart on the following page have been categorised according to the most likely effects they may exert on the central nervous system. A few of those oils categorised as 'aphrodisiac' may also have a pheromonal influence. This means they emanate subthreshold odour nuances which are reminiscent of the secretions, even excretions, of the human body. However, if the 'animal' note is consciously registered, the scent usually becomes objectionable. Sandalwood is reputedly the most potent of the aphrodisiac oils, for it embodies a musky odour nuance akin to the pheromone androsterone (see above).

But whatever your aromatic need, always remember to choose according to your aroma preference. If the aroma is disliked or conjures up unpleasant memories or feelings, the conscious mind can easily override the effect of the aroma upon the mind/body complex. It is also interesting to note that the terms 'stimulating' and 'relaxing' are not mutually exclusive states, at least not when describing the effects of essential oils. The aromas we like best are capable of relaxing and revitalising at one and the same time.

The basic methods of preparing aromatic oils for health and pleasure are to be found in Chapter 8.

AROMATIC MOOD ENHANCEMENT CHART

Stimulating
Angelica, black pepper, cardamom, carnation, cinnamon, clove, elemi, eucalyptus, ginger, grapefruit, jasmine,** lime, orange, palmarosa,** patchouli,** peppermint, pine, rosemary

Balancing
Relaxing or stimulating according to the individual's state of being.
Basil, bergamot, frankincense, geranium,* Lavender, neroli, rose absolute, rose otto,* rose phytol*

Relaxing
Cedarwood, chamomile, clary sage, cypress, hops, juniper, mandarin, marjoram, melissa (true),* petitgrain, sandalwood, valerian,* vanilla, violet leaf, ylang ylang*

Antidepressant
Basil, bergamot, carnation, chamomile, clary sage, frankincense, geranium, grapefruit, jasmine, lavender, lemon, lime, mandarin, neroli, orange, palmarosa, patchouli, petitgrain, rose absolute, rose otto, rose phytol, sandalwood, ylang ylang

Aphrodisiac
Angelica, cardamom, carnation, cedarwood, clary sage, coriander, ginger, jasmine, neroli, patchouli, rose absolute, rose otto, rose phytol, sandalwood, vetiver, ylang ylang

Anaphrodisiac
Quells sexual desire.
Camphor, cypress, marjoram, hops (men only)

Aids Clarity of Thought
Coriander, cardamom, eucalyptus, lemon, peppermint, pine, rosemary

* May be stimulating if used in concentrations above 0.5–1 per cent (see Easy Measures, page 93)
** May be relaxing if used in concentrations at or below 0.5 per cent

In the chart above asterisks following the name of an oil are explained in the footnote to the table.

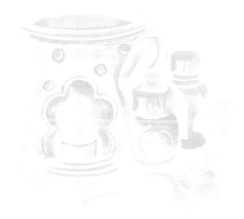

IMPORTANT

Certain floral scents are not only colloquially referred to as 'intoxicating' or 'narcotic' (in the language of perfumery the terms are synonymous), but in sufficiently high concentration they can also be intoxicating in the medical sense of the word, resulting in headache and slight nausea. For this reason, heavily scented flowers should not be left in bedrooms or sickrooms during the night. But in the right quantities (for example, what you might inhale whilst strolling in a perfumed garden for half an hour), balsamic and sweet-floral scents lull the senses into a dreamy, relaxed state. A wonderful way to nourish body, mind and soul!

LIVING AROMATHERAPY

The most natural way to enjoy the healing power of fragrance is living aromatherapy – the cultivation of fragrant plants in the home or garden. The plants in the following chart have been categorised according to the generally accepted scent groups to which they belong. There are several other groups, but they do not usually produce attractive scent. Although the response to fragrance is highly individual, the information given will be a guide for people interested in creating an aromatherapeutic garden. Those specimens marked with an asterisk are suitable as houseplants.

PLANTS FOR LIVING AROMATHERAPY

SCENT GROUP: *Aromatic*

Description and Odour Effect

There are several odour nuances within this group, including almond (intensely sweet and intoxicating); balsam (sweet and mellow with a soothing effect); aniseed (sweet, warming and stimulating); clove (warming and stimulating); nutmeg (sweet, warming and intoxicating); vanilla (soft, sweet, warming and intoxicating)

Suggested Plants

Almond: heliotrope (*Heliotropium peruvianum*), Mexican orange blossom (*Choisya ternata*), gorse (*Ulex europaeus*)

Aniseed: cowslip (*Primula veris*), magnolia (*m. soulangiana*)

Balsam: hyacinth (*Hyacinthus orientalis*),* night-scented stock (*Matthiola bicornis*), ten-week stock (*Matthiola incana*)

Clove: carnation (*Dianthus caryophyllus*), night-scented catchfly (*Silene noctiflora*)

Nutmeg: wallflower (*Cheiranthus cheiri*), tobacco plant (*Nicotiana albas*)

Vanilla: Surfina (*Petunia x hybrida*), *Clematis montana*, sweet pea (*Lathyrus odoratus*)

SCENT GROUP: *Fruit-scented*

Description and Odour Effect

Flowers having a fruit scent (other than lemon) emanate 'cheery', uplifting aromas

Suggested Plants

Apple: chamomile (*Chamamelum nobile*), rose (*Rosa wichuriana*), apple-scented geranium leaves (*Pelargonium odoratissimum*)*

Apricot: iris (*I. graminea*)

Banana: rose (*Rosa soulieana*)

Orange: rose (hybrid variety 'Wedding Day')

Pineapple: Moroccan broom (*Cytisus battandieri*)

Plum: grape hyacinth (*Muscari racemosum*), freesia (mixed varieties)

SCENT GROUP: *Hay-scented*

Description and Odour Effect

Sweetish-harsh scent with an uplifting effect

Suggested Plants

Lavender (most varieties), woodruff (*Galium odoratum*)

SCENT GROUP: *Heavy-scented*

Description and Odour Effect

Exceptionally strongly scented blooms usually possess an 'animal' undertone which becomes unpleasant when inhaled close to, or when the flowers begin to fade. The pleasing top notes carry well in the air, so enjoy the scent from a distance. The odour effect is intoxicating and erogenic

Suggested Plants

Jasmine (*Jasminium officinale* and *J. polyanthum**), Madagascar jasmine (*Stephanotis floribunda**), gardenia (*G. jasminoides**), lilac (*Syringa vulgaris*), tuberose (*Polianthes tuberosa*), lily of the valley (*Convallaria majalis*), mock orange blossom (*Philadelphus*), white lily (*Lilium regale*), honeysuckle (*Lonicera periclymenum*), azalea (*Rhododendron luteum*)

SCENT GROUP: *Honey-scented*

Description and Odour Effect

A light, sweet-floral scent with a honey/musky note which attracts butterflies into the garden. The odour effect is erogenic and mildly intoxicating

Suggested Plants

Buddleia (*B. davidii*), sweet alyssum (*Lobularia maritima*), escallonia (all varieties), honeysuckle (*Lonicera caprifolium*), olearia (all varieties), sedum (*S. spectabile*)

SCENT GROUP: *Lemon-scented*

Description and Odour Effect

A sharp, refreshing scent with an uplifting effect

Suggested Plants

Lemon balm leaves (*Melissa officinalis*), Magnolia (*M. soulangiana*), lemon geranium leaves (*Pelargonium crispum**), rose (*Rosa bracteata*), evening primrose (*Oenothera odorata*)

SCENT GROUP: *Rose-scented*

Description and Odour Effect

A soft, sweet-fruity scent with an uplifting, slightly narcotic effect. The perfume of roses themselves is highly complex, with different varieties producing a differing quality of fragrance, sometimes including citrus or spicy overtones (see also Aromatic Group)

Suggested Plants

Apothecary's rose (*Rosa gallica officinalis*), cabbage rose (*Rosa centifolia*), rose geranium leaves (*Pelargonium capiatum**), paeony (*Paeonia suffruticosa*)

SCENT GROUP: *Violet-scented*

Description and Odour Effect

Delicately sweet with a cool, moss-like quality. Soothing to a fraught nervous system

Suggested Plants

Iris (*I. reticulata*), sweet violet (*Viola odorata*), gladioli (*Gladiolus recurvus*), mignonette (*Reseda odorata*), crinum (*C. powelli*)

THE ART OF SMELLING

Rather than be over-influenced by the aromatic experiences of others, the following exercise will enable you to find your own way along the path of fragrant harmony. It will also encourage you to develop and trust your intuition, which is essential to subtle healing work of any nature.

Since none of the senses is so easily fatigued as that of smell, you will have to limit yourself to smelling just a few essences per session – certainly no more than six. Undiluted essential oils are very powerful and may cause headaches or nausea if inhaled for too long, especially in a stuffy or over-heated room. So always work in a well-ventilated area which is also moderately warm and free from cooking and other household smells.

Choose a time when you are feeling calm and receptive. Put a single drop of essential oil on to a purpose-designed smelling paper (or narrow strip of blotting paper), then waft the smelling strip around to encourage vaporisation. Hold the paper a few centimetres from your nose and inhale slowly and deeply, allowing yourself to experience its effect fully. If you find the aromas of neat essential oils too powerful (this frequently happens), dilute the test essences at around 3–5 drops of essential oil to 1 teaspoonful (5ml) of a bland (low odour) vegetable oil such as almond or grapeseed.

Having experienced the fragrance, what does it make you think of? Is it a feeling, memory or image you would like to have more often? Write down your impressions in a notebook, even if this amounts to single words like 'cheerful', 'cooling', 'earthy', 'woody', 'medicinal', or perhaps in terms of sounds, tastes, textures, colours and shapes.

It is also interesting to explore the same essential

oils at different times of the day and at intervals throughout the changing seasons. The chances are that your feelings about an individual oil may vary accordingly. Moreover, women usually find that their aroma preferences fluctuate in accordance with the rhythm of the menstrual cycle. Roman chamomile, for instance, may smell rather medicinal during the first two weeks following menstruation; but come the premenstrual phase and the oil may suddenly smell sweet and comforting. Without doubt, we are instinctively drawn to the essential oil which is right for us at a given time.

By working with the oils in this way, you will build up your own unique scent vocabulary. This is infinitely preferable to relying on a list of aroma associations compiled by an aromatherapy expert, for no two people respond in exactly the same way to the same scent. It is therefore important for professional aromatherapists to develop the capacity to step back and allow the reality of the subjective to be of sole importance to the individual concerned.

CREATIVE BLENDING

The synergistic formulas explored in the chart below demonstrate the basic principles of creative blending. It is important to emphasise that aromatherapists rarely mix purely 'physical' blends, as the chart suggests. It is in fact impossible to do so – for whatever affects the body must also affect the mind – and vice versa. A carefully blended aromatic prescription will reflect the whole person – body, mind and soul. (The latter element is believed to be closely related to aroma preference and the associated feelings and images evoked by the aromatic oil.) And yet it is common in aromatherapy to mix purely 'mental' blends (usually for stress-related problems). A 'mind' blend can be inhaled from a handkerchief, used as a personal perfume, added to the bath water, vaporised in a room or used for aromatherapy massage. Most of the 'body' formulas are suitable for massage. However, steam inhalations or compresses may be more appropriate for certain ailments (see Chapter 6).

HARMONIOUS BLENDING CHART

For reasons of space and clarity, only a few therapeutic actions of individual oils are explored. Most essences are endowed with a broad spectrum of properties (see the Directory of Healing Plants, Chapter 10).

BERGAMOT

Therapeutic Actions
Antidepressant, heals wounds, eases cold and flu symptoms.

Blending Guide: Mind
To support its antidepressant effect blend with neroli and geranium, e.g. three parts bergamot, two parts neroli, one part geranium.

Blending Guide: Body
To reinforce its wound-healing properties, blend with lavender and frankincense, e.g. two parts bergamot, two parts lavender, one part frankincense.

To support its ability to ease cold and flu symptoms, mix with orange and ginger, e.g. two parts bergamot, two parts orange, one part ginger.

CEDARWOOD (VIRGINIAN)

Therapeutic Actions
Sedative, decongestant, antirheumatic.

Blending Guide: Mind
To enhance its stress-reducing properties, mix with petitgrain and rose otto, e.g. three parts cedarwood, two parts petitgrain, one part rose otto.

Blending Guide: Body
To increase its decongestant properties, mix with sandalwood and lavender, e.g. two parts cedarwood, two parts sandalwood, one part lavender.

To support its antirheumatic properties, mix with juniper berry and rosemary, e.g. three parts cedarwood, two parts juniper berry, one part rosemary.

CHAMOMILE (ROMAN)

- **Therapeutic Actions**

Anti-inflammatory, sedative, eases muscular aches and pains.

- **Blending Guide: Mind**

To enhance its calming effect, blend with rose otto, e.g. two parts chamomile, one part rose otto.

- **Blending Guide: Body**

To support its anti-inflammatory and muscle-relaxant properties, mix with lavender and lemon, e.g. two parts chamomile, one part lavender, one part lemon.

GINGER

- **Therapeutic Actions**

Mental stimulant, relieves arthritic pain, stimulates the circulation.

- **Blending Guide: Mind**

To enhance its mental stimulant properties, mix with coriander and lemon, e.g. one part ginger, two parts coriander, two parts lemon.

- **Blending Guide: Body**

To enhance its ability to relieve arthritic pain, mix with cedarwood and lemon, e.g. one part ginger, two parts cedarwood, two parts lemon.

JUNIPER BERRY

- **Therapeutic Actions**

Sedative, antirheumatic, relieves period pain.

- **Blending Guide: Mind**

To enhance its sedative properties, mix with petitgrain and lavender, e.g. two parts juniper berry, one part petitgrain, one part lavender.

- **Blending Guide: Body**

To support its ability to ease painful periods, mix with clary sage and frankincense, e.g. three parts juniper berry, one part frankincense, one part clary sage.

To enhance its antirheumatic properties, mix with pine and rosemary, e.g. three parts juniper berry, one part pine, one part rosemary.

PATCHOULI

- **Therapeutic Actions**

Antidepressant, fever-reducing, fungicidal.

- **Blending Guide: Mind**

To enhance its antidepressant properties, mix with angelica and bergamot, e.g. one part patchouli, one part angelica, three parts bergamot.

- **Blending Guide: Body**

To reinforce fungicidal properties, mix with geranium, e.g. two parts patchouli, two parts geranium.
To support its fever-reducing properties, mix with bergamot and lemon, e.g. three parts patchouli, two parts bergamot, one part lemon.

CHOOSING THE RIGHT ESSENTIAL OILS

- When choosing an essential oil for therapy, refer to the therapeutic charts in Chapter 8. There is usually a choice of essential oils (and often more than one recommended method of application) to help any given ailment. Your final decision will depend upon price and availability as well as your aroma preference (which will change according to your physical and emotional state at a given time). You may also find it helpful to refer to the Aromatic Mood Enhancement chart on page 44. However, never let dogma override your own instincts. If you dislike a particular aroma, no matter what its 'mood-enhancing' properties may be, it is doubtful that you will respond to its subtle healing effects.

CHOOSING THE RIGHT ESSENTIAL OILS continued

- If you would like to experiment with a blend of aromatic essences, it is usual in aromatherapy to mix between two and four harmonious aromas. Advice on the aroma-compatibility of various essences is included in the Aromatherapy note to be found in the individual plant profiles in Part Three. Remember, the aesthetic element is an important part of every aromatherapy treatment. See also the Harmonious Blending Chart on pages 47–8.

- Whether you are choosing an essential oil for health or for pleasure, check that the essence is safe for you to use; for example, take extra care during pregnancy or where there is a history of allergies. Refer to the safety data on pages 86–7 and/or the CAUTION note included in the individual plant profiles in Part Three.

AROMATHERAPY MASSAGE

By combining the mood-enhancing properties of essential oils with skilled but nurturing touch we embrace every level of our being, including the spiritual aspect of self which may be nourished through our aesthetic appreciation of fragrance.

To receive a good aromatherapy massage is a truly divine experience; and giving massage can be enjoyable too. You can, of course, massage the oils into your own skin and derive benefit from them, but there is no denying that the most relaxing way is to be the recipient of a good massage from a skilled but sensitive person – someone with whom you can feel totally at ease. A professional massage once in a while is ideal if you can afford it; or you may be able to find another person with whom to exchange massage on a regular basis. By practising on each other you will begin to develop a sense of how massage should feel, and what feels good to you should also feel good to your partner.

The benefits of massage (with or without essential oils) are far-reaching. As well as improving circulation and alleviating pain and stiffness in muscles and joints, it encourages deep sleep and helps prevent insomnia; reduces high blood pressure; encourages deeper breathing and is therefore helpful for respiratory ailments and stress. It also triggers the release of 'feel good' neuro-hormones like endorphins and encephalins which in turn stimulate the body's immune defences.

Since mind and body are interrelated, when muscular tension is released negative emotions such as fear, anxiety and anger begin to melt away. You may feel deeply relaxed and peaceful afterwards, or perhaps exhilarated and more energetic than before.

The very basic strokes introduced here are meant only as a guide to enable you to develop your own intuitive style. At some point you may feel the need to attend a weekend massage workshop, or perhaps even to embark on an extended study course. Having said this, some people are superb intuitive healers and no amount of formal training will improve on their special 'touch'.

The main advantage of serious tuition is that you will be given a good grounding in anatomy and physiology. This will enable you to understand when there is a departure from the normal state; why pain may be occurring in a particular area; and when to refer the person to an osteopath or chiropractor. If you would like to learn more about aromatherapy and massage, a selection of books and training establishments are recommended at the end of this book.

CREATING A HEALING SPACE

The area where you intend to give healing massage should be aesthetically pleasing and softly lit. Work in natural daylight if possible, or under a soft lamp or by candlelight. Harsh overhead lighting will only serve to remind your massage partner of being on an operating table or in the dentist's chair! A vase of fresh flowers or a healthy houseplant will also enhance the space.

Ensure that the room is very warm and draught-free; chilled muscles contract, causing a release of the stress hormone adrenalin, something which you are trying to soothe away in the first place. If you wish, you can enhance the atmosphere by playing gentle music at low volume – preferably music which is specially composed for relaxation (see Useful Addresses). If your partner is one of the exceptional few who finds any form of music a distraction, do respect their wishes and turn it off.

THE MASSAGE SURFACE

The easiest place to give massage is on a purpose-designed massage couch. Alternatively, ask your partner to lie on a firm but comfortable surface, such as a couple of folded bath towels or a duvet on the floor. For comfort, put a cushion under the knees and a small towel under the neck. To ensure that your partner is warm and comfortable throughout the massage, cover with towels the parts of the body not being massaged.

Resist the temptation to give massage on a bed. Unless you actually get up on to the bed to massage your partner, you will have to bend from the waist and this may strain your back. Moreover, if the mattress is soft it will absorb all the pressure intended for the body.

PREPARING TO GIVE MASSAGE

Remember to remove any rings and/or the wrist watch you may be wearing. Likewise, ask your partner to remove any jewellery that may impede the massage. It is also important to ensure that your nails are not too long and likely to scratch your partner.

Most important: never give massage while feeling anxious, angry, depressed, irritable or in any other way upset. Your partner will sense your feelings and will begin to feel similarly distressed. As you become more experienced, you will realise just how easy it is to convey emotion through your hands.

Therefore, prior to giving massage, it is always a good idea to calm and centre yourself. If you are unfamiliar with such terms, the simple preparatory meditation given on page 115 can be adapted for healing work of any nature.

RECEIVING MASSAGE

To reap the full benefits of massage it is important to learn how to receive massage passively and with full awareness. If you constantly chatter, this is difficult to achieve. So close your eyes, take a few deep breaths, then exhale with a sigh and relax into the experience. Concentrate your attention on your partner's touch and enjoy the sensation. Do speak up, of course, if something hurts, or if you feel cold or uncomfortable. Also, if your neck starts to feel stiff when you lie on your front, turn it to the opposite side.

THE MASSAGE OIL

A light vegetable oil such as almond or sunflower seed will help your hands to move freely over the skin. The addition of a few drops of essential oil will enhance the experience. If you do not wish to apply an aromatherapy oil, perhaps because your partner is

---

MASSAGE CAUTIONS

- Always seek medical approval before massaging anyone with a serious health problem such as advanced heart disease or cancer

- Before massaging a pregnant woman, seek the go-ahead from her doctor or midwife

- Never massage a person suffering from a fever or infectious illness. Massage induces heat in the skin, muscles and joints which will exacerbate symptoms

- Do not massage anyone suffering from thrombosis or phlebitis. This is because blood clots are present and they could be dislodged

- Avoid massaging over skin rashes, burns, swellings, varicose veins, areas of broken skin or bruises. In short, if something hurts abandon the movement and go on to another area of the body

pregnant or has very sensitive skin, essences can be vaporised instead. This will help create a healing ambience (see pages 91–2). Put the required amount of massage oil (see page 93) into an attractive dish on the floor nearby, but do be careful not to knock it over as you work. To protect the floor covering, place the dish on some absorbent material such as kitchen roll or tissues.

ABOUT THE STROKES

The basic strokes you are about to learn can be used to relax or stimulate according to needs. Generally, slow movements are calming; fast movements are bracing. Very slow and deliberate movements can be erotic – that is to say, if both you and your partner have entered into the massage with Eros in mind. In fact, the power of intent is an integral part of any kind of massage, hence the importance of giving massage with a warm heart.

Although a professional massage may include the entire body, for the purposes of this book we shall concentrate on back massage. The body's main nerves branch from either side of the spine and supply all the internal organs. So by relaxing the back muscles and working on areas of muscle tension, stress levels can be reduced throughout the mind/body complex.

TIPS FOR GIVING A GOOD MASSAGE

- Wear something loose and comfortable and ensure that your hands are warm.

- When applying the oil, place a little in the palm of one hand, then rub your hands together to warm the oil. Apply just enough to provide a comfortable slip. Too much oil will cause your hands to slide all over the body, hindering any beneficial firmness of touch. Too little will create uncomfortable friction as a result of dragging the skin.

- Concentrate on the movement of your hands, trying not to become sidetracked with idle chatter. In so doing, the massage will become a form of meditation for both parties. Moreover, the recipient will become more aware of areas of muscular tension which can be more easily released by consciously relaxing into the experience.

- Try to work with the whole of your body. For instance, when kneading, move gently from side to side in time with your hands; when applying the long strokes on the back, lean into the movement using your body weight rather than just your hands. The more relaxed and fluid your own movements, the more relaxed and at ease your partner will become.

- To enable you to work with the whole of your body, not just your hands and arms, try to focus on your breathing. For instance, when gliding up the back, exhale slowly as you lean into the movement; inhale as you release the pressure on the return stroke. Try not to hold your breath while doing the gliding strokes (a common mistake) as this creates tension in the whole of your body, especially in your hands. This tension will then be conveyed to your massage partner.

- To improve the circulation, strokes towards the heart should be firm, whereas strokes moving away should be much lighter.

- Once you have made contact with your partner's body, try not to break it until the end of the massage. When you need to apply more oil, ensure that a knee, forearm or thigh is against their body. To break contact mid-flow can feel most disconcerting.

- Sensitivity combined with the sheer pleasure of giving nurturing massage, no matter how basic, far outweighs a full routine of complicated strokes if they are carried out in a mechanical and impersonal manner.

BACK MASSAGE (approximately 20 minutes)

Your partner will need to undress to their underpants – as they become more comfortable with receiving massage, they may be happy to undress completely. It is always best to work on a body free of the restrictions of clothing.

Ask your partner to lie on their front, head to one side, arms relaxed at the sides or loosely bent with the hands at shoulder level. Cover your partner from neck to toe with one or two bath towels. Kneel with your knees slightly apart to one side of your partner.

Attunement

1 Before oiling your hands, move to the left of your partner and allow your hands to move slowly down to your partner's body. Place your left hand lightly on the back of their head, and your right hand on the base of the spine. Remain in this position for about half a minute. When you feel you have established the initial contact, move your hands slowly away.

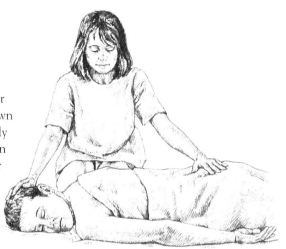

Stroking (Effleurage)

This simple movement is used at the beginning and end of a massage, and to ease the flow from one movement to another. You can sit straddling your partner's thighs if you wish. Otherwise, kneel to one side of your partner, roughly level with your partner's hips, with your knees pointing towards their head.

2 Peel back the towel, exposing the whole of the back. Begin with relaxed hands placed flat against the back, on either side of the spine, with your fingers pointing towards the head.

Never apply pressure to the spine itself, but to the strong muscles either side of the spine. Glide slowly upwards, leaning some of your weight into the stroke until you reach the neck. Fan out your hands firmly across the shoulders, easing the pressure as you glide them down. When you reach the waist, pull up gently and return smoothly to the starting stroke. Repeat several times.

3 Starting with your hands on the lower back as before, glide firmly upwards. When you reach the shoulders, move your hands in circles over the shoulder blades. Then continue to make connected circles down the back, until you reach the original position. Repeat several times.

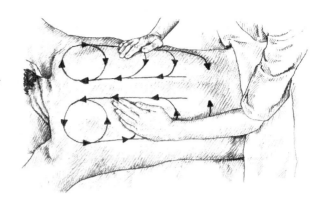

Kneading (Petrissage)

This stroke consists of alternately squeezing and releasing handfuls of flesh in a broad circular motion with the heels of the hands and fingers, rather like kneading dough. The same kneading action can also be carried out with the forefingers and thumbs in the small area between the shoulder blades. The purpose of kneading is to relax tense and painful muscles by improving the circulation, and thus the elimination of tissue wastes.

4 Position yourself to one side of your partner. Begin to knead the buttock furthest away from you. Using the whole of your hands, alternately grasp and squeeze the flesh (but do not pinch), working around the entire buttock. Keeping one hand in contact with your partner's body, move to the opposite side and knead the other buttock.

5 Continue kneading up the sides of the body and across the upper arms and shoulders, paying special attention to areas of tightness which indicate muscle tension. Move to the other side of the body and repeat.

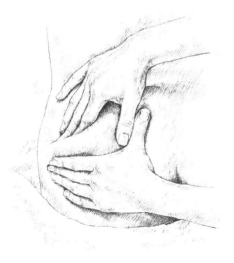

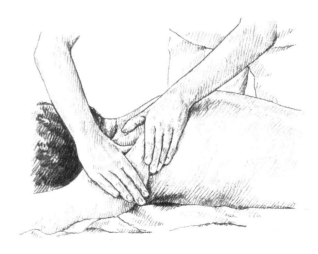

Pulling Up the Sides

This is a firm lifting stroke used on the sides of the torso.

6 Remain in position to one side of your partner's back. With your fingers pointing downwards, use alternate hands to pull steadily up the far side of the body. Ensure there is always one hand in contact with the body. Work your way slowly up to the armpits and back down again. Move to the other side of the body and repeat.

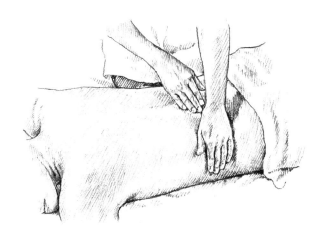

Friction

This action uses the thumbs to reach deeper into the tissue where hidden tensions lie. Only apply friction after you have relaxed your partner's muscles with the previous strokes. You can sit astride your partner's thighs for this one if you wish. Otherwise, kneel to one side of your partner at the level of their hips.

7 Place your hands on the lower back, the thumbs pointing towards each other, on either side of the spine. Keep your whole hand in contact with your partner's body, lean some of your weight into the stroke as you glide up the back to the neck. When you reach the top, fan out your hands across the shoulders, ease the pressure and slide them back down to the original position.

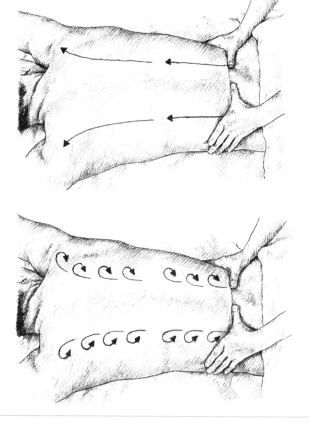

8 Starting from the small of the back, with both thumbs together on the left side of the spine, make small circular movements with your thumbs into the muscles all the way up the spine until you reach the neck. Press your thumbs briefly into the hollows at the base of the skull.

9   With your thumbs on the upper back, continue the circular movements. Work on the muscles above and around the shoulder blades. Then sweep your fingertips back down to the base of the spine. Repeat the same frictions on the right side of the body.

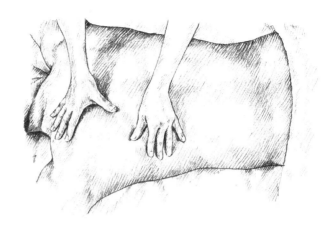

Soothe the whole back by returning to the Effleurage strokes (steps 2 and 3). Repeat two or three times before moving on to the next stroke.

Kneading the Neck and Shoulders

Position yourself to one side of your partner

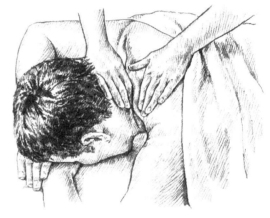

10   Using the thumb and fingertips of both hands, knead the neck muscles, working up and down the neck to include the muscles at the base of the skull.

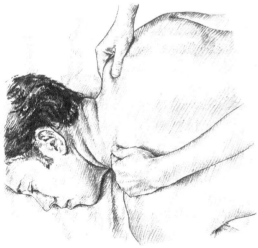

11   Place your right hand on your partner's right shoulder, your left hand on their left shoulder, and begin to knead both shoulders at the same time. Then place both hands on your partner's right shoulder and knead. Repeat the movement on the left shoulder.

Return to the long smooth stroke with which you began (step 2). Repeat several times.

Feathering

As its name suggests, feathering is an extremely light stroke which is barely perceptible to the recipient. Nevertheless, it can have a profoundly soothing effect. It can also be used to balance 'frantic' energies within the auric field, the energy surrounding the physical form (see pages 32–3), resulting in a wonderful sensation of release. Feathering is also a particularly satisfying way to end a massage.

12 With your hands very relaxed, fingers loosely separated, brush with your fingertips in long sweeping movements from the head to the buttocks. Take your hands back to the head and sweep downwards again. Gradually lighten your contact until your fingers are gliding a few centimetres above the skin. If your partner is sufficiently relaxed and focused, they will be acutely aware of your healing hands moving through their auric body. It is common to feel a pleasant tingling sensation, deep heat or even a refreshing 'breeze' around the body.

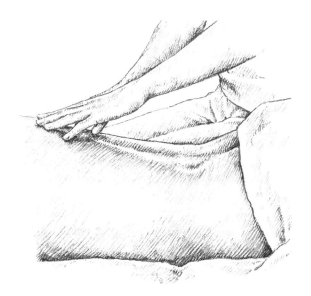

When you feel ready, cover your partner's back with a towel and return to the attunement with which you began (step 1). Then very slowly move your hands away. Allow your partner to 'come round' in their own time.

SELF-MASSAGE (approximately 10–15 minutes)

The following sequence is best carried out once or twice a week, or more often if you can spare the time. Self-massage may not be as blissful as receiving a massage from someone with 'good hands', but it is a wonderful self-nurturing activity. As well as improving the circulation and increasing vitality, self-massage can alleviate nervous tension, mild depression, stiffness and tiredness.

First cover the floor with a large towel to catch any oil splashes. Then prepare an aromatherapy massage oil to suit your needs (see page 93). It is also a good idea to begin with a bath or shower. Essential oils penetrate the skin more readily if it is warm and slightly damp.

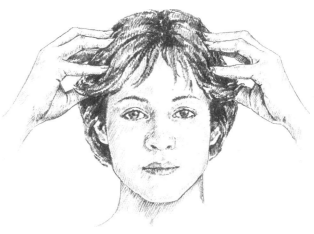

1 Sitting up, begin by massaging your head. (Unless you wish to apply oil as a pre-wash conditioning treatment, there is no need to oil the scalp.) Using the fingertips, press firmly and move the scalp over the bone. Start at the front and work over the entire head using circular movements.

2 Apply a little oil to your hands and begin massaging your face. With the pads of your fingers make circles over your entire face, working gently from forehead to chin. When you reach the throat, apply very light hand-over-hand stroking in an upwards direction.

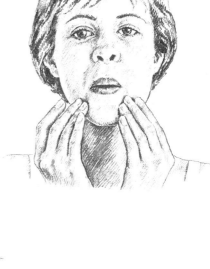

SELF-MASSAGE *continues on page 58*

3 Apply more oil to your hands. Using the flat of your hands, make circles over the sides and back of the neck and as much of the shoulders and upper back as you can reach.

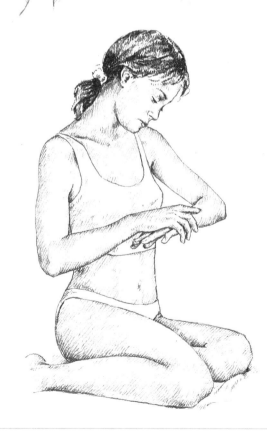

4 Massage the rest of your body with firm stroking movements. With the exception of 'feathering' (see page 56), the direction of flow should be towards the heart to improve the circulation. Begin with light strokes over your legs, arms, torso and buttocks and gradually let them become firmer and more vigorous.

5 Begin gently and rhythmically to knead the fleshy areas of your body, such as thighs, calves and upper arms (kneading is described on page 53). To knead your buttocks and hips, roll over to one side.

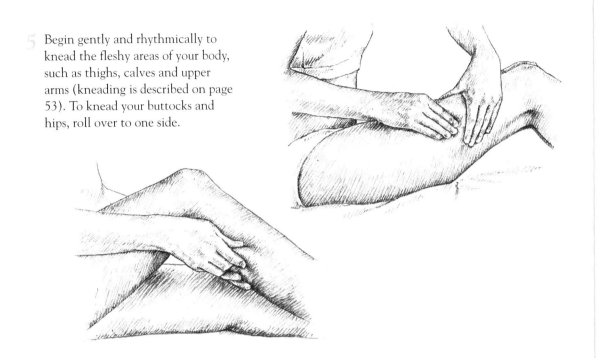

6 To massage your abdomen, lie on your back with your knees up and your feet flat on the floor. Using the whole of your hand, gently circle the area in a clockwise direction, thus following the coil of the colon. Then gently knead all over your abdomen.

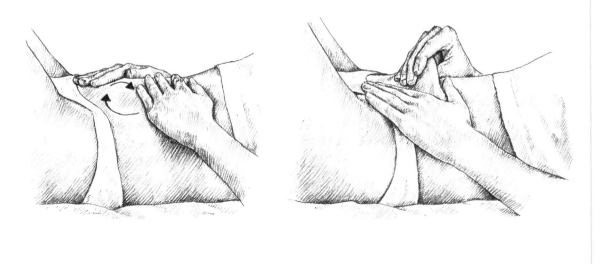

7 Sit up with your legs outstretched in front of you. Using both hands together, stroke the whole foot from the toes towards the body. Then make thumb circles all over the top of the foot.

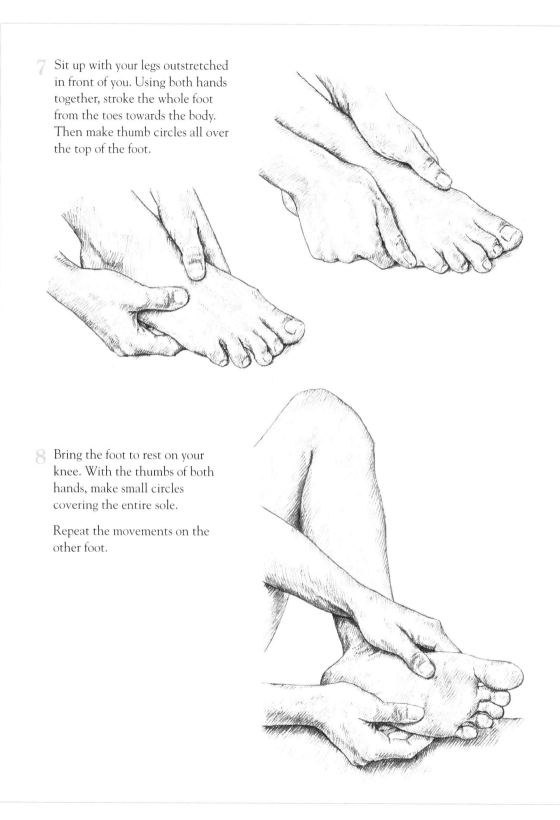

8 Bring the foot to rest on your knee. With the thumbs of both hands, make small circles covering the entire sole.

Repeat the movements on the other foot.

9 Each hand can be massaged in a similar way. Begin by stroking the whole hand, from the fingertips towards the body. Then make thumb circles all over the top of the hand, paying special attention to the finger joints. Turn up the hand and make thumb circles all over the palm and fingers, paying special attention to the fleshy area at the base of the thumb.

Repeat the movements on the other hand.

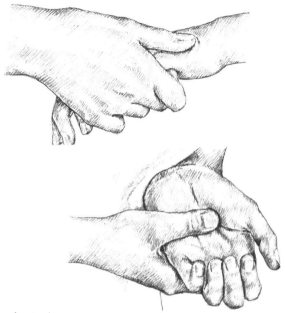

10 Standing up, apply fingertip stroking or 'feathering' (described on page 56) downwards over the parts of the body you can reach, beginning with your head and ending with your feet. Afterwards, enjoy the revitalising glow!

CHAPTER FIVE

FLOWER THERAPY

FLOWER REMEDIES, or essences as they are also called, are captured from a wide variety of tree and plant flora. Unlike ordinary herbal remedies, whose mode of action is attributable to biochemicals, flower essences are so highly diluted that barely a single molecule of the original plant material remains in the water-based liquid. This means that only the vibration or energy pattern of the original plant material is present (see Chapter 3). Since the remedies are absolutely non-toxic in their action, it is impossible to overdose on them. If an incorrect remedy is taken, it simply has no effect.

It is believed that the energetic nature of many flowers resonates in harmony with the psycho-spiritual aspect of our being. As we have seen, holistic healing is based on the premise that almost all illness is a manifestation of emotional, psychological or spiritual disharmony. By embracing the essential self, these gentle remedies help to restore a sense of balance; and in so doing, they can be instrumental in nipping the disease process in the bud.

It should be emphasised that flower therapy is not about putting on a brave face, no matter what. This only creates more tension and conflict – just as tensing up against physical pain succeeds in causing greater discomfort. Neither is flower therapy about fostering blind optimism. The remedies cannot dampen an emotion that we really need. Rather, they enable us to express our emotions honestly and assertively – and at the appropriate time. In some

people, bottled up emotion has the habit of erupting some time later, perhaps in the guise of an aggressive outburst that is usually sparked by something trivial, thus causing distress and bewilderment in those around.

The flower remedies enable us to observe our distress from a higher and wiser level of awareness. In this way, they help transmute our distress into inner strength and renewed hope. Thus they enable us to react less self-destructively to the pressures of life and to become more resilient and resourceful in the face of change and adversity.

THE PHILOSOPHY OF PRESCRIBING

Unlike the Bach remedies, many of the new flower essences are also prescribed for certain physical symptoms. This is because many people involved in flower therapy ascribe to the idea that specific negative thought processes are directly related to specific illnesses. For example, kidney problems are said to be related to deep-seated shame and disappointment; lung problems to depression; epilepsy to a sense of persecution; and menstrual problems to a woman's rejection of her femininity ('penis envy' revisited?).

While there may be a grain of truth in such assumptions, the philosophy is also dogmatic and potentially detrimental. Such a belief system can engender guilt and anger in a person who cannot overcome a physical ailment, despite their doing everything 'right'. A multi-factorial approach would seem more feasible and humane (see Chapter 7), with flower essences acting as a supportive measure.

Contrary to popular belief, Bach did not assert that different diseases are *directly* related to emotional types or temperaments. Rather, he believed that different individuals suffering from the same named disease react to the condition in their own idiosyncratic way. In other words, although physical illness may have its roots in the psycho-spiritual sphere, the specific part of the body in which it manifests is related to inherited or congenital patterns of weakness.

Moreover, the predisposing pattern can sometimes be so pronounced that, even without the additional force of negative thinking, the individual succumbs to physical and/or mental illness – as in the instance of congenital defect. There are those, of course, who would attribute such conditions to some misdeed carried out in a former life, resulting in 'negative karma' (the Eastern version of divine retribution). On the other hand, those who are blessed with good health, prosperity and happiness are supposedly reaping the benefits of 'positive karma'.

Quite apart from the elitist overtones of such a belief system (a facile revision of Buddhist doctrine), it does not explain why animals must also experience pain and suffering. After all, they are not intentionally 'evil' but simply follow their God-given instincts. While the doctrine of rebirth or reincarnation may indeed be the natural scheme of things, it is prudent to keep an open mind about its true purpose and meaning. For humanity has yet to attain a complete understanding of the life experience.

Returning to Bach's method of prescribing, he believed that flower therapy should be tailored to suit the individual pattern of emotional disharmony – the way we actually feel about life or our present condition, rather than the presenting physical symptoms. For the sake of simplicity, I have chosen to advocate the same approach. However, if you are interested in exploring both the physical and subtle healing properties of flower essences, a comprehensive manual is recommended in the reading list at the end of this book (see page 263).

CHOOSING THE RIGHT REMEDIES

On first acquaintance with the flower essence description (see pages 67–73) you may well feel that you need all of them! However, most flower therapists would agree that the vibration of one correctly chosen flower has a more profound effect than several. In practice, however, it is common to prescribe between two and six remedies at a time. The prescription is usually revised every three weeks, though it can sometimes be necessary to monitor the person's progress at weekly intervals. New remedies are prescribed, if necessary, in accordance with the changing mental state (see also Duration of Treatment, page 65).

PRESCRIBING FOR YOURSELF

Begin by writing down the remedies you feel you need, then look at each one more closely in order to prioritise. Prune back your list to four or five remedies, preferably fewer. Refining the process of selection is an important step forward. It encourages you to acknowledge your innermost needs, which all too often become stifled in the maelstrom of everyday duties and activities. Any remedies crossed off the list at this stage could perhaps be used at a later date, once you have dealt with more pressing issues.

One or two flower remedies will be strongly indicated, for they reflect your basic personality type as categorised by Bach. For example, you may be an extrovert, a natural leader, and very outspoken (Vine, Impatiens). Or perhaps you are quiet and reserved (Mimulus, Centaury, Water Violet). The type remedy is the flower that will be needed most often throughout your life. However, you may feel that two basic type remedies are required, for no single flower quite matches your essential self. Provided that you are absolutely certain about this, then so be it.

Other remedies will seem more appropriate as helpers, for they address the superficial emotional states of mind that are not characteristic but temporary. For instance, you may harbour feelings of jealousy or hatred towards a former lover (Holly), or feel nervous and apprehensive before a court hearing

(Mimulus). In such instances, of course, there is no need to take your type remedy as well – that is, unless you should feel it would help bring out the best in you. This would be important during a job interview, for example, or for public speaking.

Another way of choosing appropriate flower remedies is to consider the qualities you feel you would like to develop in yourself. For example, you may feel you need to be more patient with people and situations (Impatiens), or more courageous and self-confident (Larch). On the other hand, you may wish to become more relaxed and less intense (Vervain), or more decisive (Scleranthus). Or maybe you would like to find your true vocation (Wild Oat).

A common difficulty in self-diagnosis, especially when you are in crisis, is the inability to step back from yourself sufficiently to be able to recognise which flowers are required. This is where a close friend or partner can help. However, be prepared for a few home truths!

PRESCRIBING FOR OTHERS

It is important to develop the ability to empathise and the capacity to listen. Unlike sympathy, which hooks into your personal distress and does little to help, empathy is an intuitive response. It is about connecting both with your own and the other person's inner strength. In so doing, you help uplift their spirits and thus their ability to seek a way forward. Even though empathy is difficult to teach as a skill, provided your intentions are motivated by compassion, rather than ego, the gift of empathy will develop quite naturally.

Listen to the words the person uses and the way their story is expressed. For instance, 'I've tried everything, but what's the use' (Gorse). Or: 'I'll never be able forgive myself' (Pine). 'But there's never enough time!' (Impatiens). 'Well, I can do it, so why the hell can't she?' (Beech). Do they speak in a low and anxious voice? (Mimulus). Or do they grab your arm and swamp you with their life story including a graphic account of all their illnesses? (Heather). Maybe they seem broody, bitter and resentful: 'But it's so unfair!' (Willow). Or perhaps they come over as more actively resentful – fiery-natured, suspicious, jealous and angry (Holly).

If the person finds it difficult to express their emotional outlook, gently guide them in the right direction by asking them about their childhood, occupation and so forth. Try to establish exactly how they react to the life experience. Are they generally cautious and pessimistic (Gentian), impetuous and headstrong (Vine), happy-go-lucky (Agrimony) or perhaps constantly fearful for the welfare of loved ones (Red Chestnut)? Or are they quiet and reserved, with an air of natural dignity and superiority (Water Violet)?

Try to ascertain exactly what situation concerns them at present: an imminent operation, bereavement, a relationship problem, childbirth, a change of job, a move abroad, retirement? Then prescribe accordingly for their depression, fear, anger, guilt or whatever it might be. Most important: where there has been any kind of shock or trauma, always add Star-of-Bethlehem to the prescription (see Profound Distress below).

As the person talks, jot down all the remedies that come to mind. However, try not to let note-taking become too obtrusive. It is important to maintain a relaxed and equal relationship, an atmosphere of trust. You can always make notes immediately afterwards while the person's story is still fresh in your mind.

Above all, accentuate the positive. For example, instead of telling the person that you have prescribed Heather for their self-centred, self-obsessed behaviour, let them go away with the knowledge that Heather will help them find inner peace and security.

PROFOUND DISTRESS

Where there has been trauma such as abortion, the sudden loss of a loved one, a terrible accident, rape or some other deeply distressing experience, always prescribe Star-of-Bethlehem to disperse the shock waves. Sometimes the shock of such experiences can be so delayed that years might pass before any sign becomes apparent, perhaps in the guise of depression, inexplicable feelings of guilt, fearfulness or hostility. In such cases, Star-of-Bethlehem should be combined with other remedies accordingly. Although Rescue Remedy can be used in such cases, most flower remedy practitioners would confirm that

Star-of-Bethlehem is the finest catalyst for the healing of deep-rooted distress.

COMPLEX CASES

Whenever it seems that many remedies are required, or if there seems to be no response to treatment, Holly or Wild Oat may be the catalyst needed. The vibration of either flower will 'open' a case, bringing to the fore the predominant underlying emotions. As a result, it should be much easier to prescribe appropriately. Generally speaking, Holly is best suited to those of an active or intense nature, whereas Wild Oat works best for those of a more passive temperament.

Further insight may also be gained through Moon Sign Flower Therapy (pages 74–8) and Flower Therapy Dreamwork (pages 78–9).

PRESCRIBING FOR BABIES

Even though babies are unable to tell us about their state of mind, it is not too difficult to prescribe for them. After all, mothers instinctively know when their children are distressed and often feel the same level of emotion in themselves. The Californian flower essences Chamomile and Lavender (see Chapter 10) and the Bach remedies Cherry Plum, Holly, Mimulus, Red Chestnut and Rescue Remedy are especially helpful. They cover a whole range of emotional symptoms which are common in young children (and harassed parents!), including irritability, angry outbursts, frustration, despair, anxiety, fear and insecurity. To dissipate the trauma of the birth itself, both mother and baby will benefit from a mixture of Walnut and Star-of-Bethlehem (2 drops of each remedy can be added to the baby's first bath).

Generally, dosage is the same as for adults, though nursing mothers can take the remedies themselves, for the healing properties will be imparted to the baby through the mother's milk (see also page 101).

PRESCRIBING FOR ANIMALS

The Bach flower remedies are popular with homeopathic vets, especially Rescue Remedy which has proved most efficacious in many cases of trauma, including post-operative stress. Other flower remedies can be prescribed for deeper problems. For example, the over-possessive dog who drives his owner mad by being constantly at her heels needs Chicory. The nervous horse who jumps at the slightest sound or any sudden movement can be helped with Mimulus. The jealous and suspicious dog will benefit from Holly. While the cat with nine lives who has been hit by a car on more than one occasion needs Chestnut Bud to enable her to learn from past mistakes.

Furthermore, since animals are sensitive to the emotional states of their owners, it may be a good idea to prescribe remedies for yourself as well – possibly even the same ones! Red Chestnut (for constant fear and worry about the safety and wellbeing of another) is an excellent remedy to have at hand (animal dosage is given on page 101).

DURATION OF TREATMENT

Since treatment is tailored to individual need, it is difficult to predict the length of time the remedies should be continued. Generally speaking, with acute conditions such as exam nerves (Larch and/or Mimulus), the effects of bad news (Rescue Remedy) or violent anger (Cherry Plum) the remedy can be taken as often as required, say, every 15 minutes until you feel better.

When dealing with deeply ingrained disharmony – a domineering and aggressive personality, for example, or the lingering effects of childhood abuse or trauma – the healing process may take many months. During this time, different emotions will emerge – feelings you may have held in check for many years. Make a note of any negative change (of course, positive feelings will also surface) and change the prescription accordingly. Or simply add a new flower remedy to the existing treatment bottle.

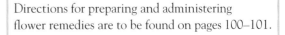

Directions for preparing and administering flower remedies are to be found on pages 100–101.

THE BACH REMEDY PROFILES

There are literally thousands of flower essences prepared from wild and exotic plants from all around the world. Since the remedies developed by Dr Edward Bach are the best known, and therefore the easiest to obtain from health shops and pharmacies, the Bach repertory is featured here in its entirety. A number of more recently developed flower essences are given a brief mention in the Directory of Healing Plants (Chapter 10).

When treating yourself or others, it is important to recognise your own or the other person's limitations. Seek professional help where necessary, perhaps in

the form of counselling (your doctor may be able to recommend an experienced person in your area) or some other therapy such as massage, herbalism, acupuncture or orthodox medicine. As mentioned earlier, flower essences work in harmony with other treatments, hastening the process of healing.

Bach grouped the remedies into seven categories: for those who have fear (Rock Rose, Mimulus, Cherry Plum, Aspen, Red Chestnut); for those who suffer uncertainty (Cerato, Scleranthus, Gentian, Gorse, Hornbeam, Wild Oat); for insufficient interest in present circumstances (Clematis, Honeysuckle, Wild Rose, Olive, White Chestnut, Mustard, Chestnut Bud); for loneliness (Water Violet, Impatiens, Heather); for those over-sensitive to influences and ideas (Agrimony, Centaury, Walnut, Holly); for despondency and despair (Larch, Pine, Elm, Sweet Chestnut, Star-of-Bethlehem, Willow, Oak, Crab Apple); and for over-care for the welfare of others (Chicory, Vervain, Vine, Beech, Rock Water). For easy reference, the flower remedies appear in this chapter in alphabetical order.

CAUTION

Anyone who talks about suicide or any other violent act should be taken seriously. He or she must be encouraged to talk to a doctor, psychiatric worker or crisis counsellor at the earliest opportunity.

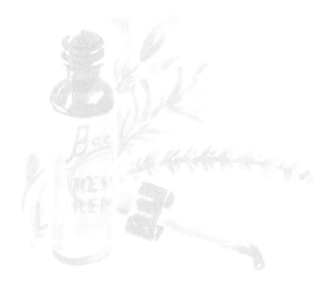

BACH FLOWER REMEDY PROFILES

AGRIMONY · *Agrimonia eupatoria*

Pattern of Imbalance

Mental torture concealed behind a cheerful façade; denial and avoidance of emotional pain; may become addicted to substances in an attempt to numb inner pain; often has trouble sleeping; even when very ill, may laugh and joke with those around; may feel suicidal at times; strives to make a good impression on other people; if on a spiritual path, may convince themselves (and others) that they have transcended pain and suffering.

Positive Potential

The ability truly to laugh at life, for personal problems are viewed from a more balanced perspective – that of the genuine optimist with a talent for creating harmony where there is discord.

ASPEN · *Populus tremula*

Pattern of Imbalance

Inexplicable fears stemming from the deep psyche; fear of some impending evil; hypersensitivity to 'bad vibes' of any nature; vague anxiety and apprehension; disturbing dreams or night terrors; may sleepwalk; possibly very psychic, but instead of tuning into joyous events, tends to focus on impending disasters; ungrounded; may demand that a light be left on all night.

Positive Potential

Fearlessness and a sense of protection; the ability to connect with the universal power of Love.

Comparison

Compare with Mimulus, whose fear is of *known* or worldly origin (fear of visiting the dentist, for example).

BEECH · *Fagus sylvatica*

Pattern of Imbalance

Intolerance, criticism and arrogance; perfectionist expectations of others; lacks empathy; pedantic attitude; overlooks the fact that everybody does not have the same advantages and potentials; finds the small habits, gestures and speech patterns of others annoying; tendency to see only what is wrong in a situation; narrow-minded; may feel isolated and lonely.

Positive Potential

Tolerance and understanding of others; the ability to see the good in everyone and everything.

Comparisons

Compare with Vine, whose need is to dominate, and with Vervain, the forceful fanatic whose need is to convert.

CENTAURY · *Centaurium erythraea*

Pattern of Imbalance

Inability to refuse the demands of others, therefore becoming a willing slave; suppresses own needs to keep the peace and to gain favour in the eyes of another; self-neglect; sapped by others; oversensitive; possibly mediumistic.

Positive Potential

A balanced recognition of own needs; ability to say 'no' when appropriate; ability to mix with others while preserving own identity; ability to be of great service to others, and yet maintain inner strength and vitality; ability to realise own true mission.

CERATO
Ceratostigma willmottianum

Pattern of Imbalance

Constantly seeks advice and counsel from all and sundry; may also imitate others, their opinions, mannerisms, style of dress and lifestyle (especially common during adolescence and young adulthood); gathers much information, but rarely acts upon it; appears foolish at times; saps others; lacks concentration; easily dominated.

● **Positive Potential**

The ability to trust own inner voice; self-confidence and certainty; highly developed intuition.

● **Comparison**

Compare with Scleranthus, who is torn between two things but, unlike Cerato, rarely bothers others with the minutiae of daily decision-making. Scleranthus eventually struggles to find the answer from within.

CHERRY PLUM · *Prunus cerasifera*

● **Pattern of Imbalance**

Fear of losing grip on sanity; uncontrolled outbreaks of temper; temper tantrums in children; fear of harming self or others; suicidal thoughts; nervous breakdown.

● **Positive Potential**

The ability to cope with inner turmoil, for the distress is healed by the balancing forces of the Higher Self.

CHESTNUT BUD
Aesculus hippocastanum

● **Pattern of Imbalance**

Failure to learn by experience, so repeats the same old mistakes; lacks observation; a slow learner; thoughts often in the future; forgetfulness; short attention span.

● **Positive Potential**

To gain knowledge and wisdom from every experience; to break free from negative patterns of behaviour.

CHICORY · *Cichorium intybus*

● **Pattern of Imbalance**

Possessive of people and things; demands sympathy, love and affection; uses emotional blackmail; prone to self-pity; anxious; self-centred; tearful; strong-willed; enjoys arguments; saps others; possibly house-proud; dislikes being alone; fussy; domineering; mentally congested; fears losing friends; may feign illness to gain sympathy.

● **Positive Potential**

Selfless love given freely; inner security and wisdom; respects the freedom and individuality of others.

CLEMATIS · *Clematis vitalba*

● **Pattern of Imbalance**

Daydreaming; indifference; little attention in the present, for thoughts are usually in the future; apathetic; unworldly; impractical; lacks ambition; welcomes the prospect of death; needs a great deal of sleep; feigns illness to escape from life; sapped by others; ungrounded; may have a poor body image and tendency to bump into things. Clematis is also for any bemused state of mind, and for unconsciousness (see page 73).

● **Positive Potential**

Emotional equilibrium; ability to experience the 'here and now'; a renewed (or new-found) sense of purpose and meaning to life.

CRAB APPLE · *Malus sylvestris*

● **Pattern of Imbalance**

A feeling of being unclean; self-disgust; may become obsessed with 'cleansing' diets and related procedures; may have an eating disorder; anxious; obsessed with imperfection; may be sexually repressed; a distaste of bodily functions such as breastfeeding and going to the toilet; possibly a history of sexual abuse; obsessive thoughts and behaviours; may have a skin complaint.

● **Positive Potential**

The wisdom to see things in their proper perspective; self-respect; freedom from obsessive thoughts and behaviours; acceptance of the physical body and material world, warts and all.

ELM · *Ulmus procera*

● **Pattern of Imbalance**

Great despondency as a result of feeling overwhelmed by responsibility; a tendency to overwork; a sense of isolation through having to rely on own resources.

Positive Potential
The ability to see problems in their proper perspective; an inner conviction that the task will be completed, for help will come at the right moment.

Comparisons
Compare with Hornbeam, whose despondency is through dislike of their work. Elm enjoys the work they are doing (and usually excels at it), but is prone to periodic feelings of inadequacy.

GENTIAN · *Gentianella amerella*

Pattern of Imbalance
Tendency to scepticism – a 'doubting Thomas' attitude; depression after a setback.

Positive Potential
The faith of the positive sceptic – one who sees difficulties, but does not fall into deep gloom over them. The strength and inspiration to try again.

GORSE · *Ulex europaeus*

Pattern of Imbalance
A sense of great hopelessness, but can be persuaded by loved ones to try again, albeit half-heartedly; may be suffering from a chronic illness.

Positive Potential
The knowledge that all difficulties will be overcome in the end. Gorse is also the remedy for those who have been ill for a long time. It engenders hope, and hope is the first step towards recovery.

Comparison
Compare with Wild Rose, whose hopelessness has descended into apathy – an emotional void.

HEATHER · *Calluna vulgaris*

Pattern of Imbalance
Over-talkative, self-centred; fears being alone; a poor listener; saps others; feigns illness to obtain sympathy; mentally congested; over-anxious for self; childish; weeps easily. The Heather state can, of course, be temporary: during illness, for example, or when enduring a crisis like bereavement, divorce or some other great loss.

Positive Potential
Great empathy as a result of having suffered; inner peace and emotional self-sufficiency.

HOLLY · *Ilex aquifolium*

Pattern of Imbalance
Feeling cut off from love; envy, jealousy, rage, suspicion, hatred; may also be physically aggressive; saps others. Almost everyone needs this remedy from time to time, though it is possible for such distress to develop into a conditioned state of mind.

Positive Potential
Feeling loved and being able to love others; great compassion.

Comparison
Compare with Willow, whose aggression has turned inwards, resulting in a brooding and bitter temperament. The Holly aggression tends to be expressed more openly and forcibly.

HONEYSUCKLE
Lonicera caprifolium

Pattern of Imbalance
Nostalgia; homesickness; absent mindedness; lives in the past; may become over-concerned with past-life theory; saps others.

Positive Potential
The ability to retain the lessons taught by past experiences, but not to cling to one's memories at the expense of the present; emotional clarity and a sense of freedom.

Comparisons
Compare with Clematis, whose thoughts are far away in the future, in happier times to come. Walnut, unlike Honeysuckle, feels the need to break with the past, but is finding the transition difficult.

HORNBEAM · *Carpinus betulus*

● Pattern of Imbalance

Tiredness, boredom, laziness, weariness, that 'Monday morning' feeling.

● Positive Potential

A renewed interest in life; energy and involvement in daily tasks.

● Comparison

Compare with Olive, whose exhaustion is complete, born of physical and emotional strain as a result of prolonged stress, a long illness or convalescence. With Hornbeam, it is only the thought of what lies ahead that causes the tiredness – the physical energy is easily mustered once the mind is motivated.

IMPATIENS · *Impatiens glandulifera*

● Pattern of Imbalance

Impatient and irritable; desires to work alone at own swift pace; overworks; has high ideals, so finds fault with others; quick in mind and body, which often results in nervous tension and muscular pain; sometimes angry and violent.

● Positive Potential

Great empathy, patience and tolerance, especially towards the shortcomings of others.

LARCH · *Larix decidua*

● Pattern of Imbalance

Lack of confidence. Although everyone can benefit from this remedy from time to time, the Larch state can become a conditioned response – an expectation of failure, reinforced by past limitation. A tendency to allow others (who are often less talented) to take the limelight.

● Positive Potential

Self-confidence, creative expression, spontaneity; perseveres even when there are setbacks.

MIMULUS · *Mimulus guttatus*

● Pattern of Imbalance

Timidity, introversion; fear of known things such as flying, travelling by water, swimming, animals and public speaking.

● Positive Potential

Quiet courage and confidence to face life's challenges.

● Comparisons

Compare with Rock Rose, whose fear is extremely acute – hysteria as a result of a terrifying accident, for example. Compare also with Aspen, whose fear stems from the deep psyche, a trembling fear triggered by dark fantasies and paranoic impulses. The Mimulus fear is less acute and of a generalised nature.

MUSTARD · *Sinapsis arvensis*

● Pattern of Imbalance

Fluctuating cycles of depression, usually without apparent cause. The remedy is also indicated for premenstrual and menopausal depression and seasonal affective disorder (SAD), also known as the 'winter blues'.

● Positive Potential

Inner serenity; the ability to transmute melancholia into joy and peace.

OAK · *Quercus robur*

● Pattern of Imbalance

Despondency as a result of obstinate, relentless effort against all odds; life is viewed as an uphill struggle; refuses to give in to illness; may suffer nervous breakdown or collapse.

● Positive Potential

Balanced strength; the ability to accept personal limits and therefore knowing when to surrender.

OLIVE · *Olea europaea*

Pattern of Imbalance
Complete mental and physical exhaustion, usually as a result of physical illness, childbirth or prolonged stress.

Positive Potential
Peace of mind; revitalisation; a renewed interest in life.

Comparison
Compare with Hornbeam, whose weariness is more of the mind – that 'Monday morning' feeling.

PINE · *Pinus sylvestris*

Pattern of Imbalance
Undue guilt, self-reproach; blaming self for the wrong-doings of others.

Positive Potential
Objective acknowledgement of own faults; self-forgiveness; ability to take responsibility with a fair and balanced attitude.

RED CHESTNUT · *Aesculus carnea*

Pattern of Imbalance
Fear and excessive concern for the welfare of others; always imagines the worst; extremely disturbed by reports of war, famine or other disasters; mentally congested; tense.

Positive Potential
The ability to send out thoughts of safety, health or courage to those who need them; to keep a cool head in emergencies.

ROCK ROSE
Helianthemum nummularium

Pattern of Imbalance
Terror, hysteria, fear and panic – at the site of a terrible accident, for example. May also help those prone to panic attacks for no apparent reason.

Positive Potential
Courage and inner stability when facing great challenges.

ROCK WATER

This is not a plant, but potentised spring water

Pattern of Imbalance
Rigid self-discipline; asceticism; denial of feelings; anxious and tense; intolerant, but rarely openly critical of others; possible tendency to eating disorders; may become fanatical about maintaining a 'healthy' lifestyle.

Positive Potential
Flexibility; an open-minded idealism; radiates joy and peace; is in touch with the emotional aspect of self; experiences sensuous pleasures; is able to relax and have fun!

SCLERANTHUS
Scleranthus annus

Pattern of Imbalance
Indecision, confusion and hesitation; wavering between two possibilities; may suffer from mood swings; unstable; tends to be unreliable; lacks concentration; lacks poise; may suffer from nervous breakdown or collapse; may have a violent temperament.

Positive Potential
Decisiveness; inner resolve; maintains poise and balance whatever the circumstances.

STAR-OF-BETHLEHEM
Ornithogalum umbellatum

Pattern of Imbalance
Shock or trauma, either recent or from a past experience; grief; emotional numbness. Although not a Type remedy (as defined by Bach), the flower essence can help those who suffer from long-term physical and emotional distress as a result of some past trauma.

● **Positive Potential**

The neutralisation of the effects of shock on the mind/body complex, whether immediate or delayed.

SWEET CHESTNUT
Castanea sativa

● **Pattern of Imbalance**

Extreme mental anguish – the 'dark night of the soul'; the utmost limits of endurance; unable even to pray; a profound sense of isolation.

● **Positive Potential**

The return of hope; the end of torment is at last within reach; personal experiences of the Godhead – or deep courage and faith stemming from the Higher Self.

● **Comparison**

Compare with Mustard, whose depression comes and goes like a black cloud, for no apparent reason. The Sweet Chestnut despair is triggered by some life-shattering event.

VERVAIN · *Verbena officinalis*

● **Pattern of Imbalance**

Strain and tension as a result of over-enthusiasm; possible tendency towards fanaticism, perhaps expressed as missionary zeal.

● **Positive Potential**

Passionate and charismatic; the ability to step back and to relax when necessary; the realisation that others have a right to their opinions; the wisdom to reach a different viewpoint through discussion and good argument.

● **Comparison**

Compare with Vine, who is pushy and domineering for egotistical reasons. Vervain is motivated by concern for the welfare of others; a desire to enthuse and convert.

VINE · *Vitis vinifera*

● **Pattern of Imbalance**

A domineering and inflexible personality who forces their will upon others; a striving for power; ruthlessly ambitious; lacks sympathy for others; may have a violent temperament.

● **Positive Potential**

Tolerance for the individuality of others; the wise and compassionate ruler, leader or teacher who inspires others; the ability to guide rather than to dominate.

● **Comparison**

Compare with Vervain, who tries to convince others through explanation and debate. Vine will not argue the matter, but simply expects others to obey.

WALNUT · *Juglans regia*

● **Pattern of Imbalance**

Great difficulty in adjusting to change of any nature, including the milestones of life such as adolescence, menopause and old age; over-influenced by the ideas and persuasions of others, or by past experiences.

● **Positive Potential**

The courage to follow own path and destiny; the ability to move with the tides of change; freedom from limiting influences.

● **Comparison**

Unlike Honeysuckle, Walnut desires to move on, but finds it difficult to break the link with the past or with certain individuals.

WATER VIOLET
Hottonia palustris

● **Pattern of Imbalance**

Pride and aloofness; disdain of social relationships; suffers in silence; physical rigidity; avoids argument; sad; radiates superiority.

● **Positive Potential**

Although remaining comfortable with own company, the desire to share with others and to appreciate social relationships; becomes a source of hope and renewal to others.

WHITE CHESTNUT
Aesculus hippocastanum

- **Pattern of Imbalance**

Persistent worrying thoughts and mental arguments, possibly resulting in headaches, physical exhaustion, disturbed sleep or insomnia. The remedy is also helpful for those whose minds are overactive as a result of excessive study.

- **Positive Potential**

Peace of mind and clarity of thought.

WILD OAT · *Bromus ramosus*

- **Pattern of Imbalance**

Confusion and indecision about life direction; boredom and frustration; inability to find work which expresses inner goals and values.

- **Positive Potential**

Profound contentment as a result of finding work (or a way of living) which harmonises with own sense of purpose and meaning.

WILD ROSE · *Rosa canina*

- **Pattern of Imbalance**

Resignation and apathy; neither happy nor unhappy; emotionally 'flat'; uncomplaining; accepts misfortune, illness and monotony as if they were a penance decreed by fate – 'for the sins of the fathers'.

- **Positive Potential**

A feeling of revitalisation; a renewed interest in life; the enrichment and enjoyment of friendship.

WILLOW · *Salix vitellina*

- **Pattern of Imbalance**

Bitterness and resentment; constantly dwells on the unfairness of life; grumpy and morose; irritable and sulky; may feign illness to obtain pity.

- **Positive Potential**

The ability to accept responsibility for own life and health; a sense of humour; the ability to see things in their true perspective.

- **Comparison**

Compare with Holly, who can more easily express anger and jealousy. Willow is much more withdrawn and depressed – the 'poor me' attitude.

RESCUE REMEDY

A composite of five Bach remedies: Star-of-Bethlehem (for shock and numbness); Rock Rose (for terror and panic); Impatiens (for great agitation, irritability and tension); Cherry Plum (for violent outbursts and hysteria); Clematis (for the bemused, faraway sensation that often precedes a faint).

As its name suggests, Rescue Remedy is for all emergencies – when there is panic, shock, hysteria, mental numbness, even unconsciousness (in which case, a few drops can be applied to the lips, temples and wrists). Although the remedy cannot replace medical attention, it can alleviate much of the person's distress whilst they await the arrival of medical aid, thus enabling the mind/body's self-healing processes to commence without delay.

Rescue Remedy is also helpful in other upsetting situations such as visiting the dentist, receiving bad news, attending court proceedings, after an argument, or when a child is distressed after seeing horror or violence on television.

OTHER DIMENSIONS

Once you have mastered the basics of prescribing as outlined earlier, you may wish to take things further. At the risk of alienating those who would dismiss as fanciful such practices as dowsing, muscle testing, astrological diagnosis and dreamwork, this section is offered as food for thought.

Although it can take time to perfect such skills, if you are drawn to this area of research you will find it both fascinating and rewarding. With regards to dowsing and muscle testing, these are just two methods of many for communing consciously with the intuitive aspect of self. As well as being tools for ascertaining the most appropriate flower remedies (and perhaps essential oils) for yourself and others, the same methods can be employed for detecting hidden allergies to foods and other substances.

DOWSING

Many flower remedy practitioners employ dowsing (using a pendulum) to ascertain the most appropriate flower remedies. The pendulum, which can be just a wooden bead, earring or wedding ring on a length of thread, is held over a number of remedies in turn. The dowser asks themselves silently whether specific essences are required. Within moments, the pendulum usually begins to swing. Most dowsers interpret a clockwise swing as 'yes', a counter-clockwise swing as 'no'. Should the pendulum swing from side to side, this indicates that the remedy may be required at a later date.

When ascertaining the most appropriate flower remedies for someone else, ask the person to place one finger on each test bottle in turn. At the same time, gently place one hand over your partner's hand to create a circuit between the two of you. Holding the pendulum in your other hand, dowse as described above.

If you have a large selection of flower essences, it may be helpful to dowse up to a dozen 'possibles' at one time – preferably with the labels turned away from you so as not to influence the outcome through auto-suggestion. The remedies to be dowsed should be determined by your own experience and knowledge of the flowers' healing properties. If the pendulum comes up with more than six remedies, simply trust your instincts and opt for those which seem especially appropriate at the time. However, should the pendulum swing particularly vigorously over just one or two remedies (as is most common), discard the 'weakly positive' essences in favour of the 'strongly positive' ones.

MUSCLE TESTING

Flower therapy practitioners employ muscle testing much less frequently than dowsing, mainly because it is more time-consuming. The method described here is just one of many exercises gleaned from the com-

prehensive system of diagnosis and healing known as Applied Kinesiology.

The subject is asked to stand erect with their right arm raised in a horizontal position (or their left arm if left-handed). With their stronger hand (left or right) the tester pushes down gently for a couple of seconds, with the palm open, on the subject's extended arm, to feel the normal muscle strength. Then the subject holds a bottle containing a flower essence in their other hand. After this, the tester reassesses the subject's muscle power by gently pressing down on the raised arm. If the oil registers as positive, the subject's arm will stay up. However, if a flower essence is unsuitable the arm may shake or give under the slightest pressure. In other words, the most beneficial essences will strengthen the muscle, or will have no effect, while those of no value at the time of the test will weaken the muscle.

Just because a remedy appears to weaken a muscle (or causes a pendulum to swing in an anti-clockwise direction), this does not mean it is 'poisonous' to the individual concerned. Rather, the subject's mind/body seems to know whether or not a remedy is going to be helpful at a given time, and communicates its response through the chosen therapeutic tool. However, when using muscle testing (or indeed dowsing) for detecting allergies to essential oils, herbs or food substances, a negative response may well indicate that a particular substance is potentially harmful.

MOON SIGN ASTROLOGY

Almost everyone has encountered Sun sign astrology, the form which has been popularised (and trivialised) in magazines and newspapers. So you probably know your Sun sign, which is dependent upon the four-week period in which you were born. For example: Aries (21 March–20 April), Taurus (21 April–21 May), Gemini (22 May–22 June), and so on through the twelve signs of the Zodiac.

The Moon, on the other hand, takes roughly two and a half days to travel through each sign. Even though it is quite possible for your Moon sign to be the same as your Sun sign, it is more likely to be different.

Naturally, serious astrology takes into account the

position of every planet at the precise moment of a person's birth, not just the position of the Sun. (Incidentally, for the sake of convenience in astrology the Sun and Moon are called 'planets', even though the former is a star and the latter a satellite.) Anyone who has taken the trouble to obtain a personalised birthchart prepared and interprseted by a professional astrologer will confirm that the information can be staggeringly accurate. None the less, most astrologers would agree that the position of the natal Moon, even when interpreted in isolation, is highly indicative of the essential self.

When astrologers refer to the Sun they are essentially referring to the conscious focused 'thinking' aspect of the personality. By contrast, the Moon reveals the deeper, more private and emotional aspects of our being. This underlying personality will reveal itself more readily when we are tired, ill or overwrought – though its positive aspects are also likely to surface, especially during peak moments in life. The natal Moon reflects how we react to situations presented to us by others and how we behave when our passions are aroused. For this reason, Moon sign astrology marries exceptionally well with flower therapy.

Moon Signs and Flower Therapy

During the earlier years of his work with flower essences, Bach took a great interest in astrology. He found that the natal Moon revealed the basic personality type; the individual's true mission in life; the lessons they had to learn; and the flower remedy (or remedies) which would most help them in that work.

However, he also believed that astrologers often place too much emphasis on fate – and, in so doing, overlook the possibility of free will. 'It is only in our earlier stages of development that we are directly influenced by the planets. . . . Once love enters into the patient, not self-love, but the love of the Universe, then we free ourselves from our stars, we lose our line of fate, and for better or worse we steer our own ship' (from *The Collected Writings of Edward Bach*). So he abandoned astrological diagnosis in favour of the direct approach: observation, spiced with intuition. He also wanted to keep everything as simple as possible, within the boundaries of common understanding and knowledge.

Generally speaking, he was right to simplify the method of diagnosis. Yet from my own experience Moon sign astrology, if applied within the context of a thorough investigation of the person's worries, fears and concerns, can impart a revealing dimension to diagnosis.

The Moon Sign Profiles which follow include a selection of possible flower remedies. Quite apart from narrowing down the process of selection, the method is especially helpful when prescribing for complex individuals who seem to have 'hidden depths' (see also Flower Therapy Dreamwork on pages 79–80).

It is important to remember that our social and cultural conditioning, along with our astrological tendencies, are not fixed. Finding the remedy which resonates most strongly with the essential self (that which is often hidden beneath the conditioned outer self) will help to release a great deal of positive potential. The remedy may even become a major catalyst in the healing process, enhancing (or revealing for the first time) a sense of purpose and meaning to the life experience.

If you do not know your Moon sign, most astrologers would be happy to provide a computerised chart of the planetary positions at the exact time and place of your birth. As long as you do not require an interpretation of the birthchart, the fee will be very modest.

Even without prior knowledge of your Moon sign, you may well recognise yourself in one of the profiles – if you can be totally honest with yourself! You will probably have less difficulty identifying the emotional patterns of other people.

Should you prefer to ignore the astrological connection, the profiles can still be used as a teaching aid. You could have fun working out the most helpful remedies for each of the twelve personality types. You may find that your own choice for a certain personality does not coincide with any of the suggested remedies. This does not necessarily mean that you are mistaken. On the contrary, you may well have hit upon something important.

Moon Sign Profiles follow on page 76

MOON SIGN PROFILES

For the sake of simplicity, most of the suggested remedies are from the Bach repertory profiled on pages 67 – 73. Those flower essences given in *italics* are from the Californian Flower Essence Society (FES) repertory. A summary of the emotional healing properties of these can be found in the Directory of Healing Plants in Chapter 10.

MOON IN ARIES

Strong desire for leadership; forceful inner drive; idealistic; inspires others; courageous, broad-minded; good sense of humour; can take a joke against self; generally warm-hearted; prepared to take risks; possibly accident-prone; acts quickly in an emergency; craves excitement and change; possibly an energetic social reformer; prone to blind optimism; short-tempered; critical and impatient; intense dislike of 'neurotic' people; over-enthusiastic; impetuous; headstrong; resents advice

Remedies Strongly Indicated: Vine, Impatiens, *Sunflower*, Vervain
Possible Helpers: Agrimony, Beech, Chestnut Bud

MOON IN TAURUS

Impulsiveness balanced by persistence and determination; a good parent; strong sense of duty; loyal; great tenacity and endurance against all odds; appreciates beauty in all its forms; quick to defend the underdog; tries hard to maintain the status quo; tendency to be over-concerned for the welfare of others; tendency to possessiveness and jealousy; self-indulgent; sometimes over-critical; intolerant of those who lack self-confidence; moody; manipulative at times; fixed opinions

Remedies Strongly Indicated: Oak, Chicory, Red Chestnut
Possible Helpers: Beech, Elm, Holly

MOON IN GEMINI

A highly complex character! Analytical mind; ambitious; good sense of humour and ability to make witty comments; indecisiveness and changeability; some conflict within the personality; hyperactive; tendency to worry over trifles; over-concern with the self; discusses own problems to excess; experiences difficulty coping with emotions of others; tense and stressed; often antagonistic; always in 'crisis'; impatient and demanding; prone to depression and exhaustion

Remedies Strongly Indicated: Scleranthus, Heather, Impatiens, *Lavender*
Possible Helpers: Rescue Remedy, White Chestnut, Chestnut Bud, Wild Oat, Olive

MOON IN CANCER

Strong need to cherish and protect; highly sensitive; empathetic and intuitive; can be trusted with secrets; moody; may indulge in emotional blackmail; clingy; lacks self-confidence, leading to jealousy and resentment; tendency to sulk; strong attachment to the past; tendency to hoard; vulnerable and weak-willed; worried and anxious; tendency to attract parasitic people; over-sentimental

Remedies Strongly Indicated: *Chamomile*, Red Chestnut, Chicory, Centaury, Willow
Possible Helpers: Walnut, Honeysuckle, Mimulus, Pine, White Chestnut

MOON IN LEO

Longs for drama, romance and excitement; leadership abilities; kind-hearted, generous and sympathetic; a good teacher; organisation skills; strong will and determination; playful, friendly and loyal; ostentatious at times; can be stubborn; occasional feelings of intense superiority, alternating with sudden loss of self-esteem; fears competition; angry and aggressive when pushed; bossy and demanding at times; craves attention and appreciation; tendency to dramatise own weaknesses in order to manipulate others

Remedies Strongly Indicated: Impatiens, *Sunflower*, Vervain
Possible Helpers: Chicory, Elm, Larch, Holly, Vine

MOON IN VIRGO

Organisational skills; logical mind; loyal and trustworthy; shy at first, but sociable when able to relax; understands others; fear of disorder and chaos; over-analytical; possibly nervous and timid disposition; tendency to overwork; self-critical; not openly affectionate; easily embarrassed; may harbour intensely critical feelings towards others, though usually keeps remarks to self; prone to pessimism; lacks self-confidence; over-concerned about own health; bottles up emotions

Remedies Strongly Indicated: Rock Water, Mimulus, Water Violet, Larch
Possible Helpers: Crab Apple, Elm, Gentian, Pine

MOON IN LIBRA

Natural charm and courtesy; a peacemaker; diplomatic; popular and friendly; strongly independent nature, yet works best in partnership; ambitious and yet lazy; logical mind; dislikes injustice of any kind; capable of putting things into action, albeit slowly; hates making decisions; possibly vain about appearance; susceptible to stress and nervous exhaustion; craves aesthetic and peaceful environment; possibly prone to travel sickness; can be duplicitous; elitist tendencies; keeps emotions under control

Remedies Strongly Indicated: Scleranthus, Wild Oat, *Lavender*
Possible Helpers: Hornbeam, Olive, White Chestnut, Water Violet, Rescue Remedy

MOON IN SCORPIO

Intense passion, combined with overwhelming need for reassurance; highly intuitive; may possess psychic gifts; hard-working and tenacious; extremely caring towards loved ones; tries to hide depth of feeling, though

usually fails; paranoiac tendencies; may channel fears and nervous energy into proving themselves sexually or materialistically; possessive and clingy; suspicious and cautious; allows feelings to fester, resulting in angry outbursts; may become silent and depressed; fearful and hypersensitive

Remedies Strongly Indicated: Aspen, *Basil*, Chicory, Willow
Possible Helpers: Cherry Plum, Holly, *St John's Wort*

MOON IN SAGITTARIUS

Restless, optimistic and cheerful; a fluent talker; sense of urgency and quickness of movement probably apparent; ability to enthuse and motivate others; can be tactless at times; finds it hard to learn from past mistakes, so repeats the same experiences; prone to blind optimism; easily bored; desires challenge; needs personal freedom and independence; broad-minded; may have an explosive temper; tendency to want something passionately, yet interest wanes once gained; often avoids facing reality

Remedies Strongly Indicated: Impatiens, Chestnut Bud, *Californian Poppy*, Agrimony
Possible Helpers: Wild Oat, Scleranthus, White Chestnut, Vervain

MOON IN CAPRICORN

Reserved, cautious and prudent; mature and practically minded; a good teacher; hard-working and tenacious; slow to anger, though overpowering and destructive when anger does erupt; over-serious and inflexible at times, relieved by a dry wit; clings to the past; old-fashioned ideas and attitudes; needs to be in control of emotions; sensitive, vulnerable and shy, though capable of overcoming this in later life; easily hurt and embarrassed; prone to gloominess and austerity

Remedies Strongly Indicated: Beech, Gentian, Oak, Walnut, Mimulus
Possible Helpers: Cherry Plum, Gorse, Honeysuckle, Mustard

MOON IN AQUARIUS

Humanitarian, eccentric and unpredictable; optimistic and cheerful; shows originality and ingenuity; inspires enthusiasm about some odd cause; desires challenge; broad-minded; detached and independent; experiences difficulty coming to terms with own emotions; intolerant of 'neurotic' people; fast thinking processes, yet also intuitive; hates to appear weak and incapable; impatient with those who are slow; can be aloof and erratic; loneliness as a result of failed emotional relationships

Remedies Strongly Indicated: Agrimony, Elm, Impatiens, Vervain
Possible Helpers: Sweet Chestnut, Water Violet, Wild Oat

MOON IN PISCES

Idealistic, creative and imaginative; intuitive and possibly psychic; empathic and patient; good with children and 'let's pretend' games; natural teacher and counsellor; dislikes any form of injustice; fears making people angry; hypersensitive and sulky; tendency to martyrdom; attracts parasitic individuals; easily depressed; a worrier; superstitious and fearful of inexplicable 'dark forces'; senses impending disaster; often gloomy and pessimistic; prone to boredom and laziness; low self-esteem; possibly reclusive

Remedies Strongly Indicated: Aspen, Centaury, Mimulus, Pine, Wild Oat
Possible Helpers: Clematis, Water Violet, Larch, Gorse, Hornbeam, Gentian

HEALING DREAMS

Since the beginning of time primitive people of many cultures have revered dreams, regarding them as a means of understanding themselves and nature. It was not until 1900, however, when Sigmund Freud published his ground-breaking *Interpretation of Dreams* that the subject was deemed worthy of serious study. 'Dreams', he wrote, 'are the royal road to the unconscious.' He saw all dreams as wish fulfilments, an expression of repressed, sexual, 'forbidden' desires in a disguised form.

The Swiss psychiatrist Carl Gustav Jung, who broke ranks with Freud in 1913, disagreed with him about the wish-fulfilment and sexual nature of dreams. He also believed that Freud's 'disguise' was too elaborate and preferred to take the dream at face value. He did, however, share the view that dreams put the dreamer in touch with parts of the self which are usually concealed during waking life. Jung also saw dreams as a way of attaining self-knowledge, which in turn (together with religious or spiritual experiences) is a path towards 'self-realisation'. Self-

realisation is the ultimate aim of the personality: a lifelong process attained by very few individuals, Jesus and Buddha being notable exceptions. Nevertheless, Jung acknowledged that not all dreams are equally significant in this respect.

While Freud assigned fixed meanings to dream symbolism, Jung was much more fluid in his approach. He also advocated the study of dream series, that is, several dreams recorded over a period of time by the same individual. Above all, he looked for archetypal images.

Jung believed that all human consciousness is linked – that the consciousness of each person is like a small pond which trickles into the ocean of a shared 'collective unconscious'. The contents of this collective unconscious contain the archetypes. These are cross-cultural imprints, images and ideas which are intrinsic to the human psyche – patterns, themes, symbols and beings which appear in myth, fairy tales and world religions. Jung identified a large number of archetypes, including themes such as birth, death, rebirth, power and magic; also visual patterns such as the spiral, circle and five-pointed star; and beings such as Earth Mother, the Wise Old Man, the Demon, or God. According to Jung, the appearance of archetypal imagery in dreams signifies that the dreamer has transcended the boundaries of the personal self and is in direct contact with the collective unconscious, which in turn signifies a major step forward in the quest for self-realisation.

Following the works of Freud and Jung, many other psychoanalytic theories and methods have emerged and continue to evolve. One notable example is the work of Frederick (Fritz) Perls, founder of Gestalt therapy in the 1950s. Perls believed that dream images contain aspects of the dreamer's own personality and that we are the sum of the characters that dwell within us all.

In 1966 Calvin S. Hall described dreams as 'a personal document, a letter to oneself'. Like Jung, he advocated the study of dream series rather than single, isolated dreams.

However, it would seem that no single theory has the monopoly on truth. For this reason many therapists today favour the eclectic approach – that is, taking the best from the many psychotherapeutic systems and discarding anything that runs counter to their own belief systems.

It is a well-known phenomenon in psychotherapy that where there is a genuine desire for growth, whatever dreamwork method is adopted – be it Jungian, Freudian, Gestalt or perhaps the simple method you are about to learn – the client will dream to suit. Moreover, they need not even understand the theory. It appears that the unconscious, or Higher Self, is an all-knowing entity forever striving to enlighten the relatively naive conscious mind by whatever means it can muster, even if it means communicating through a mediator – the therapist and their chosen frame of reference!

FLOWER THERAPY DREAMWORK

The dreamwork method proposed here dispenses with the intricacies of dream symbolism and interpretation, which can be misleading (and unnecessarily complicated) for beginners. None the less, it has proved to be an invaluable tool for the flower therapy practitioner. It is also a method which can be employed in self-diagnosis and, when you have gained experience, in the diagnosis of others.

While many dreams are nothing more than a rehash of the day's events, others represent situations and patterns that need resolution. Occasionally a dream may provide an answer to a pressing problem, or it may even turn out to be precognitive. More often, dreams pose questions and invite responses.

The aim of flower therapy dreamwork, therefore, is to encourage you to focus on the feelings and responses your dreams evoke in you, and to prescribe accordingly. For example, you may be shocked by an expression of jealousy and violence in a dream (Cherry Plum, Holly), or some other powerful reaction rarely expressed in waking life. You might feel embarrassed, ashamed or guilty about being caught doing something untoward, or something you would normally regard as private (Crab Apple, Pine). You may feel overwhelmed by something or someone (Elm, Oak). Another dream may leave you feeling tense and anxious (Chamomile, Mimulus); depressed (Gentian, Gorse, Mustard, Sweet Chestnut); or trembling with fear (Aspen, Rescue Remedy).

As most dream therapists would verify, what we do not deal with in life will eventually come up in our dreams. Recurring dreams, or those which evoke familiar patterns of emotion, are particularly significant in this respect. Likewise the inability to sleep, or to remember our dreams, is sometimes due to a resistance to processing repressed material requiring expression.

If your dream reactions are similar to those in your outer life, this indicates that you have attained a certain degree of self-awareness. If they are very different, however, this suggests a great deal of repressed emotion to be dealt with. Interestingly, those who lead miserable or monotonous lives sometimes have wonderful dreams in vivid colour as a form of compensation.

Flower essences tend to activate the dream life, which is why it is useful to keep a record of your dreams for about a month whilst taking the remedies prescribed in the normal way. Once you can identify recurring themes and emotions, you will be in a good position to begin deeper work with the remedies. You can even ask for a significant dream just before falling asleep. As mentioned earlier, the unconscious or Higher Self is always willing to progress the course of self-knowledge.

Keep beside the bed a pen and notebook or a tape recorder, and immediately on waking (for dreams fade very quickly) write down all you can remember about a significant dream – there is no need to record every dream. Any dream which triggers a definite emotion might be significant, especially if it is an emotion or mode of action rarely expressed in the waking life. If a dream does evade you, record the particular emotion or mood it evoked. Then try to answer the following questions which are based on the work of the Jungian therapist and dreamwork expert Strephon Kaplan-Williams. Do not be concerned if you cannot answer every question fully; simply deal with as many issues as you can. The purpose of the exercise is to enable you to view your dreams from the flower remedy perspective.

1. What am I doing and why am I doing it?

2. What do I most need to deal with in this dream?

3. Would I react this way in the waking life, or am I reacting in a very different way?

4. What in this dream is related to things in other dreams I have had?

5. What in this dream is related to what is going on in me or in my life at present?

6. Why did I have this dream? What do I need to look at or make a choice about?

The purpose of writing is to externalise or make more concrete that which hitherto has had the advantage of being able to work in the dark of the unconscious. It is by viewing a disturbing feeling, memory or image in the light of conscious awareness that it becomes less threatening, perhaps totally disempowered. However, should your dreams be overwhelming, perhaps stemming from some half-forgotten childhood trauma, it would be advisable to seek the aid of an accredited counsellor who will help you work through the feelings, enabling you to release them.

CHAPTER SIX

THE GREEN HEALER'S APPRENTICE

THIS CHAPTER describes the basic methods of preparing and administering herbal remedies, aromatic oils and flower remedies. As many people have discovered, the primordial satisfaction of preparing plant remedies can be a healing experience in itself. Moreover, if you have a garden and can grow a variety of medicinal plants using sustainable methods of husbandry, without the use of artificial fertilizers and poisonous sprays, you will find as much joy in giving to the Earth as in reaping her precious gifts. However, because the practice of organic gardening requires a volume to itself, a few excellent manuals have been recommended in the reading list on page 263.

A wide choice of herbal remedies and essential oils, many of which have been produced from organically grown crops or from wild plants, can also be obtained from retail outlets specialising in herbal medicine and aromatherapy. Should you experience difficulty in obtaining any of the plant remedies explored in these pages, a list of mail order companies can be found in the Useful Addresses section on page 264.

COLLECTING MEDICINAL PLANT MATERIAL

The healing potential of a plant varies (at times considerably) according to many interrelated factors, particularly the age of the plant, the time of picking, the nature of the soil and the climate. Hence there are a number of rules which must be respected. But rather than confound you with a host of complicated recommendations for individual medicinal plants, the following guide will be sufficient for most purposes.

Harvest only fresh and healthy material. Generally speaking, plant material should be collected during warm, dry weather, after the dew has evaporated but before the greatest heat of the day. However, bark and roots are collected in a different manner.

BARK

This is collected either in spring or in autumn, when the sap is at a maximum and the bark can be readily detached from the trunk or thick branches. The bark will separate even more readily during damp weather. To prevent injury to the tree, be careful to gather only very small pieces here and there.

ROOTS AND RHIZOMES

These should be dug up from cultivated plants in the autumn or spring. This is because they are storage organs for the plant and accumulate medicinal constituents during the summer months.

LEAVES

These can be gathered throughout the growing period, though young leaves are thought to contain the highest-quality medicinal agents.

HERBAGE (THE AERIAL OR TOP PARTS OF THE PLANT)

The flower-bearing stems are cut off well above the ground, just before or at the beginning of the flowering stage.

FLOWERS

Gather at the beginning of the flowering stage when they are at the peak of perfection. Discard any blooms that have started to fade.

FRUITS AND SEEDS

These are collected when the seed pods have reached maturity, that is to say, as soon as they begin to darken and dry out.

WARNING

- Medicinal plants should only be gathered when identification is certain. Where there is the slightest doubt, buy a commercially produced remedy from a reputable supplier.

- Never gather plants that have been exposed to traffic fumes, factory emissions, artificial fertilisers or poisonous sprays.

- When gathering wild plants, always remember that conservation is of prime importance. A stand of plants should never be harvested in its entirety.

- Rare plants are protected by law and should never be collected from the wild. In such instances, a warning note has been included in the CAUTIONS section of the respective plant profiles (see Chapter 10).

- In Britain, it is illegal to uproot without permission any wild plant on land that does not belong to you, irrespective of whether it is a protected species.

DRYING AND STORING MEDICINAL PLANT MATERIAL

While it may be desirable to use fresh medicinal plant material, it is also important to dry some of it for use throughout the year. If carried out with care the medicine will remain potent for about a year – that is to say, from one harvest to the next.

NATURAL DRYING

This method is suitable for leaves, flowers and delicate herbs. Never wash the plants before putting them to dry as this will encourage the development of mildew. The material should be spread out on clean paper (not newsprint) in a shady, well-ventilated place, and turned over from time to time. Alternatively, bundles of herbs can be placed in paper bags, tied at the neck to keep out both sunlight and dust. Herbs are dry when they feel brittle and are easy to crumble. This may take 3–7 days for leaves, 7–14 days for bunches. Store in airtight glass jars, and crumble or rub the herbs through your fingers as you need them.

OVEN DRYING

Hard plant material like roots and bark needs to be dried out by heating. Remove any loose soil clinging to the roots and then rinse thoroughly in cold water. Do not scrub with a brush as this may cause the loss of precious constituents. Thick, tough roots and rhizomes may need to be cut in half lengthwise and then into small pieces in order to dry out properly.

IMPORTANT

Stored herbs should be frequently checked for signs of moisture, mould or insect attack and be discarded if necessary. Storage jars (preferably dark glass) should always be clearly labelled with the name and part of the herb, the date collected and the date bottled. It is essential to keep the jars in a cool, dry, dark place.

Cover a baking sheet with baking parchment and place the plant material on top. Put the tray in a very low oven, no higher than 50 degrees C (120 degrees F). Leave the oven door slightly ajar to prevent the build-up of moisture. Turn the plant material frequently. When the pieces can be easily broken they are ready to store in airtight glass jars.

Berries, for example elderberries, are dried in the same way. However, because they are so juicy they will need to be forked off their stalks when half dry. Turn them frequently during the drying process. Once the berries are completely shrivelled, store them in airtight glass jars.

DRYING AND STORING SEEDS

Choose a dry day for collecting ripe pods and for shaking larger seeds off the plant and into paper bags. Herbs like evening primrose and thyme produce minute seeds which must be collected before they fall to the ground. Cut the whole flowerhead on its stalk, tie the heads in bunches and hang them from hooks over a tray to catch the seeds. Alternatively, catch the seeds by inverting the heads into a paper bag and then tying the bag round the stems with string. Seed pods can also be dried on paper indoors for two weeks to remove all traces of moisture (see Natural Drying above). Dried seeds and/or seed pods must be stored in airtight jars as usual. Seeds intended for propagation can be stored in clearly labelled envelopes.

PREPARING HERBAL REMEDIES

Even though most medicinal herbs are available in tablet or capsule form, with the possible exception of valerian (a foul-tasting medicine), my own feeling is that it is preferable to use fresh or dried herbs. Smelling and tasting the herbal remedy can be an important part of the treatment, especially when dealing with digestive upsets. For example, certain constituents collectively known as bitters (found in peppermint and sage) promote the flow of saliva and gastric juices in a complex way via the taste buds and a reflex action in the brain. This action is bypassed when the remedy is taken in tablet or capsule form.

Many herbal remedies are also available as tinctures or alcohol-based extractions (see pages 84–5). Alcohol is an excellent medium for extracting both water-soluble and oil-soluble constituents. However, it can be tricky to prepare high-quality tinctures at home. Some plants take longer than others to impart their healing properties to alcohol, so there is little point in offering generalised instructions. There is also the difficulty of obtaining medicinal-grade alcohol (ethyl alcohol). In Britain (and in many other countries) it is not generally available as an over-the-counter commodity. Vodka or brandy could be used instead, though the resulting extract is generally regarded as inferior. All in all, it is best to obtain your herbal tinctures from a health shop or specialist mail order supplier.

CAUTION

Seek professional advice if there is any doubt about the interactions of herbal remedies with other medications that are already being taken. Advice should also be sought if there is any doubt about the safety of a herbal medicine intended for a child, pregnant woman or nursing mother. For babies and very young children, again seek professional guidance. The standard dose for children between the ages of five and twelve is one-quarter to one-half of the adult dose.

INFUSION (TISANE OR TEA)

Put 15g dried herbs into a warmed china, enamel or ovenproof glass vessel. Pour 600ml boiling water over the herbs, cover to prevent loss of volatile oils in the steam, and allow to steep for 10–15 minutes. If using fresh herbs, you will generally need three times as much. Seeds such as angelica and coriander should be bruised in a pestle and mortar to release the essential oils before being made into an infusion. The usual dosage is one teacup three times daily for chronic conditions, and up to six times daily for acute ailments.

DECOCTION

This method is used for hard woody plant material such as roots and bark, for instance ginger root and cinnamon bark. Break 15g dried plant material, or 45g fresh, into small pieces and place in an enamel or other heatproof vessel. Never use aluminium, as it will react toxically with the plant's chemistry. Pour 300ml water over the material and bring to boiling point; then turn down the heat and simmer with the lid on for 10–15 minutes. The usual dosage is one teacup three times a day for chronic conditions, and up to six times daily for acute ailments.

LOTIONS AND COMPRESSES

Cooled infusions of herbs like calendula, chamomile, lavender and violet can be applied externally as a soothing lotion for itchy or inflamed skin. They can also be used as a compress: pieces of lint are moist-

---

LET YOUR TASTE BUDS GUIDE YOU

Certain herbal infusions and decoctions, particularly those of flowers, fruits and spices like chamomile, elderflower, rosehip, lemon and ginger, may be sweetened with a little honey if desired. Others, like sage, rosemary marjoram and dandelion, have a strong savoury taste which does not marry well with honey. Simply allow your taste buds to guide you in this matter.

CAUTION

It is unwise to store infusions and decoctions for longer than 12 hours (even when kept in the fridge); mould spores develop within a surprisingly short space of time.

---

ened and applied to a bruise, skin rash, inflammation or injured area. They can be loosely bandaged into place if necessary, say when treating a swollen ankle (see also Aromatic Compress, page 91).

HERBAL BATH

Aromatic herbs like lavender, rosemary, chamomile and peppermint can be added to the bath to soothe, refresh or relax according to need. Simply fill a square of muslin with a generous handful of fresh herbs (or a couple of tablespoons of dried) and tie it on to the hot tap. For itchy skin or eczema, fill the muslin bag with a handful of oatmeal – oats are incredibly soothing to distressed skin. (Incidentally, a small muslin bag of moistened oatmeal can be used as a gentle facial 'scrub' for smoothing dry, flaky skin.) Alternatively, make an infusion of 55g dried herbs to 1 litre water. Allow to steep for 20 minutes, strain and pour into the bathwater.

HERBAL TINCTURES

The advantage of herbal tinctures is that they are quick and easy to administer. The usual dosage is 10–25 drops in half a teacup of water three times a day. The dosage varies according to the specific plant used and the strength of the tincture. Always read the label.

Certain tinctures, like calendula and sweet violet, can also be applied externally to treat skin rashes and eruptions. Add 10 drops to a 50ml dark glass bottle, then top up with distilled or boiled water and shake well. However, alcohol can be drying and slightly irritant, so avoid tincture-based lotions if your skin is exceptionally dry or sensitive. However, tinctures are less likely to dry out the skin if incorporated into a cream or ointment base. For example, to every 30g of shop-bought unperfumed cream or ointment, stir in 1 teaspoon of an appropriate tincture.

Tinctures should be stored in a cool, dark place away from damp. Although they are generally reckoned to remain potent for up to five years, once the bottle has been opened the shelf-life begins to decrease due to the process of oxidation (see page 89). Therefore, it may be prudent to use up your tinctures within two years of purchase.

HERB PILLOWS

The herb pillow (a form of aromatherapy) is an old remedy for facilitating restful sleep. Pillows stuffed with hops and other relaxing herbs become more strongly fragrant the longer they are lain on, because the warmth and pressure of the body help to release the essential oils. The method is simple: make a muslin bag to fit inside the pillow case and fill it loosely with dried, crushed herbs, so that it lies flat across your ordinary pillow.

When mixing different herbs, remember that lavender is a wonderful relaxant but the scent does not blend harmoniously with that of hops (though your nose is free to disagree!). Instead, try blending the hops with marjoram, lemon balm or linden blossom (or a little of each). Lavender blends especially well with lemon balm and chamomile. You could also dust the herbs with a little orris powder (the ground root of *Iris florentina*). It acts as a fixative, prolonging the staying power of the aromatic herbs, and imparts its own soothing, violet-like scent to the mixture.

You will need about 200g of herbs to perfume an average-size pillow. Although the aroma will still be detectable after a couple of years, the pillow will be more efficacious if the muslin bag is replenished once a year.

INTRODUCTION TO THE USE OF ESSENTIAL OILS

Essential oils are excellent healing agents, but they also highly concentrated and potentially hazardous if misused. So before you begin experimenting with the oils please read the safety guidelines given here.

AROMATHERAPY DURING PREGNANCY

During pregnancy the skin becomes more permeable and also more sensitive, so essential oils need to be used with great care. Moreover, certain essential oils, especially citrus essences, are able to cross the placental barrier. Citrus essences are also more likely to irritate sensitive skin. And yet these are the very oils which many aromatherapists promote as being among the safest to use during pregnancy!

Other potentially risky essential oils are those which have a stimulating effect on the uterus, the central nervous system, liver or kidneys. Examples of such oils include common sage, nutmeg, rosemary and juniper respectively. Even so, you may still come across an aromatherapy book which promotes the use of such oils during pregnancy.

Having painted such a confusing picture, it is important to get everything into perspective. There is no evidence whatsoever to suggest that pregnant women have been harmed by *therapeutic* applications of essential oils. If this were not the case, aromatherapy would have been banned years ago. In reality, a woman would need to apply (or swallow) a high concentration of essential oil in order to cause

---

CAUTION

Due to the soporific properties of hops, they should be avoided by people suffering from depression.

---

miscarriage, as the few reported cases in the USA of attempted abortion by ingestion of essential oils would verify.

Nevertheless, before using any essential oil do please check that it is safe to do so. Refer to the Directory of Healing Plants (Chapter 10). Where appropriate, a CAUTIONS note is included at the end of individual profiles (see also Essential Oil Precautions below).

For the record, my own approach is to advise against the use of essential oils on the skin during pregnancy because of the increased risk of sensitivity.

It is far better to use mood-enhancing room scents, perhaps complemented with gentle massage using plain vegetable oil.

Some people express doubts about the safety of *inhaling* low concentrations of essential oils during pregnancy. But considering that many pregnant women are exposed to petrol fumes, cigarette smoke, synthetic odorants, electromagnetic radiation and other pollutants, it would seem ludicrous to suggest that a few drops of essential oil (chosen according to personal preference) in a vaporiser could be harmful. On the contrary, many pregnant women have found

---

ESSENTIAL OIL PRECAUTIONS

- Keep bottles out of reach of children.

- Unsupervised skin application of essential oils on babies and young children is not recommended. It is safer to use plain almond or olive oil for massage, and/or to vaporise low concentrations (2 or 3 drops maximum) of any of the following oils according to need: citrus essences, frankincense, Roman chamomile, lavender, sandalwood, rose, neroli, petitgrain. For children over the age of five, use one-quarter to one-half the usual adult concentration of essential oil. Where there is the slightest doubt, please seek the advice of a qualified aromatherapist.

- There are many essential oils which should be avoided during pregnancy, including basil, cedarwood, clary sage, juniper and rosemary (see Chapter 10). The following oils have not been profiled in this book but are strongly contra-indicated: bay, birch, tagetes, hyssop, fennel, nutmeg, parsley, sassafras, spikenard, tarragon, thyme (see also pages 87–8).
  Generally, use essential oils in the lowest recommended quantities (see Easy Measures, page 93). Alternatively, avoid skin applications and use mood-enhancing room scents instead.

- Nursing mothers should use essential oils in the lowest recommended quantities (see Easy

Measures, page 93). Strong aromas can cause sleeplessness and irritability in babies. Remember, essential oils rubbed into the skin and/or inhaled can end up in the body fluids, including breast milk. Although there is no evidence to suggest that babies have been harmed by ingesting aromatic molecules through the breast milk, it is important to be especially careful. If in doubt, seek the advice of a qualified aromatherapist.

- People with epilepsy should avoid the following essential oils: fennel, hyssop, rosemary, sage. There is a remote chance that these oils may provoke a seizure.

- Generally, do not apply neat essential oils to the skin. Two exceptions are the occasional use of neat lavender on minor burns, scalds and cuts, and neat tea tree oil applied directly to pimples. In my experience, however, an alcohol-based product such as calendula tincture is best for zapping spots (applied neat) because it is very drying.

- Keep essential oils away from varnished surfaces as they may dissolve the coating. Despite this alarming fact, when correctly diluted as advocated in this chapter, essential oils are harmless to human tissue.

essences of ginger or peppermint helpful for early morning sickness.

Skilled but sensitive massage with olive oil (preferably the 'extra virgin' grade) is soothing to both mother and baby. The oil is also a wonderful preventative of stretch marks. A more finely textured and less odoriferous alternative is cold-pressed sunflower seed oil. Favourite essential oils can be vaporised into the room during the massage and at other times according to need, though smaller amounts are usually preferred. During pregnancy (particularly during the first trimester) many women experience a heightened sense of smell and taste. Undoubtedly this is a natural safety mechanism to deter the mother from ingesting (or inhaling) potentially toxic substances which might harm the unborn baby.

POTENTIALLY HAZARDOUS ESSENTIAL OILS

The essential oils profiled in this book represent just a fraction of those available to therapists. For this reason, the cautions given are not exhaustive. However, certain oils should not be used at all in

---

ESSENTIAL OIL PRECAUTIONS continued

- Keep essential oils away from the eyes. Should any get in, rinse it out at once with plenty of cool water.

- Never take essential oils by mouth, rectum (suppository) or vagina (pessary or douche). Although such methods are advocated by French aromatherapy doctors, unsupervised self-treatment is not recommended. Always seek medical advice beforehand.

- Citrus oils, especially bergamot, increase the skin's sensitivity to sunlight, so do not use on the skin shortly before exposure to sunlight (or a sunbed) as they can cause unsightly pigmentation. Other strongly photo-sensitising oils include angelica (root) and tagetes. However, it is possible to obtain a rectified bergamot oil labelled 'Bergamot FCF' (see page 221) which is virtually free of photosensitising agents.

- Avoid prolonged use of the same essential oil (i.e. daily for more than three months) as there is a slight risk of developing a sensitivity to it. Take a two-month break before using it again.

- If you suffer from sensitive skin, it is advisable to carry out a skin test before using an essential oil for the first time (see page 88). However, allergy sufferers are advised to seek constitutional treatment from a fully accredited medical herbalist or homeopath. This is especially important if you suffer from a chronic condition such as asthma, eczema, allergic rhinitis or food allergies.

- If you are undergoing homeopathic treatment, do seek the advice of your homeopath before embarking on the use of essential oils. Most aromatic substances have the potential to negate the effect of homeopathic remedies; coffee, cannabis, camphor, peppermint, tea tree and eucalyptus are believed to be particularly problematic. Additional known antidotes include spicy food, paint fumes, immunisation, dental work, emotional shock, acupuncture, shiatsu, deep tissue massage, antibiotics and other drugs. Always store essential oils well away from homeopathic remedies.

- Professional advice should always be sought if there is any doubt about the interactions of essential oils with other medications that are already being taken.

- Above all, never use an essential oil about which you can find little or no information.

aromatherapy. Some are highly irritant to skin and mucous membranes, whereas others are generally toxic. While such oils may be safe when used in minute quantities (as employed by the perfume and flavours industries), the quantities used in aromatherapy are comparatively high and therefore pose a greater risk.

Just because a herb or spice may be perfectly safe to take by mouth, it does not follow that the essential oil of the same plant, especially when applied to the skin, is equally benign. For this reason, the following essential oils are unsuitable for home use: aniseed, cinnamon (bark), clove (bud, stem and leaf), pennyroyal, elecampane (*Inula helenium*), fennel (bitter), origanum, sage (not to be confused with clary sage which is safe for home use), sassafras, savory and wintergreen.

Although the essences listed above can be used in a vaporiser, say as fumigants when infectious illness is around, skin applications must be avoided at all costs. Cinnamon bark, for example, is a powerful sensitiser. Once sensitised, the body will always react to the same substance (whether the essential oil or the culinary spice), no matter how tiny the quantity. Symptoms can vary from an itchy rash through to more widespread reactions such as streaming eyes, swollen tissues and wheezing.

Skin Test

When using an essential oil for the first time it is advisable to carry out a skin test, especially if you have sensitive skin. Mix up to 3 drops of the test essence in a teaspoon of almond oil. Rub a little of the mixture behind your ears, in the crook of your arm or on the inside of the wrist (ultra-sensitive spots). Leave uncovered and unwashed for 24 hours. If there is no redness or itching, the oil is safe for you to use.

In fact you can test up to six oils at the same time using this method, but you will need to keep a record of the oils used and where they were applied. For example, ginger behind the right ear, ylang ylang in the crook of the left arm, and so on.

Quality Control

With the increase in demand for essential oils has come the growing problem of adulterated products being sold to an unsuspecting public. Essences may be tampered with at source or somewhere else along the line before reaching the retail outlets. They may be diluted with an alcohol, for example, or perhaps blended with a less expensive oil with a similar-smelling aroma. There are also BP grade essential oils – those that have been modified in some way to meet a pharmaceutical standard. Far worse, an oil may be entirely synthetic, despite it being labelled 'natural'. While impure aromatic oils may have some therapeutic potential, say as antiseptic agents, they are much more likely to provoke allergic reactions like skin rashes, wheezing and sneezing.

The 'tricks of the trade' are difficult to detect unless the oil is analysed by costly high-tech methods such as gas-liquid chromatography. Yet it is possible for an experienced human nose with many years of training to detect quite sophisticated forms of adulteration.

Clearly it is vital to buy your oils from a reputable supplier, preferably a company whose oils carry a recognised certificate of purity awarded by the Essential Oil Trade Association (EOTA) or the Aromatherapy Trade Council (ATC) – see Useful Addresses, page 264. Organically produced oils will carry the seal of approval awarded by bodies like the Soil Association in Britain (see opposite). The same companies also market their products through good health food stores.

But do ensure that an essential oil labelled as such is in fact 100 per cent essential oil. You may come across an oil which is actually a mixture of about 2–3 per cent essential oil in a carrier such as grapeseed or almond oil. Such blends are fine as ready-mixed massage oils, though they are an expensive way to enjoy aromatherapy. It is less costly in the long run to purchase undiluted essential oils from which you can create your own aromatherapy blends.

ORGANIC ESSENTIAL OILS

Not all essential oils are produced by organic methods, that is to say, extracted from plants grown without the use of chemical fertilisers and poisonous sprays. However, a number of oils are distilled from wild trees or extracted from disease-resistant species, for example cypress, juniper, frankincense, pine and myrrh. Or they may be produced in areas where chemical sprays and fertilisers are not in general use, for example sandalwood oil from Mysore in India.

In Europe, organic growers meeting the desired standards are awarded certificates by bodies such as the Soil Association in Britain, Biofanc in France and Demeter in Germany. The symbol of the respective associations will be clearly visible on the label.

CARING FOR YOUR OILS

Essential oils evaporate readily and are easily damaged by light, extremes of temperature and exposure to oxygen in the air. This is why they are sold in well-stoppered dark glass bottles. The usual capacity is 10ml, though expensive oils like rose and neroli may be sold in quantities of 5ml and 2ml.

Most essential oils will keep for a few years, depending on how often you open the bottle and expose the contents to the air. However, with the exception of bergamot, citrus oils may deteriorate rather sooner – within 6–9 months. A few oils improve with age, rather like some good wines; examples are sandalwood, patchouli and frankin-

cense. But the more often you open the bottle, the greater the chance of oxidation – a process whereby a substance is chemically combined with oxygen so that its original structure breaks down, as reflected in the deterioration of the aroma.

To prolong the shelf-life of your oils, keep them in a dark, dry place in normal to cool temperatures. Essential oils can be stored in the fridge, but not in the freezer. Put the bottles into an airtight food container and keep in the salad compartment which is less cold than other parts of the fridge. Although many essences turn cloudy when kept cold, they become clear again after an hour or two at room temperature. Citrus essences, however, are the exception and may become irreversibly cloudy if stored in very cold conditions. Nevertheless, this will not affect their therapeutic properties. Incidentally, rose otto (not rose absolute) is unusual because it is semi-solid at low temperatures, but becomes liquid with the slightest warmth, so rub the bottle between your hands for a few seconds before use. Oils kept in the fridge should be removed an hour before use.

Although undiluted essential oils have a long shelf-life, once they are diluted in a base oil such as almond or sunflower seed the aroma will quickly deteriorate – along with the oil's therapeutic properties. Massage blends should be stored in the same conditions as concentrated essences but for no longer than about 6 weeks. However, it is far better to mix just enough massage oil for a single treatment, rather than to store it for any length of time.

CONSERVATION WARNING

Avoid using rosewood (also known as bois de rose). At present the principal supplies of this oil come from trees torn down from the rain forests of Brazil. Even though a replanting programme has been attempted, the new trees are unable to grow healthily in the impoverished soil whose nutrients have been leached by exposure to the elements. For the same reason, it is also advisable to avoid supplies of rosewood from other areas of South America and Africa.

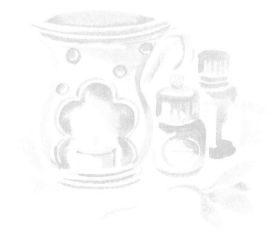

DIFFERENT WAYS TO USE ESSENTIAL OILS

There are many ways of using essential oils for promoting health and a sense of wellbeing. For the purposes of this book, we shall concentrate on the most popular and useful methods.

AROMATIC BATH

Essential oils can be added to the bath simply for pleasure, to aid restful sleep, to help skin problems, relieve muscular pain, ease cold and flu symptoms, and much more. Quite apart from their capacity as healers of an ailing body, they can also be used to subtly influence mood.

Add 4–8 drops of essential oil after the bath has been drawn. Agitate the water to disperse the oil. If you add the essences whilst the water is running, much of the aromatic vapour will have evaporated before you get into the bath. If you have dry skin, you may wish to mix the essences with a couple of teaspoons of a vegetable base oil, such as almond or sunflower seed.

FOOT/HAND BATH

This method can be used for athlete's foot and other skin complaints of the hands or feet – or just for the sheer joy of it! An aromatic foot bath at the end of a tiring day can be as relaxing as a soak in a full-size bath.

Put 5–6 drops of the appropriate essential oil in a bowl of hand-hot water, then agitate the water to disperse the oil droplets. Soak feet or hands for about 10 minutes. Dry thoroughly and massage into the skin a little vegetable oil (or cream) containing a few drops of the same essence(s).

INHALATIONS

As well as being helpful for respiratory ailments, aromatic inhalations can help bolster a flagging memory and uplift the spirits (see Aromatic Mood Enhancement on page 44).

Dry Inhalation

For mood enhancement, or to aid clarity of thought for study purposes, add a few drops of an appropriate essential oil to a handkerchief and inhale as required.

To help clear nasal congestion, put 5–10 drops of essential oil such as eucalyptus, tea tree or peppermint on a handkerchief and inhale as required. This method can be used to supplement the benefits of steam inhalation (see below).

Essential oils like lavender, rose otto and sandalwood can also be sprinkled on your pillow to help you breathe more easily when suffering from respiratory ailments. The same oils promote restful sleep too. However, certain pigmented oils like rose absolute and patchouli will stain linen. In such instances, it is preferable to put the oil on to a clean handkerchief and leave it nearby.

For nervous indigestion, put a few drops of peppermint oil on to a handkerchief and inhale every few minutes until you experience relief.

Steam Inhalation

This is a much more powerful decongestant for the respiratory ailments mentioned above. Researchers at Exeter University in the UK have produced scientific validation of old-fashioned steam inhalation as a treatment for colds and flu. The viruses responsible for these conditions are very sensitive to steam, which can actually kill them off. If done at the onset of symptoms, steam inhalations can prevent the condition from developing further. Adding a few drops of an antiviral essential oil like tea tree or eucalyptus increases the efficacy of the treatment.

CAUTIONS

Overuse of steam treatments, say more than twice weekly over a period of a few months, may result in a condition known as 'jungle acne'. If you have broken capillaries (thread veins) it is best to avoid the method altogether because the intense heat may exacerbate the condition. Avoid steam inhalations if you suffer from asthma: concentrated steam may trigger an attack.

Pour about 500ml of near-boiling water into a bowl and then add 2–4 drops of essential oil. The quantity depends on the strength of the aroma. Peppermint, for example, is extremely powerful and will make you catch your breath if you use too much. Inhale the vapours for about 5 minutes, but no longer than 10. In order to trap the aromatic steam more efficiently, drape a towel over your head and the bowl to form a 'tent'. You can take steam inhalations two or three times a day over a short period if you are suffering from a cold or flu.

Facial Steam

The same method can be used as a weekly deep cleansing facial. Stay under the steam for just a few minutes. Afterwards, splash your face with plenty of cool water (preferably bottled) to close the pores and remove tissue wastes which have been drawn to the surface. Apply an aromatic skin tonic if desired (see page 100).

AROMATIC COMPRESSES

A compress is a valuable first-aid measure for such problems as muscular aches and pains, skin eruptions, swellings, bruises and menstrual cramps. The most useful essential oils here are lavender or chamomile (Roman or German), for they are endowed with a wide range of therapeutic properties. However, it is important to know when to apply a hot compress and when to apply a cold one.

Hot

These are for old injuries, muscular pain, toothache, boils and abscesses. They can also reduce pain and congestion in internal organs and are therefore helpful for menstrual cramp.

To make a hot compress, add about 6 drops of essential oil to a bowl containing about 500ml of water as hot as you can comfortably bear. Place a small towel, or a piece of lint or cotton fabric, on top of the water. Wring out the excess and place the fabric over the area to be treated. Cover this with a piece of plastic clingfilm, then lightly bandage in place if necessary (for an ankle or knee, for example). Leave on until the compress has cooled to body temperature; renew at intervals as required.

Cold

These are for recent injuries such as sprains, bruises, swellings and inflammation, and for headaches and fever.

For a cold compress, use exactly the same method as above, but with very cold, preferably icy, water. Leave in place until the compress warms to body heat; renew at intervals as required.

VAPORISATION

This method can be used to purify the air when infectious illness is around. It can also be used to create a subtle mood-enhancing ambience in the home or workplace. Although there are many ways to vaporise essential oils, including adding a few drops to a radiator humidifier, the purpose-designed essential vaporiser, diffuser or 'burner' is by far the most effective.

The essential oil burner is usually earthenware, with decorative openings cut out of the sides to facilitate a free flow of air for the night-light candle which is placed inside. A small, sometimes detachable, reservoir which fits over the night-light is filled with water and a few drops of essential oil floated on the surface. This is gently heated by the flame. As the water evaporates, the room becomes permeated with fragrance. However, do ensure that the model you choose has a reservoir deep enough to accept at least 2 tablespoons of water. Otherwise, if you forget to refill the reservoir after the water has evaporated (which can be quite soon with some vaporisers) you may be left with a sticky, blackened residue of burnt oil which can only be removed with an alcohol-based solvent like surgical spirit.

Electric diffusers are also available. Since they do not pose a fire risk they are particularly suitable for the workplace, and certainly much safer than night-lights for use in the bedrooms of children and elderly people.

Generally, you will need between 4 and 15 drops of essential oil, depending on the odour intensity of individual oils used (let your nose be your guide), the capacity of your particular vaporising equipment and the purpose for which the oil is intended. For mood enhancement, less is certainly more. Even when the aroma can no longer be detected, the essential oil will carry on working on a subtle level (see page 41). As a fumigant, however, a stronger brew is recommended.

You can also vaporise floral waters (the by-products of the distillation process) such as rosewater, orangeflower water and lavender water. Simply fill the vaporiser vessel with the floral water instead of plain water. To strengthen or enhance the aroma, you may wish to add a couple of drops of an aroma-compatible essential oil (see the Aromatherapy note in the appropriate plant profile in Chapter 10).

Unfortunately, most of the floral waters available from the high street chemist are prepared from aroma chemicals. But genuine floral waters (also known as hydrolats or hydrosols) can be obtained from reputable essential oils suppliers.

MASSAGE OILS

Essential oils intended for massage need to be diluted in a natural base oil like olive, almond, peach kernel or sunflower seed, preferably labelled 'unrefined' or 'cold-pressed'. Ideally, the oil will also be described as 'organic'. While a refined oil (one which has been subjected to intense heat, bleaching agents, deodorants and possibly petroleum-derived solvents) will not actually harm the skin unless you have an allergy to the plant from which it derives, unrefined oils are

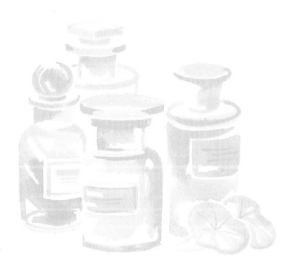

superior. They contain naturally occurring nutrients such as vitamins D and E, essential fatty acids (those which the body cannot manufacture for itself) and trace minerals, all of which are beneficial to the skin whether taken internally (as salad oil) or applied topically.

Never use mineral oil (often available as 'baby oil') as a base for essential oils. Not only does it lack the health-giving properties of unrefined vegetable oil, it also tends to clog the pores of the skin, contributing to the development of blackheads and pimples. Also, when used as a base for essential oils it hinders their absorption through the skin. Above all, the use of synthetic oil of any nature runs counter to the philosophy of aromatherapy.

SHELF-LIFE OF BASE OILS

With the possible exception of the highly stable extra virgin olive oil, other unrefined vegetable oils should be stored in the fridge. Even though the oil will turn cloudy, this will not damage its therapeutic properties.

It is important to remember that once an unrefined oil has oxidised (which can happen very quickly if the oil is kept in poor conditions) it will have a detrimental effect on the skin. During the oxidation process, oil molecules break down to produce what are known as free radicals. These substances, if left unchecked, can damage and destroy cells. They have also been implicated as a primary cause of the ageing process itself, so it is imperative to buy unrefined oils in small quantities and to use them up quickly, preferably even earlier than the 'best before' date stamped on the bottle.

MIXING MASSAGE OILS

Essential oils should be diluted at a rate of 0.5–3 per cent (see Easy Measures opposite), depending on the odour intensity of the oil in question and the purpose for which it is being used. The lowest concentrations (0.5–1 per cent) are best for facial oils, for pregnant and breastfeeding women, and for those with sensitive skin, including children under the age of twelve. I rarely use concentrations above 2 per cent for adults, even those with 'normal' skin. However, 3 per cent concentrations of certain oils like lavender or marjoram can be helpful when there is a great deal of muscular tension in the legs, back, neck and shoulders.

Certain essential oils emanate much stronger aromas than others, which means they will predominate your blends unless used in tiny amounts. Although your blending skills will develop with experience, it may be helpful to know that the fol-lowing oils are especially odoriferous and are best used in high dilution. The same oils will not necessarily irritate the skin if a little more is used (except perhaps if you have very sensitive skin); the quantities recommended below are ideal from the aesthetic viewpoint, an important consideration in aromatherapy. In the chart below those oils printed in *italics* have not been profiled in the plant directory, but are included here because they are widely available.

THE CORRECT DILUTION

Very Low Dilution (0.5 per cent or even less)

Angelica, basil, *galbanum*, ginger, valerian, *cardamom*, *fennel* (sweet), hops, *lemongrass*, melissa (lemon balm), *nutmeg*, rose otto, rose phytol, *vetiver*.

Blend Percentage	Essential Oil in Drops	Base Oil in Teaspoons (1tsp = 5 ml)
0.5	1	2
1	1	1
2	2	1
3	3	1

Low Dilution (1 per cent)

Black pepper, chamomile (Roman or German), clary sage, coriander, *elemi*, frankincense, geranium, jasmine, neroli, patchouli, peppermint, rosemary, ylang ylang.

Easy Measures

If you intend to mix enough oil for a single massage, use a 5ml plastic medicine spoon (available from pharmacies) to measure the base oil, as ordinary teaspoons generally hold less than 5ml. For a full body massage, you will need about 6–8 teaspoons of oil (a little more if the skin is hairy or very dry).

For a facial massage, you will need as little as 1–2 teaspoons. Since the skin of the face is usually more sensitive than the rest of the body, it is important to make up a separate facial oil with a higher dilution of an appropriate essential oil (refer to the Skin Care chart on page 99).

Just in case you are not quite sure where to begin, a selection of massage blends for specific conditions can be found in Part Two.

Mixing Larger Quantities of Massage Oil

Inexpensive dark glass bottles suitable for storing aromatherapy massage blends are obtainable from pharmacies. The capacity in ml (millilitres) is usually imprinted into the glass on the base of the bottle. The 50ml and 100ml sizes are the most useful. When filling the bottles with base oil, a small kitchen funnel will ease the process. Having filled the bottle almost to the top with base oil, add the essential oil; replace the cap and shake well to disperse.

Blend Percentage	Essential Oil in Drops (for a 50 ml bottle of base oil)
0.5	5
1	10
1.5	15
2	20
2.5	25
3	30

AROMATHERAPY PERFUMES

Many essential oils and absolutes make delightful skin perfumes when used singly or blended with other essences. They may be used purely for pleasure or to complement other aromatherapy treatment for healing emotional disharmony (refer to the Aromatic Mood Enhancement chart on page 44).

Natural perfumes can be diluted in light coconut oil (available from essential oils suppliers) or refined almond oil. As well as having a long shelf-life, these oils have very little odour of their own – an important consideration in perfume-making. Commercial perfumes are usually diluted in ethyl alcohol, but this is not generally available in Britain due to restrictions imposed by Customs and Excise.

The usual quantity is between 10 and 20 drops of essential oil to 10ml of base oil. The exact quantity will depend on the odour intensity of your chosen aromatics. Jasmine, for example, is highly odoriferous, whereas sandalwood has a much less intense aroma. Let your nose be your guide.

CAUTION

The quantity of essential oil in perfume blends is very much higher than for massage oils. Always carry out a skin test (see page 88). However, if you have sensitive skin it is advisable to avoid this method of use, though you could perhaps perfume the ends of your hair.

BLENDING PERFUMES

While it is enjoyable experimenting with blends of aromatic oils, you may also discover that a certain essence smells wonderful all by itself. The most popular oils suitable as perfumes in their own right include rose, neroli, patchouli, ylang ylang, cedarwood and sandalwood. Other possibilities (available from a few specialist suppliers) are the following precious absolutes: beeswax, jasmine, linden blossom and carnation.

When blending different aromatics, it is helpful to know that 'families' of essences generally harmonise: florals (rose/ neroli/ ylang ylang); citrus (bergamot/

PERFUME BLENDS

Here are some interesting perfume blends just to inspire you. As your blending skills develop, no doubt your aromatic good taste will take you in many other directions. The therapeutic properties of the blends will reflect the psychotherapeutic value of the oils used. However, it is much more important to follow your own instincts, to choose an oil (or a blend) that makes you feel good. Quantities are given in drops for a 10ml bottle of base oil.

Aytar
Deeply relaxing and sensuous
10 drops sandalwood
3 drops rose otto (or 6 drops rose absolute)

Earth Spirit
Reminiscent of an ancient forest
4 drops clary sage
4 drops petitgrain
1 drop patchouli
8 drops cedarwood (Virginian)

Fleur
Intoxicating and voluptuous
5 drops ylang ylang extra (or ylang ylang complete)
2 drops jasmine absolute
3 drops rose absolute
2 drops neroli

Serenade
Uplifts the spirit
8 drops bergamot FCF
3 drops orange
3 drops lemon
2 drops geranium
4 drops ylang ylang extra

orange/lemon); woods (sandalwood/cedarwood); spices (coriander/ginger); herbs (lavender/clary sage). Other compatible blends are spices with citrus (coriander/bergamot/orange); woods and flowers (sandalwood/rose); flowers, spices and citrus (ylang ylang/black pepper/mandarin).

Or why not be wild and creative and try mixing some unlikely-sounding aromas, such as voluptuous jasmine with a trace of holy frankincense; mature and earthy patchouli with the youthful green fragrance of clary sage; or the jolly scents of orange, lemon and bergamot with the sobering influence of juniper. You may well be delighted with the results! if you would like to know more about the art of blending and natural perfumery, see the Suggested Reading section on page 263.

How to Apply Perfume

Perfume is usually applied to the pulse points – behind the ears, at the sides of the neck, on the inside of the wrists, in the elbow creases, behind the knees and around the ankles. These points are traditionally believed to help to radiate the fragrance, perhaps because they are marginally warmer than other parts of the body.

Perfume can also be applied to the ends of your hair (if you have enough hair, that is!) for extra scent. Hair acts as a fixative for perfume (it increases its staying power); it also enhances the fragrance. Indeed, the slightly musky odour nuance of clean hair combines well with any perfume, but especially with citrus essences (the main ingredients of classical eau de cologne). Try to avoid getting perfume on the scalp, as the skin is sensitive there.

Home Distillation

Distilling essential oils at home may not be possible, for vast amounts of plant material are required to obtain a tiny quantity. However, you may be able to distil your own aromatic waters if you have an abundance of fragrant plants and plenty of time. The resulting liquids make excellent skin fresheners, or they can be vaporised in an essential oil diffuser to perfume a room subtly.

Half-fill a large enamel kettle with your chosen aromatic plant material – elderflowers, lavender, rosemary or strongly scented rose petals, for example. Pour in as much water as the kettle will hold. Place on the heat and attach a length of rubber tubing (available from good pharmacies) to the spout. Fill a bowl with ice and put this on a low kitchen stool or chair next to the cooker. Place a jug on the floor, near the stool or chair. Bend the tubing somewhere in the middle, resting the kink in the ice, then put the end of the tubing into the jug on the floor.

Bring the water to the boil, then reduce the heat so the water is kept at a very low simmer for a couple of hours or until the kettle is nearly, but not completely, dry. The steam that travels along the tubing will carry the essential oil droplets. The steam is cooled by the ice, which acts as a condenser, and the resulting aromatic water drips into the jug.

Infused Oils

Even though you can obtain a variety of infused oils from retail outlets specialising in natural remedies, it is much more satisfying to make your own. By macerating fresh aromatic plant material in a high-quality vegetable oil, it is possible to obtain a solution of the essential oil in the vegetable oil base. This can be used undiluted as a massage oil, or mixed 50/50 with a further quantity of vegetable oil. The diluted version is best for children, pregnant women and those with sensitive skin. Infused oils can also be incorporated into home-made creams and ointments (see pages 97–8).

CAUTION

It is advisable to carry out a skin test before using an infused oil for the first time (see page 88).

A SELECTION OF INFUSED OILS TO MAKE YOURSELF

The oils suggested here are some of the most useful and easiest to make. Lilac is not profiled in the Directory of Healing Plants, but the infused oil has a delightful mood-elevating fragrance. Interestingly, lilac is rarely used in European herbalism, though it features in Russian folk medicine, primarily for treating arthritic and rheumatic pain.

CHAMOMILE
Chamaemelum nobile

Parts Used: Flowerheads
Uses: General skin care (most skin types), skin rash, nervous tension
Suggested Blend: To increase the oil's anti-inflammatory and relaxant properties, mix 50/50 with infused oil of lavender

ROSE-SCENTED GERANIUM
Pelargonium graveolens

Parts Used: Leaves
Uses: Inflamed skin conditions, poor circulation, nervous tension
Suggested Blend: To enhance the oil's ability to soothe the nerves and calm itchy skin conditions, blend with equal quantities of infused oil of lavender and lemon balm

MARIGOLD · Calendula officinalis

Parts Used: Flowerheads
Uses: Inflamed skin conditions, including nappy rash, sore and cracked nipples, and eczema. Also helpful for healing scar tissue and encouraging stretch marks to fade
Suggested Blend: To increase the oil's skin-healing properties, mix 50/50 with infused oil of St John's wort

ST JOHN'S WORT
Hypericum perforatum

Parts Used: Flowering tops
Uses: For sunburn, bruises and haemorrhoids, and to ease the pain of sciatica, fibrositis and rheumatism
Suggested Blend: To increase the oil's ability to ease rheumatic pain, mix 50/50 with infused oil of meadowsweet or lavender (see CAUTION, page 97)

LILAC · Syringa vulgaris

Parts Used: Flower spikes (divided into florets)
Uses: For rheumatic pain and for uplifting the spirits
Suggested Blend: To increase the oil's antirheumatic properties, mix 50/50 with meadowsweet

MEADOWSWEET
Filipendula ulmaria

Parts Used: Flowering tops
Uses: Rheumatic and arthritic pain, nervous tension
Suggested Blend: To enhance the oil's ability to soothe nervous tension, blend 50/50 with infused oil of lavender

LAVENDER · Lavandula angustifolia

Parts Used: Flower spikes and leaves
Uses: Rheumatic aches and pains, headache, skin rashes, nervous tension and insomnia
Suggested Blend: To enhance the oil's ability to soothe skin rashes, mix 50/50 with infused oil of marigold

LEMON BALM · Melissa officinalis

Parts Used: Flowering tops
Uses: Nervous indigestion, anxiety, headache and insomnia
Suggested Blend: To enhance the oil's relaxant and anti-depressant properties, mix 50/50 with infused oil of lavender

MAKING AN INFUSED OIL

Pick the healthiest-looking flowers and/or leaves on a warm, sunny day, after the dew has evaporated. This is the time when the essential oil is at its highest concentration (with the exception of night-scented flowers such as jasmine and honeysuckle). You will need about 60g of fresh plant material to 600 ml of vegetable oil. To help release the essential oils, bruise the plant material by placing it on a wooden chopping board and crushing it with a rolling pin or a wooden mallet. Half-fill a large glass jar with the herbs, then cover with a good-quality vegetable oil. Place the jar outside in the sun for 2–4 weeks, weather permitting, but bring it indoors at night. Remember to shake the jar hard whenever you pass by.

IMPORTANT

Unrefined olive oil is one of the few natural oils capable of withstanding high temperatures. Most other cold-pressed oils, such as sunflower seed, safflower or hazelnut, are especially vulnerable to oxidation and must never be subjected to hot sun. The best grade of olive oil to use as a base for infused oils is virgin olive, but not the 'extra' grade as its pungent aroma may overpower that of the herb. If you would prefer to use a cheaper base oil, buy refined olive oil or some other reasonably stable refined oil such as corn, sesame or soya.

The ability to judge when the infused oil is ready comes with experience, but intensity of colour and aroma are good indicators. When ready, press the mixture through a few layers of muslin, then bottle the oil. After a while, there will probably be a separation of oil and herbal liquid (the oil will float on top): simply decant the oil into another bottle. If stored in a cool, dark place, your herbal oils will keep for about one year – from one harvest to the next.

AROMATIC OINTMENT

An aromatic ointment can be used for cuts, grazes, insect bites and stings, athlete's foot, ringworm, cold sores and chilblains. Simply 'doctor' 30g of an unperfumed shop-bought cream or ointment with up to 20 drops of essential oil. For example: 10 drops of tea tree, 5 drops of lavender, 5 drops of geranium. Put the cream in a little sterilised glass pot, and stir in the essences with the handle of a teaspoon. The ointment will keep for at least 6 months if stored in a cool, dark place.

MAKING YOUR OWN SKIN CREAMS

Most natural remedy suppliers carry a range of unperfumed skin care products suitable for 'doctoring' with essential oils and/or flower remedies. The usual quantity is 4–8 drops of essential oil (depending on the odour intensity of individual oils) to 30g of base cream. Flower remedies are added at the rate of 4 drops to 30g cream base, though precise quantities are not at all crucial.

You may prefer to create your own creams for soothing and nourishing stressed skin. Home-made skin creams are richer and heavier than the super-light creations available at the cosmetics counter, but they are extremely effective and economical. The recipe below makes a fairly soft cream which will harden slightly if kept in the fridge (to halt the formation of mould), but nevertheless melts on contact with the skin. You will find that a tiny amount will go a long way. The cream can be used anywhere on the body, though it is especially beneficial where the skin is flaky, chapped or cracked.

You can experiment with other base oils in the blend, such as hazelnut, apricot kernel or sunflower seed, or perhaps an infused oil such as lavender or marigold. But do ensure that the oil adds up to 120ml in all. Your creams will keep for three months if stored in a cool, dark place, preferably the fridge. Since home-made skin creams do not contain preservatives, it is advisable to use a cosmetic spatula (or perhaps the back of a clean teaspoon) to dispense the cream. Even the cleanest fingers harbour micro-organisms which can accelerate the deterioration of home-made cosmetics.

Yellow beeswax (used in the recipe opposite) is more natural than white beeswax. However, if you are prone to allergies the refined white version is less likely to irritate, but it is always a good idea to skin test it first (see page 88). Both kinds of beeswax can be obtained from herbal suppliers. If possible, try to obtain beeswax granules (rather than a hard block) as they are much easier to use. Should you wish to include in the basic recipe an essential oil suitable for your skin type, refer to the Skin Care chart on page 99.

As an alternative to beeswax you could use cocoa butter (the solid fat derived from roasted cocoa beans), but you will need to double the quantity as it is much softer than beeswax. It is also advisable to carry out a skin test first. As well as being good for drier skins, cocoa butter has the reputation for helping to prevent stretch marks during pregnancy.

Flower remedies can also be added to the cream base, especially the flower(s) you know you will need for as long as the cream lasts – for example your 'type remedy' (see page 63). If you are prone to nervous tension and anxiety, it is certainly worth adding a few drops of any one of the following Californian flower essences: Chamomile, Lavender or Valerian. Or, how about making a 'No Regrets' face cream? According to New Age psychotherapists, the negative emotion of regret accelerates the ageing process of the skin. So, if you regret the passing of time, the star ingredient of all your beauty creams should be the Bach flower remedy Honeysuckle!

BASIC SKIN CREAM

15g yellow beeswax (or 30g cocoa butter)
120ml almond oil
30ml distilled water
4–8 drops essential oil (optional)
4 drops flower remedy (optional)

Melt the beeswax with the oil in the top of an enamel double boiler or heatproof basin over a pan of simmering water. Meanwhile, heat the distilled water in another basin over a pan of simmering water until it has warmed. Begin to add the warm water, drop by drop at first, to the oil and wax, beating with a rotary whisk, balloon whisk or electric food mixer set at the lowest speed. After you have mixed about two teaspoons of the water into the oil and wax, remove from the heat and continue adding the water a little at a time until you have incorporated it all. As soon as the mixture begins to set, stir in the essential oil and/or flower remedy. Divide the mixture among little sterilised glass pots, cover tightly and label.

Variations

1. You could replace 1 teaspoon of the distilled water with the same quantity of a herbal tincture. Excellent choices for most skin types are marigold (calendula), lavender or chamomile. However, leave out the essential oil and/or infused oil, otherwise the cream may be too strong and likely to irritate rather than heal the skin.

2. Instead of plain vegetable oil, use the same quantity of infused oil according to need (see page 96). In this instance, leave out the essential oil and/or herbal tincture.

SKIN CARE CHART

You can prepare your own skin care blends from the choice of essential oils. Dilutions for facial treatment (see Easy Measures, page 93) that greatly exceed 1 per cent should be avoided. Best results are achieved if the oil is applied after a bath or shower, because warmth and moisture facilitate the absorption of essential oils. For oily skin, the ideal carrier for the essential oil is jojoba (a liquid wax derived from a desert plant native to South America). When massaged into the skin it combines with sebum and acts as an emulsifier, gently unclogging the pores and freeing embedded grime. It also contains myristic acid, which has anti-inflammatory properties.

Skin Type NORMAL

Description
Soft, smooth and finely textured. Few problems like spots and flakiness
Essential Oils
Chamomile (Roman or German), lavender, rose otto

Skin Type DRY

Description
Close-textured and fine, but can feel tight after washing with soap. May also flake and is predisposed to developing facial lines
Essential Oils
Chamomile (Roman or German), rose otto, sandalwood

Skin Type OILY

Description
Has a characteristic shiny look with large pores; prone to developing blackheads and pimples
Essential Oils
Frankincense, juniper berry, lavender, patchouli, rosemary

Skin Type COMBINATION

Description
The chin, nose and forehead form an oily T-zone on the face, whereas the skin around the eyes and on the cheeks and neck is dry
Essential Oils
Chamomile (Roman or German), frankincense, geranium, lavender, rose otto

Skin Type SENSITIVE

Description
Can be of any type, and may become sensitive from exposure to harsh soaps and cosmetic materials. Always carry out a skin test before using any skin care product (see page 88). Use essential oils in very low concentration, e.g. 0.5 per cent or even less
Essential Oils
Chamomile (Roman or German), lavender, neroli, rose otto

Skin Type THREAD VEINS

Description
Broken veins usually occur around the nostrils and across the cheeks. Can affect all skin types, especially sensitive skin
Essential Oils
Frankincense, geranium, neroli, rose otto

Skin Type MATURE

Description
In need of nourishing and toning
Essential Oils
Frankincense, geranium, neroli, sandalwood, rose otto

AROMATIC WATER

An aromatic water can be used in the same way as a commercial skin tonic or aftershave – splashed on after washing or shaving. Cider vinegar is included in the basic recipe given below because it helps to restore the skin's natural acid mantle. If you wish to use rosewater or orange flower water in the blend, do ensure that it is the genuine product (synthetic substitutes abound) by purchasing from a reputable essential oil supplier (see Useful Addresses, page 264).

METHOD

1 teaspoon cider vinegar
2–3 drops essential oil
Distilled water, rosewater or orange flower water

Put the cider vinegar into a 100ml dark glass bottle. Then add the essential oil, or a blend of essences amounting to no more than 3 drops altogether, chosen according to your skin type (refer to the Skin Care chart on page 99). Top up with distilled water (not tap water as this quickly develops mould), rosewater or orange flower water, and shake well to disperse the oil droplets.

For very oily skin or acne, you could use a more astringent base such as witch-hazel (the distilled extract of the leaves and twigs of the woodland shrub *Hamamelis virginiana*). This could be made slightly less astringent by mixing with an equal volume of distilled water.

Keep in a cool dark place and use up within 6 weeks. Remember to shake the bottle each time before use to disperse the essential oil droplets.

FLOWER REMEDIES

These come in little dropper bottles of what is known as stock concentrate. While the Bach flower remedies can be obtained from health shops and good pharmacies, most other flower essences (such as those profiled in the Directory of Healing Plants) are more easily obtained by mail order (see Useful Addresses on page 264). You may also enjoy learning the art of potentising your own flower essences (see pages 101–104).

SHELF-LIFE

If stored in a cool, dark place away from damp, the bottles of stock concentrate have a shelf-life of at least 5 years. Although the drops can be taken undiluted from the dispensing bottle, as is most common with Rescue Remedy, the usual method is to dilute flower remedies in a quantity of spring water (see below). Once diluted, the mixture will keep for no longer than 3–4 weeks.

PREPARATION OF THE TREATMENT

The standard dilution is 2 drops from each chosen bottle of stock (preferably no more than six different essences at a time) to a 25–30ml dropper medicine bottle (available from most pharmacies) three-quarters filled with spring water or mineral water. The bottle is then topped up with brandy or cider vinegar, which acts as a preservative. Tap water can be used if no other water is available, but it does turn stale sooner than bottled water, unless boiled and allowed to cool before use. A 30ml treatment bottle will be enough for a 3–4 weeks' course. Always label the treatment bottle with the date and the flower remedies used.

CAUTION

When prescribing for a recovering alcoholic, never add brandy to the treatment bottle. Always preserve the mixture with cider vinegar, for this masks the faint brandy taste of the diluted remedy. Alternatively, the diluted remedy from the treatment bottle can be added to half a cup of hot water and left to stand for 2 minutes, after which time the alcohol should have evaporated. Another method is to apply flower remedies externally to the pulse points, or else you could incorporate them into a skin cream or massage oil and/or add them to the bathwater (see also page 101).

DOSAGE

The standard dosage is 4 drops of the diluted remedy on the tongue three or four times daily. Or you may prefer to add the drops (diluted or neat) to fruit juice or herb teas. Shake the bottle each time before use to activate the remedy. If you are using a single flower essence you could take the remedy neat, 2 drops at a time. However, when taking a composite remedy it is far easier (and economical) to dilute the remedies as described above.

The most beneficial times to take the remedy are upon rising and at bedtime. But if you are in acute distress the remedy can be taken as often as required until you feel better. If preferred, the drops (either the stock concentrate or the diluted remedy from the treatment bottle) can be taken in a small glass or cup of spring water, herb tea or fruit juice.

USING THE BACH RESCUE REMEDY

If no water is available, the remedy can be used neat. Bach suggested taking 4 drops directly on the tongue several times a day. In extreme states of distress, such as hysteria or numbed shock, the remedy can be taken every 15 minutes until you experience relief. On an unconscious person, the neat or diluted remedy can be applied externally. Moisten sensitive areas of the body such as the temples, the back of the neck, the inner wrists, the backs of the knees, or behind the ears.

PREGNANCY, BABIES AND BREASTFEEDING MOTHERS

Flower essences are perfectly safe and beneficial for the expectant mother and her unborn child. The method and treatment are no different from usual. Moreover, the remedies can be given to newborn babies (as well as older children). Indeed, even though babies are unable to tell us about their state of mind, it is still possible to prescribe flower remedies for them, as discussed in Chapter 5.

The dosage is the same as for adults. Add 4 drops of the diluted remedy (without the additional brandy or cider vinegar preservative) to the baby's bottle or to a teaspoon of boiled water or fruit juice, and give this three to four times a day. Breastfeeding mothers can take the diluted remedies themselves: the flower vibrations will be imparted to the baby through the milk. Alternatively, moisten the baby's lips's with the diluted remedy and/or add flower essences to the baby's bathwater (see External Treatment).

ANIMAL TREATMENT

Diagnosing animals is discussed in Chapter 5. The normal dosage for domestic pets is 4 drops of Rescue Remedy (or 2 drops of any other flower essence) in drinking water or milk, and some of this can also be sprinkled over the animal's food. The remedy can be used directly from the stock bottle or diluted and dispensed from a treatment bottle (as described earlier for human dosage). For larger animals such as horses, 10 drops of Rescue Remedy (5 of any other flower essence) to a bucket of water; or, if easier to administer, 4 drops of undiluted Rescue Remedy, 2 of any other chosen flower, on a sugar lump.

EXTERNAL APPLICATIONS

The flower remedy vibrations can also be absorbed through the skin. Add 4 drops of flower essence to every 30g of cream or ointment base. An unperfumed shop-bought product can be used for this purpose, or you may prefer to make your own cream as described earlier. The same number of drops can be added to 30–50ml of skin lotion, aromatherapy massage oil or distilled water. For best results, apply to sensitive areas of the body such as the temples, palms of the hands, backs of the knees, wrists and solar plexus area (midriff). Alternatively, add up to 6 drops of a flower essence to the bathwater, preferably, to help activate the remedy, whilst the water is still running.

MAKING YOUR OWN FLOWER ESSENCES

It may not be possible to track down all the flowers profiled in this book, but you should be able to make a few selected essences. If you intend to use wild flowers, remember that many wild plants are protected by law. If in doubt, look up the plant in the profiles section (see Chapter 10) and check the

CAUTIONS note (if applicable) to see if a conservation warning has been included.

Never gather flowers that have been exposed to traffic fumes, factory emissions, artificial fertilisers or poisonous sprays. It may also be advisable to avoid flowers growing close to power lines: electromagnetic radiation is said to weaken the therapeutic potential of many plants.

If you have a garden, you could grow a variety of herbs and flowers suitable for making your own essences, though it is essential to employ organic methods of husbandry. Some of the most useful garden essences are Lavender, Lemon Balm, Roman Chamomile, Marigold (Calendula), Sunflower and Rosemary.

Bach devised two methods of potentisation: the Sun Method and the Boiling Method. The flower essences developed in more recent years are invariably potentised by the first method, though sometimes modified so that the flowers do not have to be picked. Here we shall concentrate on the methods employed by Bach.

SELF-PREPARATION

Although Bach did not mention the importance of preparing ourselves physically and emotionally before making flower essences, in view of what we have already learned about the power of thought and its influence upon the vibrational quality of substances (see Chapter 3), it would seem essential to do so. If you are experienced in meditation, you will know exactly how to calm and centre yourself. Otherwise, carry out the following simple procedure.

First take a bath or shower and put on some clean clothes. Just before collecting the flowers, find a place where you can sit quietly for a few minutes (it is always a good idea to bring with you a small blanket to sit on). Adopt a comfortable but poised position, such as a simple crossed-legged pose. Or you may find it more comfortable to kneel down with your buttocks resting on your heels.

Close your eyes and become aware of the rhythm of your breath as it flows in and out. Do not try to control the breath in any way, simply become aware of its movement. Then begin to focus on each part of your body in turn – your legs, buttocks, trunk, shoul-

ders, arms, hands, neck, face and scalp – letting go of any tension you might find there. Now focus entirely on your breathing, allowing all the stresses and strains of life to ebb away on the out-breath. Whenever your mind begins to wander (as frequently happens) do not let it be a source of irritation; gently redirect your attention to the ebb and flow of the breath.

Once you feel totally relaxed, imagine that you are centred along a straight line running from the top of your head, down the front of your body and into the earth. This will help to engender a sense of inner peace and stability. When you feel ready, slowly stand up and begin to prepare the flower remedy.

THE SUN METHOD

The essences must be prepared on a cloudless, sunny morning, preferably before 9 a.m. If the sky should cloud over at any time during the potentisation of the remedy, the preparation will have to be discarded.

The Bach remedy Rock Water is best obtained from the supplier recommended in Useful Addresses on page 265. This is because the remedy needs to be prepared from pure water obtained directly from a natural spring. Sadly, unpolluted spring water is increasingly difficult to find.

Equipment

- Clear glass bowl, the size of a sugar bowl for most flowers, though a much larger vessel will be necessary for sunflowers

- Small heatproof glass or china jug

- Dark glass 100ml bottle with screw cap

- Dark glass 30ml dropper bottle. If you cannot obtain a dropper bottle, you will need to use a separate pipette (available from most pharmacies)

- Small bottle of brandy

- Bottled mineral or spring water (preferably a brand which comes in a glass bottle rather than a plastic one)

- Labels for bottles

Method

1. To sterilise the small glass bowl, bottles and jug, first place them in a large pan of cold water. Bring the water to the boil and simmer gently for 20 minutes. Then wrap the sterilised bowl and jug in a spotlessly clean tea towel. It may not be possible to sterilise an extra-large bowl suitable for a sunflower head. Instead, wash the bowl in hot, soapy water, then rinse it under a running tap until it is sparkling. Dry with a freshly laundered tea towel, then wrap the bowl in a clean cloth.

2. Half-fill the sterilised 100ml bottle with brandy. Screw down the cap and label it Mother Tincture, along with the name of the flower to be potentised.

3. Fill the sterilized 30ml bottle with brandy and label it Stock, along with the name of the flower included on the larger bottle.

4. Take all the equipment except the Stock bottle to the plants you intend to use, and place the bowl on level ground where it can remain in full sun for 3 hours. Fill the bowl with spring water.

5. To ensure that no plant is depleted, pick the flower heads from as many different plants of the same species as possible. Choose only those flowers which are at the peak of perfection, avoiding any which show signs of fading.

6. Place the flowers one by one on the surface of the water in the bowl, so that they overlap and the surface is completely covered. Avoid casting a shadow over the bowl, or touching the water with your fingers.

7. After 3 hours, or sooner if the blossoms begin to fade, remove the flowers. The best way to do this is to flick out the spent flowers with a stalk or leaf from the parent plant, thus avoiding skin contact with the potentised water. Transfer the now potentised water to the jug.

8. Top up the bottle labelled Mother Tincture with potentised water. Replace the cap securely and shake well.

9. Once you return home, add just 2 drops of the Mother Tincture to the brandy-filled bottle labelled Stock. Replace the cap securely and shake well to disperse. Although the drops can be taken directly from the Stock bottle, it is more usual to dilute the remedy further by preparing a Treatment bottle (see page 100).

THE BOILING METHOD

Once again it is important to gather plant material (which in this instance will include twigs, buds young leaves and flowers) on a bright morning, preferably before 9 a.m.

Incidentally, just why Bach included this comparatively harsh method of capturing the energies of certain flowers is something of a mystery. It is commonly believed that the Boiling Method was devised for plants, bushes and trees which flower in early spring (a time when the sun is at its weakest strength). While this is true for early-flowering trees like Aspen, Cherry Plum and Elm, the same cannot be said for plants like Honeysuckle, Mustard, Wild Rose and Sweet Chestnut, all of which bloom during the height of summer. It may have been that the English summer was exceptionally overcast the year Bach found these particular remedies. As a matter of interest, I have potentised Honeysuckle and Wild Rose using the Sun Method and have found the remedies to be just as efficacious.

Equipment

- Large enamel or stainless steel saucepan and lid
- Two small china or glass jugs
- Dark glass 100ml bottle with cap
- Dark glass 30ml dropper bottle (or a similar-size bottle with a screw cap and a separate pipette)
- Bottled mineral or spring water (preferably a brand sold in glass bottles)
- Coffee filter papers
- Labels for bottles
- Secateurs for collecting plant material

Method

1. Sterilise the jugs and bottles, then wrap the jugs in a clean cloth. When the bottles are cold, add the brandy and label (see Sun Method, steps 1–3).

2. Take the saucepan, covered with its lid to keep out the dust, to the chosen spot.

3. Fill the pan three-quarters full with the flowering sprays, young leaves (if open) and twigs. If you have a camping stove, you can prepare the remedy out in the open. Otherwise, return home as quickly as possible.

4. Cover the plant material with a generous litre of bottled water. Place the pan, uncovered, over the heat and bring the water to the boil. Stir the mixture occasionally with a twig from the parent tree or plant. After half an hour, remove the pan from the heat and cover it.

5. When the pan is cold, remove the plant material with a twig of the same tree or bush. Allow the pan to stand for a further period to allow the sediment to settle.

6. Cover one of the jugs with a coffee filter paper. Fill the other jug carefully from the pan without disturbing the sediment, then pour the liquid a little at a time through the filter paper. When sufficient has been filtered, continue as for the Sun Method (steps 8–9).

PART TWO

THE
MULTI-DIMENSIONAL
APPROACH

Medicines and food have a definite chemical action upon blood and tissues... They are useful so long as the material consciousness in man is uppermost. They have their limitations, however, because they are applied from outside. The best methods are those that help the Life Energy to resume its internal healing activities.

PARAMAHANSA YOGANANDA

CHAPTER SEVEN

TOWARDS WHOLE HEALTH

THE TERM 'HOLISTIC' has been used many times already, but so far we have barely scratched the surface of its meaning. The word itself is derived from the Greek *holos*, meaning whole. It was first used in 1926 by the South African statesman and soldier J.C. Smuts (1870–1950) to describe the tendency in nature to produce wholes from ordered groups of units.

Unlike conventional medicine, which regards the human being as a machine composed of disparate parts, holistic medicine aims to strengthen the vital or organising force which permeates the mind/body complex, thus triggering into action the person's innate self-healing capacity. This is also known as homeostasis, a process whereby organisms strive to maintain a steady internal state. The aim of holistic medicine is to strengthen the body's immune defences. Just as an impoverished soil weakens the growth of plants and encourages the development of disease and infestation, a poorly functioning immune system allows viruses to take root and pathologies to develop.

Since conventional medicine regards its practitioners as body technicians rather than healers, treatment is geared towards such things as destroying abnormal cells, removing diseased tissue, replacing dysfunctioning parts – or perhaps kick-starting, slowing down or blocking the action of aberrant processes. No one would argue that such measures can sometimes be vital. Yet it is also true that conventional medicine tends to weaken the body's immune defences by suppressing conditions without removing the cause. At the same time, chemical drugs cause side-effects which the body then has to deal with as well as the disease. This can lead to iatrogenic disease (doctor-induced), a problem which may be far more widespread than is generally realised.

Holistic medicine places a greater emphasis on prevention of disease. Instead of regarding the patient as a passive recipient of the health practitioner's administrations, it demands a great deal of time and commitment from ourselves. While recognising that heredity plays an important part (some people are born healthier than others), it is also true that most of us can take steps to improve our health and possibly prevent the development of chronic illness. This is not as easy as surrendering your body to the doctor and simply taking the medicine, nor can you expect an overnight cure. But the long-term results in terms of increased vitality and life enhancement are well worth the effort.

The holistic practitioner recognises that health is largely dependent upon the quality of the food we eat, the water we drink and the air we breathe. Perhaps even more important, we need to nurture the spiritual aspect of self; for we are more than a body and a mind. The spiritual aspect is hard to define, but is an integral part of our relationship with ourselves and with other people, of our sense of purpose and meaning – and, indeed, of the health of our planet.

MODES OF THINKING

As well as taking steps to improve our diet and way of living, wherever feasible, it may be necessary to explore the inner self. For example, are your attitude and/or conditioned responses to the life experience contributing to any emotional or physical symptoms? If so, what steps can you take to nurture your inner being?

Even though we cannot always change our outer situation, it is possible to change our attitude to it – although it takes time to develop positive responses. Doing so makes all the difference to the way we cope with pain, suffering and setback: 'Two men look out of prison bars; one sees mud, the other stars.' (Anon).

But a word of warning: there are pitfalls for the over-enthusiastic health professional, or well-meaning friend, partner or relative. Certain individuals are particularly vulnerable to feelings of guilt. If such a person is allowed to go away with the idea that their illness or harrowing life situation is entirely their own fault (a misunderstanding of the philosophy of holism) this is likely to hinder the healing process. From my own observations, it would seem that it is much easier for humans to succumb to negative patterns of thinking than to be genuinely positive.

Trying too hard to be positive may result in suppression of powerful emotions like anger, grief and jealousy. If left to fester beneath the surface, such emotions are likely to exacerbate any existing health problems. So we must think most carefully about our approach to extolling the virtues of 'positive thinking', lest it should have the opposite effect. There is also the possibility that the pattern of imbalance may be too deeply ingrained for it to be within the range of conscious control. As mentioned earlier, heredity plays a major part in the manifestation of ill health (perhaps including inherited modes of thinking), along with many other interrelated factors.

It is far better to develop a positive acceptance of our own limitations, maybe with the help of flower essences, than to attempt against all odds to overcome every possible failing. Flower essences like Oak, Chamomile, Californian Poppy and Sage may prove enlightening. Positive self-acceptance, which is quite different from the state we call resignation, is an essential part of the quest for self-knowledge. It is enriching because it makes us slower to criticise the faults of others. Above all, it can lead to the experience of *true* healing (see page 35). Paradoxical as it may seem, the attainment of self-knowledge is the key to understanding the purpose and meaning of life itself.

Before we explore some of the ways in which we can improve our health and sense of wellbeing, it would seem appropriate to take a closer look at the bane of modern living: the condition we call 'stress'.

THE NATURE OF STRESS

The word 'stress' is increasingly being used as a blanket term for every conceivable state of emotional disharmony. The classic definition of stress, however, singles out the instinctive 'fight or flight' response. When our early ancestors were faced with a ferocious beast they had to make a split-second choice between fighting the animal and running for their lives. Exposed to any unpleasant stimulus, the body reacts by producing a chemical called adrenalin, which increases the heart and pulse rate and causes blood pressure to rise. Extra blood sugar is released into the bloodstream, the muscles tense and breathing becomes more rapid – a response designed to give added speed of thought and action in the face of adversity.

In modern society we may never encounter a ferocious beast, but whenever we find ourselves feeling fearful or pressurised precisely the same physical changes take place. For the most part it is socially unacceptable to put up a fight or run away, and so we bottle up our true feelings. As a result, there is no direct outlet for the physical and emotional effects of adrenalin. The longer the 'stressed out' feeling remains, the more potentially harmful it can be to our long-term health.

Not all stress, however, is bad. On the contrary, we actually need a certain level of stimulation to motivate us and keep us going. Indeed, without the 'spice of life' we become despondent, depressed or apathetic. Stress only becomes a problem when it develops into *distress*, especially if the feeling is prolonged. Whether we are suffering from the strain of living in the fast track or from the despair of a monotonous existence, in either situation we feel we have no control over life and we fear there is no way out.

It is also true that our physical and emotional responses to stress are largely idiosyncratic. It is not so much the outside pressures and problems which impinge upon us, but rather how we react to those things. We all know people who remain cool, calm and collected under the most trying circumstances (and indeed seem to thrive on such experiences), and we know others who collapse under the strain of relatively minor difficulties. The trick is to maintain just the right level of stimulation to make life interesting and fulfilling, and of course this balance is different for each of us.

PROMOTING HEALTH AND VITALITY

The rest of this chapter is devoted to outlining some of the ways in which we may begin to create favourable conditions within every level of our being. In so doing we will enhance the action of plant remedies – and, indeed, the efficacy of any other method of healing we may choose to employ. For without attention to such things, the action of natural remedies is curtailed.

Unlike powerful drugs, which can generally override biochemical processes, the gentle-acting plant remedies explored in this book work in harmony with the mind/body complex, supporting its self-healing capacity. However, a body congested with cigarette smoke, junk food and the debris of a generally unhealthy way of living responds less readily to natural remedies. This is not to undermine the ultimate superiority of the psycho-spiritual aspect of self – indeed, some people fail to respond to treatment despite their doing everything 'right' (see page 63). Rather, it is to say that the physical aspect, being an interrelated part of the whole, needs to be nurtured by material as well as spiritual means.

FOOD

Arguments abound as to what constitutes a 'well-balanced diet'. One minute we are told to avoid all animal fat because it is bad for the heart, and to eat polyunsaturated vegetable oils and soft margarines instead. The next moment we are told that, far from being healthy alternatives, many highly refined vegetable oils and margarines actually contribute to heart disease and ill health in general. This is because they contain trans fatty acids which are not found in nature but are formed during the manufacturing process.

And while most nutritionists are of the opinion that sugar in any shape or form is the number one enemy of teeth and gums, there are those who believe that unrefined muscovado (not the refined, artificially coloured kind which masquerades as the real thing) actually prevents tooth decay! This view was formerly advocated by health food pioneers in the 1950s. As if this were not surprising enough, researchers in California have recently declared as healthful a combination of red wine and dark chocolate! These former 'baddies' are now deemed to be protective against heart disease – that is to say, if consumed in moderation and as part of a sensible wholefood diet.

Yet despite the mass of contradictions surrounding diet, the old adage 'You are what you eat' still holds true. In fact, it has even wider implications than is generally realised. Apart from the physical benefits of good nutrition, it influences emotional stability. This is because the brain is made entirely of food molecules such as complex essential fatty acids, vitamins, minerals, proteins and other nutrients. Even as far back as the 1960s, Canadian researchers Dr Hoffer and Dr Osmond were able to demonstrate that certain forms of schizophrenia could be effectively treated through specific diets and nutritional supplements. Moreover, mental health research over the last few decades has proved that food allergies or intolerance can also result in mental and emotional symptoms.

Serious mental imbalances aside (for their treatment requires expert intervention), everyone can benefit from the mood-enhancing (and therefore stress-reducing) effects of food. The first step in balancing brain chemistry, and thus our mental outlook, is to alkalise the blood and keep blood sugar levels up. The first can be achieved through a diet largely comprising fresh fruit, salad greens, culinary herbs and other vegetables (see pages 110–11). The latter depends upon timing of meals. Some people need to eat little and often – maybe five small meals a day – in order to keep their emotions on an even keel. This is particularly important for women dur-ing the pre-menstrual phase and at menopause. Moreover, certain foods have been found to influence the secretion of sex hormones and have proved efficacious in the treatment of problems associated with the female life-cycle (see page 146).

Of course, our moods are not entirely governed by what we ate for lunch. They are always both chemical and psychological, moving in response to the dictates of our own guiding impulse. Indeed, even when people are suffering from a biochemically based depression they must still learn psychological skills in order to cope with life, moods and feelings.

Sifting the Wheat from the Chaff

Despite the merits of individual foodstuffs, there is no one ideal diet suitable for everyone. We are each very different, with varying physical needs and personal philosophies. Whatever we may believe about diet, certainly our food should be as free as possible from the potentially harmful effects of modern food production. As well as containing potentially harmful additives and the toxic residues of agrochemicals, some foods today (powdered spices, dried culinary herbs and tomatoes, for example) may have been irradiated – exposed to controlled levels of radiation in order to destroy micro-organisms and slow down the process of decay.

Moreover, through biotechnology scientists are mixing and matching DNA material – isolating a gene from one kind of organism and joining it with another species – in order to 'improve' a plant or farm animal. So we have corn genes in rice, chicken genes in potatoes – even human genes in fish, pigs and rapeseed.

Genetically modified foods have been associated with increased incidence of allergies, most recently when a strain of soya bean was joined with the brazil nut. Genetically engineered plants are also better able to tolerate high levels of agrochemicals which, of course, is another cause for concern. At the time of writing, no testing and no labelling is required for foods containing genetically engineered ingredients (similarly, no labelling is required for irradiated food). Clearly, scientists have not learned from the BSE scandal in the UK – undoubtedly the result of adding recycled meat products (including beef) to cattle feed.

However, there is a glimmer of light on the horizon. In response to public pressure, the European Commission has finally agreed to a package of proposals on the regulation of genetically engineered foodstuffs. Foods with characteristics which raise ethical or safety concerns for certain people will be labelled. For example, if foods normally eaten by vegetarians contain genes of animal origin, or foods contain genes from known allergens such as nuts, these will be labelled. These proposals do not go far enough, of course, so we must continue to voice our opinions to government health officials requesting that the practice be banned.

Nutritional Supplements

Although nutritional supplements undoubtedly have a place in holistic healing, they should never be regarded as an alternative to a healthy diet. A factory-produced vitamin C tablet, for example, is not as welcome to the digestive system, nor as pleasing to the psyche, as a bowl of fruit salad. Generally, it is fine to take a well-balanced multivitamin and mineral supplement as a health insurance measure if you so wish. Such formulas are also helpful in the short term to help boost your immune system during periods of ill health or prolonged stress, and perhaps for a month or two afterwards to aid recovery.

But if you feel run-down, despite eating a healthy diet and leading a fairly sensible lifestyle, do not dose yourself with all manner of expensive supplements but seek the advice of a nutritional therapist who will devise a supplement programme to suit your personal needs (see Useful Addresses on page 265). Without such attention to detail you could be wasting your money, for not everyone absorbs nutrients to the same degree. Of greater concern is the fact that you might end up creating a biochemical imbalance in your system, thus compromising your long-term health.

CAUTION

Pregnant women should always seek professional advice before taking vitamin supplements. Also, there is some evidence to suggest that high doses of vitamin C (more than 1g a day) can cancel out the healing effects of high-potency homeopathic remedies. Similarly, some herbalists are of the opinion that megadoses of vitamins can hinder the healing potential of certain herbal remedies.

GUIDE TO HEALTHY EATING

The following steps outline a wholefood diet as recommended by many aware nutritionists. Of course, it cannot take into account individual food intolerances – some people feel unwell if they eat dairy products, nuts or wheat, for example – or if you wish to avoid animal foods altogether (veganism). It should, however, serve as a useful guide that can be adapted to suit individual needs. Aim to alter your diet gradually over a period of 6 months. Drastic overnight changes will almost certainly lead to digestive discomfort or upset.

- Buy organically grown food if you can, but don't fret if you can't. Worrying too much about your diet will only lead to stress, which can be more harmful than a less than perfect diet.

- Eat wholemeal bread and other complex carbohydrates such as dried beans, lentils, nuts, seeds (e.g. sunflower, pumpkin and sesame), wholemeal pasta, oats, brown rice and other wholegrain cereals. If dried beans and pulses cause excessive flatulence, try sprouting them in a purpose-designed salad sprouter (available from health food stores) to break down the chemicals responsible for causing intestinal gas. Sprouted beans, lentils and seeds are packed with vitamins and minerals. They are best eaten raw in salads, though they can be added to soups, stews and casseroles.

- Eat plenty of fruit and vegetables – preferably unpeeled, well scrubbed and raw in salads or lightly steamed. Many elderly people and babies, however, cannot digest raw vegetables, though they can derive nourishment from vegetable soups and purees. Frozen fruits and vegetables are fine as a standby, especially during the winter months when fresh produce may be in short supply, but they should not form the basis of your diet.

- Cut down on all fats, particularly those from animal sources, especially lard, suet, double cream, butter and full-fat cheese. As much as possible, reject any product that has been hydrogenated or highly processed. Use moderate amounts of cold-pressed vegetable oils such as extra virgin olive, sesame and sunflower seed (about 1 tablespoon each day) in salad dressings. If you intend to cook with oil, the most stable is olive (both the extra virgin and virgin grades). It does not break down during storage or cooking to create substances which harm essential fatty acids in the body. But keep it in the fridge and use up before the recommended date.

- Cut down on milk, whether full-fat or skimmed. The most digestible is probably organically produced goats' milk, which people normally allergic to dairy products (eczema sufferers, for example) can usually tolerate. Live, full-fat plain yoghurt (preferably organic) is good for most people, whether it comes from the cow, goat or sheep.

- Sweeten your foods sparingly with honey (preferably raw or unheated) or a little unrefined muscovado sugar, or more lavishly with dried fruits such as dates, figs, sultanas and raisins.

- Cut down on salt (even sea salt should be used sparingly), and use more herbs and spices to flavour your food. A high-salt diet can be a contributing factor in the development of high blood pressure and oedema (fluid retention).

- Buy free-range eggs if possible.

- Eat red meat only occasionally, if at all. Instead, eat free-range poultry and fish, particularly oily fish such as mackerel.

- Try to avoid processed foods in cans and packets because they are usually laden with chemical additives. They will do no harm as an occasional standby but should not form the basis of your daily diet.

- A little red or white wine (preferably organic) is good for the digestive system and can help normalise blood cholesterol levels. One to two glasses a day is the recommended quantity.

- Drink plenty of water (bottled or filtered), herbal tisanes and diluted fruit juices. Try to limit your caffeine intake to no more than two cups of coffee a day (preferably organic ground coffee rather than additive-laden instant), or three cups of tea. Decaffeinated versions may be laden with chemicals employed in the process – unless, that is, the label states that the caffeine has been removed by water extraction. It is probably better for your sense of wellbeing to enjoy the rounded flavour of an occasional cup of ordinary tea or coffee than to grin and bear a decaffeinated version!

- It is fine to err once in a while – to indulge in a bar of chocolate, cream cake or fry-up. And there is no need to feel guilty about it either. It is only when such indulgences become a daily habit at the expense of more nutritious foods that they constitute a health hazard.

- Throw away the scales and forget about counting calories, especially if you are stuck in a diet/binge cycle. Enlightened nutritionists now realise that people have very different ways of utilising calories – while there are those who can eat vast quantities and retain a normal body weight, others certainly cannot. If you are genuinely overweight – that is to say, substantially more than nicely rounded – for no apparent reason, and lacking in vitality, you may be suffering from hidden food sensitivities. If so, seek the advice of a holistic nutritionist.

- Eat slowly in convivial surroundings, and above all enjoy your food!

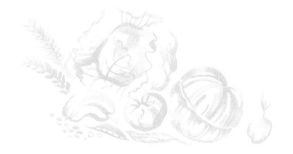

MOVEMENT

Moderate but persistent activity has a wonderful effect upon our sense of wellbeing. Unlike a machine that breaks down with use, we become stronger and more flexible if every muscle and joint is used frequently. Exercise also strengthens the heart and lungs, stimulates circulation, improves the quality of sleep and reduces stress levels throughout the body/mind complex.

Any form of movement which is perceived as a pleasure rather than a chore is infinitely superior to that which is so taxing that you ache from head to toe afterwards. Swimming, cycling, walking, dancing (any style to suit your taste and stamina) are some of the most enjoyable forms of physical activity. You may also enjoy yoga, Tai Chi, Kung Fu or some other mind/body system.

Some people, especially those in sedentary occupations, feel they benefit most from vigorous outdoor sports like football, rugby or tennis. However, if you have a high-powered job which encourages you to compete in the marketplace, it may not be advisable to take up a competitive sport. The stress if you lose will negate the benefits of the exercise.

If you are elderly, physically disabled or too ill to take much exercise (or perhaps cannot exercise at all), regular aromatherapy massage can be of enormous benefit and need not be carried out by a professional. Sensitive, nurturing massage given by a friend or loved one can improve your circulation and enhance your inner sense of wellbeing.

NATURAL LIGHT

Light is as much a nutrient as food and water, yet few of us even realise it. It is absorbed by our bodies and used in a wide range of metabolic processes, including the photochemical response in the skin – tanning and the synthesis of vitamin D from ergosterol. This vitamin is essential for the absorption of calcium and other minerals, which are central to the growth of healthy bones. Light also has an indirect effect through photo-receptors in our eyes. The type and quality of light entering our eyes can affect our hormonal balance and body chemistry as a whole, influencing energy levels and mood.

Artificial light is vastly inferior, lacking the full spectrum of the ultra-violet rays of daylight, and has been blamed for a number of ailments suffered by indoor workers. The most common problems associated with light deprivation are lethargy, headaches, irritability, lack of concentration and a seasonal state formerly known as 'winter depression', now seasonal affective disorder (SAD).

Light manufacturers have taken notice of reports about the importance of full-spectrum lighting and have introduced lights that simulate natural sunshine (see Useful Addresses on page 265). While these are undoubtedly better than ordinary electric bulbs, they cannot replace the revitalising effect of light as nature intended. It is important to get outside for at least an hour a day, particularly during the winter months. As a matter of interest, the skin of the face and hands of white people has become super-efficient at absorbing ultra-violet rays. It is believed that as little as twenty minutes' exposure can supply the minimum level of vitamin D required for a whole day. However, dark-skinned people require much more light than this to maintain adequate levels of vitamin D.

What about sunbathing? True, excessive exposure to natural or simulated sunlight is the principal cause of skin cancer – although holistic practitioners feel that sunbeds are potentially more harmful than natural sunlight. It may come as a surprise to learn, however, that sun-worshippers using proprietary sun-screens run an increased risk of malignant melanoma – possibly triggered by the synthetic chemicals used in these products (*British Medical Journal* 1996: 312 7047).

Most naturopaths (those who employ 'nature cure' methods such as hydrotherapy, mud packs, massage and dietetics) still believe in the health benefits of *moderate* exposure to sunlight – that is to say, beginning with as little as 15 minutes' exposure on the first day, gradually increasing the time to one hour maximum. But it is important to take your sun bath at the most favourable time of day – in the morning before midday, or after four o'clock in the afternoon, when the sun's rays are longer and weaker and therefore less likely to burn. Apply a moisturising and protective oil such as extra virgin olive or sesame (not the dark version prepared from roasted seeds). These oils are believed to afford a low sunscreen factor of around 3 or 4. Unlike high factor commercial preparations, they do not block the synthesis of vitamin D.

If you have very fair or sun-sensitive skin, you can still benefit from the mood-elevating and health-giving properties of sunlight by sitting in the shade covered from head to toe in cotton garments.

Unfortunately, there are few dietary sources of vitamin D; foods containing appreciable amounts are eggs, tuna, salmon, egg yolks and fish liver oils. Vegans who are unable to enjoy adequate sunlight may have to supplement their diet with a synthetic formula from non-animal sources. However, it is advisable to consult a nutritional therapist because excessive amounts of the nutrient can be toxic.

DEEP BREATHING

Many of us are shallow breathers (especially if we are feeling stressed); we use only the upper part of our lungs, which means that toxic residues are not completely removed. As a result the blood is deprived of much of the oxygen it needs to feed the body tissues, so we may end up feeling listless or suffering from vagueness of thought. At the same time the oxygen deficit hinders the assimilation of nutrients from the food we eat.

One of the easiest ways to begin learning to breathe fully is to practise the yoga Complete Breath. This exercise is also beneficial to people prone to respiratory ailments such as asthma, hay fever and bronchitis. If possible, do deep breathing outside in the fresh air; otherwise, it can be performed in a well-ventilated room. Best results are achieved if the exercise is carried out twice daily, perhaps when you get up and just before you go to sleep, and at other times when you feel stressed.

If practising indoors, you may wish to vaporise an essential oil (or a blend) to enhance the experience. Frankincense, cedarwood and sandalwood are traditional choices. They act to deepen the breathing, which in turn facilitates contemplation and meditation. Other helpful essences include lavender, juniper berry and pine.

THE COMPLETE BREATH

1. Lie on a rug on the floor (or on the ground if outside, perhaps in the garden), or alternatively on a firm bed, with your arms at your sides, palms facing down.

2. Close your eyes and begin to inhale very slowly through your nose. *Without forcing the breath*, expand your abdomen slightly, then become aware of the air rising up into your ribcage and then your chest. Hold for a few seconds.

3. Now begin to breathe out slowly through your nose in a smooth, continuous flow until your abdomen is drawn in and your ribcage and chest are relaxed. Hold for a few seconds before repeating two or three times.

4. Now breathe in slowly as before, but this time gradually raise your arms overhead in time with the inhalation until the backs of your hands touch the floor. Hold your breath for 5–10 seconds (according to your own capacity) while you have a really good stretch from fingertips to toes. Slowly breathe out as you bring your arms back down to your sides. Repeat two or three times.

Variation
The Complete Breath can also be performed whilst standing. To enhance the stretch as you raise your arms overhead on the in-breath, stand on tiptoes, your heels coming back down again as you breathe out.

DEEP RELAXATION

Having mastered the Complete Breath, you will be ready to learn the art of deep relaxation. Studies in hospitals have shown that, as well as dissipating excess nervous energy and promoting tranquillity, deep relaxation improves sleep, lowers high blood pressure, releases tension in the muscles, improves digestion, helps certain skin complaints and strengthens the immune system.

Find a quiet, well-ventilated room with a pleasing decor. Wear loose, comfortable clothing and take off your shoes. If you live in a noisy area, it may also be helpful to play a tape or CD of gentle music, but keep the volume down very low (just enough to mask unwanted sounds) as your senses will be especially acute. Most important: ensure that you will not be disturbed for at least 15 minutes.

Initially, deep relaxation should be performed once or twice a day. However, once your body and mind have become accustomed to the process you may find that just two sessions a week have the desired effect. It can be helpful to record the instructions on to tape, although after a few sessions you will be able to move through the sequence unaided.

To facilitate deep relaxation and encourage the mind to drift into a dreamy state, you may wish to vaporise any of the following essential oils: cedarwood (Atlas or Virginian), chamomile (Roman), clary sage, geranium (but in very low concentration, otherwise it has the opposite effect), lavender, marjoram (sweet), neroli, patchouli (in very low concentration), petitgrain, rose, sandalwood, ylang ylang.

DEEP RELAXATION SEQUENCE

1. Lie down on the floor, supported by pillows if you like – one under your head and another under your knees. Alternatively, lie down on a firm bed.

2. Close your eyes, take one or two deep breaths, then exhale through your mouth with a deep sigh. Have a really good stretch from fingertips to toes.

3. Now become aware of your feet. As you inhale through your nose, flex your feet towards your body. Hold on to that tension for a few seconds. Then, as you breathe out, this time through either your nose or mouth (whichever feels most comfortable), let go of your feet. Say to yourself silently: 'My feet are feeling heavy, heavy and relaxed. They are sinking through the floor.' Allow enough time to experience the heaviness.

4. Now think of your calves. As you breathe in through your nose, tense your calves, hold for a few seconds, then, as you exhale, release them. Say to yourself silently: 'My calves are getting

heavier, heavy and relaxed. They are sinking into the floor.'

5. Now concentrate on your thighs. Breathe in, tense your thighs, hold on to the tension for a few seconds, then, as you exhale, let them go. 'My thighs are getting heavier, heavy and relaxed. They are sinking into the floor.'

6. Continue moving over your whole body, tensing and releasing the muscle groups in turn, and allowing yourself to sink deeper and deeper into relaxation. As well as relaxing your hands, arms and legs, do not forget your buttocks, abdomen, face and even your tongue, jaws and eyes.

7. Now become aware of the whole of your body and 'feel' around with your mind for any areas that may still be tense. Repeat the tightening and releasing of the muscles until you feel deeply relaxed and at peace.

8. When you feel it is time to come back (after at least 5 minutes of lying quietly and breathing normally), say to yourself: 'I am going to get up now and I will feel happy and refreshed.' Open your eyes and have a good stretch from fingertips to toes before slowly getting up.

CREATIVE IMAGERY

Current biofeedback research into the benefits of creative imagery has shown that simply imagining ourselves in a warm nurturing situation has the same effect as actually being there. For some this place might be a sun-drenched beach, for others a beautiful garden. Wherever the place may be, the focus is on making the image as real as possible. Guided imagery imparts a magical dimension to the basic deep relax-ation technique described above. It can be incorpo-rated at the point where you feel you have released all muscular tension, and thus feel deeply relaxed.

GUIDED IMAGERY AND VISUALISATION

What is the difference between guided imagery and visualisation? Visualisation is an important, but specific, aspect of imagery. Studies have shown that the form of imagery which most powerfully connects with the deeper levels of the psyche involves all of the senses. In addition to visualising or 'seeing' a sun-drenched beach, for instance, the aim is to feel it, smell it, hear it and even taste it. For example, you might touch a rock and become acutely aware of its rough texture, perceive the aroma of seaweed, hear the cry of a gull, and taste the saltspray on your lips. Kinesthetic evocation is important too – the sense through which you are aware of your body and its movements.

You will also discover that one or two of your senses are more highly developed than the others. For most people, visual imagery is the easiest to evoke, odours the most difficult. Mastery of the tech-nique comes with practice; the imagination, just like our muscles, becomes more powerful and limber through frequent use.

CREATING AN INNER SANCTUARY

You may like to make your own tape of a guided imagery sequence with appropriate pauses and a soft voice. Otherwise, work with a sympathetic friend or partner, someone with whom you can exchange roles of narrator and explorer. Of course, guided imagery tapes on the 'inner sanctuary' theme are commer-cially available, but it can be difficult finding a recording that captures your own personal idea of a spiritually uplifting place. When creating your own guided imagery sequence, here are a few guidelines.

- Your sequence should be written in the present tense, beginning with a walk along a well-worn path leading up to a hilltop idyll, perhaps, or down to a secluded cove. For example: 'You are walking along a path through a wide green swathe. It is a warm, sunny afternoon and your senses are alive with expectation …'. A little later in the sequence: 'The path meanders down to a sun-drenched beach. …'

- Try to bring all your senses into play. What can you see around you? What is on the ground? What does the ground feel like underfoot? Is the air warm, cool, moist, dry or breezy? Are there any scents wafting on the air? And when you look up, what does the sky look like? What sounds can you hear? What can you taste? Can you sense the movement in your limbs as you wander through your inner landscape?

- Always begin and end your journey in exactly the same place. This imparts a sense of completeness.

- At the end of the sequence (after about 15 minutes), say farewell to your inner sanctuary, but remind yourself that you can return any time you wish. It is always there for you whenever you need to relax, to be by yourself and to be nourished spiritually.

FIRST STEPS IN MEDITATION

The aim of deep relaxation and guided imagery is to allow the mind to drift into a pleasant, dream-like state. Meditation, on the other hand, is a state of relaxed alertness, of becoming fully focused in the present moment. The beneficial effects of meditation are similar to those of deep relaxation and imagery work, but with the ultimate aim of facilitating communication with the Higher Self – the all-wise aspect that manifests itself in those rare moments of inspiration and clarity.

There are many forms of meditation, some of which require an extremely high degree of dedication. Other methods, such as the simple technique you are about to learn, are delightfully simple and yet highly beneficial. As little as one (perhaps two) 10–15-minute sessions a day will be enough to refresh your mind and replenish your energies. Initially you may have to glance at the clock to remind yourself when to stop. However, once accustomed to the process you will assuredly find yourself moving out of meditation at the appointed time, without any external help. It is just like setting the bedside alarm, only to wake up the next morning seconds before it sounds.

To help create a conducive indoor atmosphere in which to meditate, you may wish to vaporise any of the following classic meditation essences: frankincense, cedarwood (Atlas or Virginian), sandalwood or juniper berry – perhaps blended with a little lavender to lift the aroma.

SIMPLE MEDITATION ON THE BREATH

Find a quiet place where you will not be disturbed – a pleasant, airy room, or perhaps outside in the garden, or maybe by a stream or bubbling fountain. Remember to wear comfortable clothing so as not to restrict your breathing, and take off your shoes. If you are accustomed to sitting on the floor or ground in a cross-legged position, then by all means adopt this pose. Otherwise sit in a straight-backed chair (which should support your back) with your feet flat on the floor and your hands resting in your lap. Your position needs to be comfortable, but poised in order to facilitate your breathing.

1. Close your eyes. Empty your lungs by exhaling through your mouth with a sigh. Now begin to breathe through your nose, allowing your abdomen to extend slightly with each inhalation and to sink in again as you exhale.

2. Become aware of your feet, thinking relaxation into them. Then move over every part of your body in turn, letting go and relaxing every part.

3. Now focus on your breath. Breathe naturally without strain, making no effort to control the breath. It does not matter if your breath is uneven – longer one moment and shorter the next. Simply enjoy the sensation, becoming aware of the still point between the in-breath and the out-breath.

4. Now, on every out-breath count 'one', and then 'two', and so on up to ten. Remember, count only on the out-breath. Once you reach ten, go back to one again. If you lose count or thoughts come crowding your mind (as they surely will), do not become irritated but gently push them aside and start counting again from one.

5. After about 10 minutes, stop. Imagine that you are centred along a straight line running from the top of your head to your feet. This imparts a sense of completeness, composure and peace.

6. Open your eyes, shake out your limbs and have a good stretch from fingertips to toes. When you are ready, get up and resume your everyday activities with renewed energy and awareness.

HEALING THE SOUL

Many of us live in cities, which means our feet barely touch the living earth. Instead, we are subjected to concrete, tarmac, synthetic carpets, vinyl floor coverings and many other artificial materials, most of which generate electrostatic fields which tend to sap our vitality. Even without knowing it, we can become very much out of balance when divorced from the natural earth currents.

So, whenever you can, walk on springy turf and breathe in the scents of flowers, trees and grasses. Listen to the birds, moving water, rainfall or the moaning wind; touch the rough bark of a tree; contemplate the beauty of your favourite animal; stroll barefoot on the seashore, feeling the wind and salt-spray in your hair and on your skin.

To engender a sense of freedom, gaze up at the sky and make meaningful shapes out of clouds. At nightfall, contemplate the starry firmament and freewheel into eternity! Watch the waxing and waning of the Moon. Reflect on how the lunar cycles pull on the seas and oceans, and the tides of our own body fluids and moods, our time of receptivity and creativity.

When we experience the wonder of nature and the cosmos, we invoke a sense of the sacred. Sacredness is bound up with our innate need to acknowledge the specialness of life, a transcendent quality that is all but lost in an increasingly desacralised world. We find sanctuary in the midst of chaos, calm in the eye of the storm. Far from encouraging escapism, however, we emerge revitalised and clear-minded, and thus better able to deal with the demands and challenges of everyday life. And in coming close to the earth we 'sit in the lap of Mother', as the Native Americans would put it, and reconnect with the primal source of human contentment.

CHAPTER EIGHT

THE PRACTICE OF GREEN HEALING

MANY OF THE botanic remedies explored in this chapter act quickly to alleviate acute conditions like headache, muscular aches and pains (due to over-exertion), digestive upset, minor burns and so forth. But in the treatment of long-term disorders such as asthma, eczema, arthritis and PMS the action of plant remedies is slow, gentle and cumulative, working to strengthen the various body systems over many months.

There may also be a brief period known as 'the healing crisis', at which point the body begins to throw off accumulated toxins in its attempt to restore equilibrium. Symptoms of the healing crisis may include offensive breath, a white-coated tongue, headache, spotty skin and loose bowels. Rest assured, the crisis will subside within a week or two, after which time there is usually a wonderful sense of renewed vitality.

To prevent your body from becoming too accustomed to an aromatherapy or herbal formula, thus rendering the remedy less effective (a common problem), it is advisable to cycle the treatment over a period of 3–6 weeks. For example, begin with one herb (or a simple mixture) for a few weeks, then change to another for the same period, before resuming with the original prescription. With essential oils, it is also beneficial to allow for one week's break after 6 weeks of continuous use.

Unless otherwise stated, the suggested herbal remedies can be taken long-term without risk of toxicity – that is to say, provided the recommended dosages are not greatly exceeded. However, the ideal is to reach a stage at which your body has learned to exercise its own healing powers unaided. Once you begin to experience increased vitality, try tapering off the dose gradually over a 4-week period. If your condition worsens, return to the original dose and try to reduce it again later, until you have established a

---

MOST IMPORTANT

If you are suffering from a serious condition like asthma, chronic fatigue, or deep-rooted anxiety or depression, it is advisable to seek the advice and cooperation of a qualified health practitioner before embarking on any of the self-help treatments advocated in this chapter.

It can also be helpful to employ the conventional health service as a means of diagnosing any condition about which you may be concerned. You can then choose to embark on a holistic healing programme – incorporating dietetics, herbs, aromatherapy and other natural methods – should you so wish, perhaps under the guidance of a qualified holistic therapist. However, with certain conditions such as chronic high blood pressure and heart disease, natural treatments may have to be used in conjunction with prescribed medication as a means of buffering the adverse effects of stress, thus promoting personal happiness and wellbeing.

maintenance dose. Eventually, you may be able to stop using the plant remedy because improvement has become permanent. In this way health can be maintained solely through good nutrition and a sensible lifestyle.

ESSENTIAL OILS OF EUCALYPTUS, TEA TREE AND GARLIC

Although these oils have not been profiled in Chapter 10 they are excellent additions to the green pharmacy. They have antibiotic, antiseptic and antiviral properties and are especially helpful for respiratory ailments like colds and flu, and for treating wounds, infestations and infections.

Unlike other essential oils, however, garlic oil is taken internally in the form of capsules (available from chemists and health food stores). It boosts natural immunity, improves the circulation and speeds the healing of infected skin conditions. Since the potency varies from one brand to another, always follow the manufacturer's recommended dose. However, garlic in any shape or form should be avoided by those suffering from a dry cough, eczema, or irritation of the stomach or intestines, and by breastfeeding mothers (it may cause colic in the baby).

A WORD ABOUT FLOWER ESSENCES

Flower essences are a wonderful adjunct to any healing programme. But since the remedies are best prescribed in accordance with the ever-changing emotional state of the individual, rather than the named physical condition, flower essence blends are not included in the charts. To enable you to refine the process of selection, a comprehensive repertory of emotional/psychological states can be found on pages 240–44. This should be used in conjunction with the information given in Chapters 5 and 6. Having chosen the required flower essences, remember that they can be added to herbal infusions, decoctions, tinctures and aromatherapy blends to support the healing process.

INTRODUCTION TO THE THERAPEUTIC CHARTS

For ease of treatment, the following charts will enable you to devise a healing plan for whatever state of mind/body disharmony you may be experiencing. While plant remedies can help many other disorders, the common ailments included on the charts respond especially well to self-help measures.

PREPARING THERAPEUTIC REMEDIES

Instructions for preparing essential oils and herbs for therapeutic applications are in Chapter 6. Where aromatic blends are suggested in the charts, the quantity of essential oil is given in drops per 25ml of base oil. The same number of drops can be used in the bath and/or an average-sized vaporiser.

THE INTERACTIVE NERVOUS SYSTEM

Experts in the field of psychoneuroimmunology have come to realise that the nervous system, endocrine (hormonal) system and immune system interact at many levels. The skin, too, has an important role to play in the body's defence system (see page 125). So there are obvious pitfalls in attempting to separate the parts that make up the whole. The state of our body chemistry is influenced by the food we eat, our level of physical activity (or lack of it), and, above all, our thoughts and emotions. Indeed, every thought, emotion and action is reflected in a cascade of biochemical responses throughout the whole organism. Little wonder that emotional disharmony is a contributing factor in almost all illness.

A common manifestation of psychophysical stress is chronic muscular tension and perpetual tiredness. Aromatherapy massage is extremely beneficial for such problems, especially when combined with restorative herbal remedies and soul-caressing flower essences. The following charts offer treatments for a number of ailments which are commonly regarded as 'stress-related'. The principal aim of treatment sis to restore energy levels and promote a sense of wellbeing.

ANXIETY AND STRESS-RELATED PROBLEMS

The most common flower essences for embracing the mind/body states in this section include Agrimony, Aspen, Chamomile, Cherry Plum, Gentian, Gorse, Holly, Impatiens, Larch, Lavender, Mimulus, Mustard, Olive, Red Chestnut, Rescue Remedy, Rosemary, Scleranthus, St John's Wort, Vervain, Wild Oat, White Chestnut and Valerian.

ANXIETY

SUGGESTED ESSENTIAL OILS
Angelica, bergamot (and other citrus oils), chamomile (German and Roman), clary sage, frankincense, juniper berry, lavender, melissa (true), neroli, petitgrain, rose, sandalwood, ylang ylang

Methods of Use
Bath, massage, vaporiser, personal perfume, dry inhalation (drops on handkerchief)

Aromatic Prescription
Massage/bath/vaporiser: 2 drops neroli, 1 drop petitgrain, 4 drops orange (see also aromatic recipes for Stress, page 124)

SUGGESTED HERBS
Calendula, Californian poppy, chamomile, honeysuckle, hops, lavender, lemon balm, linden blossom, oats, orange blossom, rose petal, valerian, violet (sweet)

Botanic Prescriptions
1. Infusion: equal parts linden blossom, orange flower and chamomile
2. Infusion: 1 part lavender, 2 parts rose petal, 2 parts calendula
3. Infusion of lemon balm. Add 15 drops hops tincture per teacup

FURTHER ADVICE
Nervous apprehension and acute distress are normally triggered by some harrowing life experience. Chronic anxiety (sometimes accompanied by depression and/or insomnia and panic attacks) needs professional help as it may be linked to food intolerance, excessive caffeine, the side-effects of certain drugs, or an underlying physical or psychiatric disorder. Reduce stress (see Chapter 7). A professional aromatherapy massage is highly beneficial. Your doctor may be able to recommend a local accredited counsellor.

DEPRESSION

SUGGESTED ESSENTIAL OILS
Basil, citrus essences, clary sage, coriander, frankincense, geranium, jasmine, juniper berry, lavender, neroli, pine, rose, rosemary, sandalwood, ylang ylang

Methods of Use
Bath (except basil), massage, vaporiser, personal perfume, dry inhalation (drops on handkerchief)

Aromatic Prescription
Massage/bath/vaporiser: 2 drops rosemary, 2 drops lavender, 1 drop geranium, 1 drop clary sage

SUGGESTED HERBS
Lavender, lemon balm, linden blossom, ginseng, honeysuckle, oats, rosemary, St John's wort, vervain

Botanic Prescriptions
1. Infusion: equal parts honeysuckle and lemon balm. Add 20 drops St John's wort tincture per teacup
2. Infusion: equal parts rosemary and vervain. Add 15 drops tincture of oats per teacup
3. Infusion of lemon leaves or decoction of lemon peel (organic). Add 15 drops tincture of linden blossom per teacup

FURTHER ADVICE
Depression is a normal response to crisis, emotional upheaval or excessive stress. But chronic depression usually indicates an underlying physical or psychological illness, and needs professional help. Your doctor may be able to put you in touch with a counsellor or psychotherapist. If possible, consult a holistic nutritionist as well. Milder depression can be greatly helped with herbs, aromatic oils and flower essences. Energetic exercise triggers 'feel good' brain hormones.

FATIGUE/TIREDNESS

SUGGESTED ESSENTIAL OILS
Angelica, bergamot (and other citrus oils), coriander, geranium, ginger, juniper berry, lavender, melissa (true), patchouli, pine, rose, rosemary

Methods of Use
Bath, massage, personal perfume, dry inhalation (drops on handkerchief), vaporiser

Aromatic Prescription
Bath/massage/vaporiser: 1 drop angelica, 2 drops orange, 2 drops bergamot, 2 drops lemon

SUGGESTED HERBS
Agrimony, angelica, basil, echinacea, ginger, ginseng, lemon balm, oats, rosehip, rosemary. As part of holistic treatment for post viral syndrome (ME), herbalists have found the following plants helpful: centaury, echinacea, garlic (can be taken as capsules), St John's wort, vervain

Botanic Prescriptions
1. Decoction of angelica root or seed mixed 50/50 with infusion of lemon balm. Add 15 drops oats tincture per teacup
2. Infusion: equal parts basil and rosemary. Add 10 drops St John's wort tincture per teacup

FURTHER ADVICE
There are many possible causes of perpetual tiredness. Some are obvious: prolonged physical and emotional stress, overwork, lack of sleep or convalescence. Fatigue is also symptomatic of ME (post-viral syndrome), anaemia, hormonal change at menopause, poor diet, air pollution, incorrect breathing, lack of exercise, excessive caffeine, cigarette smoking, the effects of certain drugs, or an underlying illness. If there is no improvement after several weeks of home treatment, or the cause is unknown, have a medical check-up. If you have ME, it is certainly worth consulting a medical herbalist or homeopath.

HEADACHE

SUGGESTED ESSENTIAL OILS
Chamomile (German and Roman), clary sage, lavender, marjoram, melissa (true), peppermint, rose, rosemary

Methods of Use
Cold compress, massage (especially to head, neck and shoulders), dry inhalation (drops on handkerchief), headache balm (see Aromatic Prescription)

Aromatic Prescription
30g unperfumed skin cream, 3 drops marjoram (sweet), 3 drops rosemary, 4 drops lavender. Stir essential oils into cream. Apply to temples and back of neck as required

SUGGESTED HERBS
Basil, chamomile, feverfew, hops, lavender, lemon balm, marjoram, peppermint, rosemary, sage, valerian, vervain, violet (sweet)

Botanic Prescriptions
1. Infusion: 1 part lavender, 2 parts lemon balm, 2 parts chamomile
2. Infusion of marjoram (sweet). Add 10 drops valerian tincture per teacup

FURTHER ADVICE
There are numerous causes of headache, including nervous tension, eye strain, high blood pressure, food allergy, lack of sleep, muscle spasm at the base of the skull, and constipation. Generally, try to reduce stress. Persistent headaches must be investigated by a medical practitioner.

INSOMNIA

SUGGESTED ESSENTIAL OILS
Chamomile (German and Roman), clary sage, lavender, marjoram, melissa (true), neroli, petitgrain, rose, sandalwood, ylang ylang

Methods of Use
Bath, massage (especially back), vaporiser, drops of essential oil on pillow (or on handkerchief placed nearby)

Aromatic Prescription
Massage/bath/vaporiser/pillow: 2 drops clary sage, 2 drops lavender, 2 drops neroli (or rose)

SUGGESTED HERBS
Basil, Californian poppy, chamomile, hops, lavender, lemon balm, linen blossom, oats, orange flower, rose petal, valerian

Botanic Prescriptions
1. Infusion: equal parts lemon balm and Californian poppy
2. Infusion: 1 part lavender, 2 parts chamomile, 2 parts linden blossom
3. Infusion of orange flower. Add 10 drops hops tincture per teacup

FURTHER ADVICE
Try to reduce stress and to get plenty of fresh air and exercise. Persistent insomnia, especially if it results in chronic fatigue, must be investigated by a medical practitioner. As well as being a wonderful remedy for insomnia, regular aromatherapy massage is an excellent preventative measure.

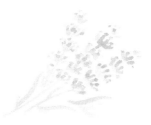

JETLAG

SUGGESTED ESSENTIAL OILS

To calm: chamomile (German and Roman), clary sage, frankincense, geranium (lowest recommended quantity), juniper berry, lavender, melissa (true), neroli, petitgrain, pine, rose, sandalwood, ylang ylang
To enliven: bergamot, geranium (maximum recommended quantity), lemon, orange, peppermint, pine, rosemary

Methods of Use

Massage bath, dry inhalation, personal perfume, vaporiser

Aromatic Prescriptions

1. Massage/vaporiser/bath/ inhalation (balancing blend): 1 drop frankincense, 1 drop juniper berry, 4 drops bergamot FCF, 2 drops lavender
2. Bath: 225g sea salt, 4 drops pine, 2 drops petitgrain, 2 drops lemon

SUGGESTED HERBS

To promote sleep: Californian poppy, hops, valerian
To enliven: sage, rosemary, vervain
To balance nervous system: oats

Botanic Prescriptions

1. Infusion (restorative): Equal parts vervain, peppermint, chamomile, marjoram
2. Infusion (restorative): 1 part sage, 2 parts rose petal. Add 15 drops oats tincture per teacup

FURTHER ADVICE

Symptoms of jetlag may include fatigue, insomnia, swollen ankles, menstrual disturbance, general malaise. During the flight avoid alcohol, which is dehydrating and contributes to jetlag; drink plenty of bottled water instead. Elevate your feet by resting them on a holdall to help prevent swollen ankles. Gentle massage above and beneath swelling, always towards the heart. The salt in the bath in Aromatic Prescriptions helps to ease aches and pains (see also Epsom salts bath, page 142). A course of ginseng taken a few months before a long flight helps to strengthen the nervous system.

MENTAL FATIGUE

SUGGESTED ESSENTIAL OILS

Specifics: basil, peppermint, pine, rosemary
General: angelica, coriander, geranium, lavender, lemon, melissa (true), rose

Methods of Use

Specifics: vaporiser, dry inhalation (drops on handkerchief)
General: massage (especially head, face, neck and shoulders), baths (except basil)

Aromatic Prescription

Vaporising blend (to facilitate clarity of thought): 3 drops peppermint, 2 drops clary sage, 2 drops lavender

SUGGESTED HERBS

Angelica, basil, peppermint, rose petal, rosemary

Botanic Prescription

Decoction of angelica (root or seed) mixed 50/50 with infusion of rose petals

FURTHER ADVICE

Take regular breaks. Provide for compensatory physical exercise, preferably in the fresh air. Do something practical like gardening, cooking or perhaps a blitz on the housework. Laughter is a wonderful antidote, so watch a funny film or play – or meet up with some jovial friends and have a good belly laugh! Possible flower essences: try the Californian FES Lemon, or the Bach remedy White Chestnut.

MIGRAINE

SUGGESTED ESSENTIAL OILS

Angelica, chamomile (German and Roman), clary sage, coriander, lavender, marjoram (sweet), melissa (true), peppermint, rose otto, rosemary

Methods of Use

As a preventative: regular aromatherapy massage, especially to head, neck and shoulders
During an attack: warm or icy compress, whichever gives most relief. This varies from one person to another

Aromatic Prescription

30g unperfumed base cream, 3 drops rose otto, 6 drops lavender. Stir essential oils into the cream. Apply to temples and back of neck as often as required (see also Aromatic Prescription for Headache, page 121)

SUGGESTED HERBS

Basil, chamomile, feverfew, ginseng (as a preventative during periods of prolonged stress), hops, lavender, linden blossom, marjoram, peppermint, rosemary, valerian, vervain

Botanic Prescriptions

Infusion: 1 part lavender, 1 part feverfew, 2 parts lemon balm
Infusion: equal parts of basil, vervain and marjoram
Infusion: Equal parts lemon balm and rosemary. Add 10 drops valerian tincture per teacup

FURTHER ADVICE

Try to reduce stress. Migraine can be symptomatic of structural misalignment, muscle spasm at base of skull, depression, hormonal change (menopause, the pill), food intolerances, extremes of temperature, and more. Seek professional advice from a medical herbalist, holistic nutritionist or homeopath. Other helpful treatments are acupuncture and osteopathy.

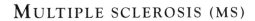

MULTIPLE SCLEROSIS (MS)

SUGGESTED ESSENTIAL OILS

Generally choose according to aroma preference (to uplift the spirits). Rosemary in a base of St John's wort oil (see page 96) may help numbness and tingling

Methods of Use

Massage

Aromatic Prescriptions

1. 50ml infused St John's wort oil, 10 drops rosemary
2. 50ml extra virgin olive oil, 12 drops rosemary, 6 drops geranium

SUGGESTED HERBS

As for Anxiety, Stress, Depression. Many sufferers feel that evening primrose oil makes a remarkable difference. Dosage: 4 × 500 mg daily

FURTHER ADVICE

MS is a disease of the central nervous system: the myelin sheath which insulates the nerve fibres is destroyed. Symptoms vary dramatically, though often include limb weakness, numbness and tingling, sometimes leading to paralysis and incontinence. Symptoms relapse and remit, apparently without reason. As there is no known cause nor cure, plant medicine can help nurture the spirit, and alleviate depression and exhaustion. If possible, seek the advice of a holistic nutritionist as diet can help the symptoms.

STRESS

SUGGESTED ESSENTIAL OILS

Bergamot (and other citrus essences), cedarwood, chamomile (German and Roman), clary sage, frankincense, geranium, jasmine, juniper berry, lavender, marjoram, neroli, patchouli, peppermint, petitgrain, pine, rose, rosemary, sandalwood, ylang ylang

Methods of Use

Massage, bath, vaporiser, personal perfume

Aromatic Prescription

Massage/bath/vaporiser: 2 drops juniper berry, 2 drops pine, 4 drops sandalwood, (see also Aromatic Prescription under Anxiety)

SUGGESTED HERBS

As for Anxiety. Also ginseng (tonic for whole system), echinacea (if prolonged stress has resulted in increased susceptibility to colds and other infections)

Botanic Prescriptions

1. Infusion: equal parts lemon balm and orange leaves (or flowers). Add 10 drops ginseng tincture per teacup
2. Infusion: 1 part sage, 3 parts marjoram. Add 10 drops echinacea tincture per teacup. (See also recipes for Anxiety)

FURTHER ADVICE

The longer the stressed-out feeling remains, the more harmful it can be. Try to reduce stress through deep relaxation (perhaps with a relaxation tape), meditation, yoga or Tai Chi (enquire about classes in your area). Take plenty of fresh air and exercise, and make time in your life for something frivolous and enjoyable. A professional aromatherapy massage now and again is one of the finest treatments available.

VDU STRESS

RECOMMENDED ESSENTIAL OILS

As for Stress

Methods of Use

Massage (especially to neck, shoulders, hands and arms), bath, vaporiser

Aromatic Prescriptions

As for Stress

SUGGESTED HERBS

Botanic Prescription

As for Jetlag (see also Epsom salts bath, page 142)

FURTHER ADVICE

The symptoms of VDU stress vary from one person to another. Common problems are eye strain, skin rash, nausea, muscular aches and pains, palpitations, insomnia, irritability or a general feeling of malaise. Take a break every 2 hours.

Get up and walk around, or do some gentle stretching. Provide for compensatory outdoor physical activity. The column cactus (*Cereus peruvianus*) is said to absorb radiation, so place one near your computer. Studies have shown that quartz crystals placed around the computer terminal can 'fight back' radiation. Try the flower essence composite known as Radiation Remedy (see page 246).

THE SKIN

The skin is the body's self-renewing outer covering and has many functions. It protects the inner tissues and skeletal structures from damage, shaping and holding together the body with the minimum restriction, maximum stretch and resilience. It protects the rest of the body from excessive loss of water, salts and organic substances, insulates from too much heat or cold, manufactures vitamin D, and is the vehicle of our sense of touch.

In the East the skin is known as 'the third lung', for it continuously expands and contracts, in a sense, 'breathing', excreting waste matter and acting as the body's first line of defence against disease organisms. Indeed, the skin is an essential part of the immune system. It is laced with Langerhans cells, whose function is to interact with the body's helper T cells (a type of white blood cell) to assist the body's immune responses.

Along with the kidneys, lungs and colon, the skin is an organ of elimination. So dysfunction in any of these organs will manifest as spots, rashes, scaling, pallor, dark circles around the eyes, and puffiness, or perhaps the skin will take on an unhealthy waxy appearance. In natural medicine, this is considered to be the result of accumulated poisons being pushed to the surface of the body. Paradoxically, the skin is also capable of absorption (see page 39), a function which is of special importance to aromatherapists.

Even though conventional skin therapists recognise that anxiety and stress can exacerbate skin problems, especially eczema and psoriasis, they persist in treating the skin locally as though it were a separate entity. For example, they may prescribe antibiotics to clear up acne or a hydrocortisone cream to calm down eczema. The danger with this approach is that, by suppressing the condition without removing the cause, the ailment may go deeper and perhaps manifest as a more serious complaint such as asthma, arthritis or weakened immunity.

It is important, therefore, to be careful when attempting treatment of chronic skin complaints. If the cause is not dealt with (be it a hidden food allergy or prolonged stress), treatment with herbs and essential oils (more especially the latter) can be little better than suppressive orthodox treatment. At best, the symptomatic approach offers only partial or temporary relief. Bearing all this in mind, the following charts offer treatments for a number of common skin problems.

CAUTION

Always carry out a skin test (see page 88) before using essential oils, vegetable oils, ointments and external applications of herbs. Apart from idiosyncratic allergic reactions to certain plants, fatty oils and ointments are not always tolerated because they can cause the skin to overheat.

SKIN PROBLEMS

If skin problems make you feel self-conscious or 'unclean', take the Bach flower remedy Crab Apple and/or incorporate the remedy into aromatherapy and herbal skin care preparations.

ACNE

SUGGESTED ESSENTIAL OILS
Cedarwood (Atlas), chamomile (German and Roman), frankincense, geranium, juniper berry, lavender, patchouli, rose otto, rosemary, tea tree. Internally: garlic oil capsules

Methods of Use
Warm compress, facial steam, full body massage (to balance nervous system), aromatic water (see page 100)

Aromatic Prescription
1 teaspoon cider vinegar, 2 drops frankincense, 1 drop lavender, 50ml distilled water, 50ml witch-hazel. Dissolve the essential oil in the vinegar, top up with water and witch-hazel. Shake well to disperse the oil droplets. Apply with cotton swabs twice daily after cleansing

SUGGESTED HERBS
Calendula, dandelion, echinacea, nettle, rose, sage, violet (sweet)

Botanic Prescriptions (internal)
1. Decoction of dandelion root mixed 50/50 with infusion of nettle. Add 10 drops of echninacea tincture per teacup
2. Infusion of sage mixed 50/50 with decoction of lemon peel (organic)
3. Infusion: equal pats rose and chamomile. Add 10 drops violet tincture per teacup

FURTHER ADVICE
Sunbathe (one hour a day maximum) and take plenty of fresh air and exercise. Take 2 × 500 mg capsules evening primrose oil daily. If PMS exacerbates the condition, increase to 4 × 500 mg premensturally (or Efamol premenstrual formulation from pharmacies). Drink two wineglasses organic carrot juice a day to help the body synthesise vitamin A. If no improvement after 3 months, consult a medical herbalist, holistic nutritionist or homeopath.

ATHLETE'S FOOT

SUGGESTED ESSENTIAL OILS
Lavender, patchouli, pine, tea tree

Methods of Use
Foot bath, aromatic ointment (see Botanic Prescription). For small patches, apply neat tea tree or lavender

Aromatic Prescription
4 teaspoons cider vinegar, 6 drops patchouli, 10 drops lavender, 30 ml distilled water. Dissolve the essential oil in the vinegar, then top up with water. Shake well to dispense the oil droplets. Using damp cotton wool, or a cotton bud if only a tiny area is affected, apply three times daily

SUGGESTED HERBS
Internally (to boost the immune system in stubborn cases): echinacea

Botanic Prescription
30g shop-bought unperfumed skin cream, 2 teaspoons calendula tincture, 3 drops lavender, 5 drops tea tree. Stir tincture and essential oils into cream. Apply three times a day

FURTHER ADVICE
A fungal infection between the toes, sometimes spreading over the whole foot. Expose feet to fresh air and sunlight whenever possible; keep them very clean and dry well after washing; avoid hosiery made from synthetic fibres. if the condition is recurrent, despite treating with herbs and essential oils, consult a medical herbalist or homeopath who will offer constitutional treatment.

BOILS

SUGGESTED ESSENTIAL OILS
Chamomile (German and Roman), lavender, lemon, tea tree
Internally: garlic oil capsules

Methods of Use
Warm compress, followed by aromatic ointment or neat tea tree or lavender

Aromatic Prescription
4 teaspoons cider vinegar, 30 ml distilled water, 4 drops Roman chamomile (or 2 drops German chamomile). Dissolve the essential oil in the vinegar, then top up with water. Shake well to disperse the oil droplets. Apply with damp cotton swabs three times daily

SUGGESTED HERBS
Internally: nettle, echinacea
Externally: calendula ointment (see recipe under Athlete's Foot)

FURTHER ADVICE
A tendency to boils often indicates physical neglect and/or emotional disharmony; also with acne and diabetes. Have a medical check-up, then consider holistic treatment from a medical herbalist or homeopath.

CHILBLAINS

SUGGESTED ESSENTIAL OILS
Chamomile (German and Roman), lavender, lemon, marjoram (sweet)

Method of Use
Foot/hand bath, aromatic ointment

Aromatic Prescription
30g unperfumed base cream, 8 drops marjoram (sweet), 5 drops lemon. Stir the essential oil into the cream. Apply two or three times daily

SUGGESTED HERBS
Internally (to improve circulation): ginger (including culinary uses), lemon balm, nettle, peppermint
Externally: calendula ointment (see recipe under Athlete's Foot)

FURTHER ADVICE
An inflammatory condition of the skin, whereby the affected area (fingers, toes, ears or nose) becomes swollen and itchy, sometimes leading to ulceration. Chilblains are associated with sluggish circulation (see page 136).

COLD SORES (HERPES SIMPLEX)

SUGGESTED ESSENTIAL OILS
Chamomile (German and Roman), melissa (true), tea tree

Methods of Use
Aromatic water. To reduce stress, full body massage with any oil(s) of your choice

SUGGESTED HERBS
Internally: chamomile, echinacea, lemon balm
Externally: lavender (diluted tincture), walnut (decoction of leaves). Also, calendula and St John's wort ointment (see Botanic Prescription)

Botanic Prescription
30g unperfumed shop-bought aqueous ointment/cream, 1 teaspoon calendula tincture, 1 teaspoon St John's wort (hypericum) tincture. Put ointment into sterilised glass pot, then stir in tincture. Apply several times daily

FURTHER ADVICE
The virus lies dormant in certain individuals, flaring up whenever you feel stressed, tired or run-down. Strong sun, excessive cold or food intolerances can also trigger it. Avoid foods containing the amino acid arginine (e.g. chocolate, nuts, mushrooms, tomatoes, green peppers). Do eat foods rich in the amino acid lysine (e.g. beansprouts, soya products, yoghurt, brewer's yeast). If possible, consult a holistic nutritionist, medical herbalist or homeopath.

ECZEMA

SUGGESTED ESSENTIAL OILS
Chamomile (German and Roman), geranium (weeping eczema), juniper berry (weeping eczema), lavender, rose otto

Methods of Use
Lukewarm or cold compress, hand/foot baths (localised eruptions), bath, full body massage if possible (to reduce stress) but not if eczema is widespread and/or weepy. Massage where skin is clear. Aromatic ointment if tolerated

SUGGESTED HERBS
Internally: calendula, chamomile, echinacea, heartsease (wild pansy), nettle, oats, rose petal, violet (sweet)
Externally: calendula, violet (sweet)

Botanic Prescriptions
1. Infusion: equal parts rose petal and calendula. Add 10 drops of violet tincture per teacup
2. Infusion of nettle. Add 15 drops echinacea tincture per teacup

FURTHER ADVICE
There are two main types of eczema: atopic (chronic) and contact dermatitis. The first is usually hereditary, associated with a family history of asthma, hay fever or migraine. Food intolerances may also be implicated, especially to dairy products. In contact dermatitis there may be local reaction to household/industrial chemicals, certain plants (e.g. primrose), cosmetics, nickel etc. Contact allergy is also highly likely to occur in people with atopic eczema. Evening primrose oil is highly beneficial (6 × 500 mg capsules daily). If possible, seek constitutional treatment from a holistic nutritionist and/or medical herbalist or homeopath.

HEADLICE

SUGGESTED ESSENTIAL OILS
Eucalyptus, geranium, lavender, rosemary

Method of Use
Hair oil (see Aromatic Prescription)

Aromatic Prescription
100ml vegetable oil (e.g. olive), 25 drops geranium, 25 drops lavender, 25 drops rosemary. Put essential oils into a dark glass bottle, add vegetable oil and shake well. Apply to wet hair and massage into scalp to reach hair roots. Leave on for 2 hours, then shampoo out. Remove eggs (nits) with a regulation fine-toothed comb (essential oils destroy the lice but not the eggs). Repeat the treatment twice more at three-day intervals to ensure infestation is completely cleared

NAPPY RASH

SUGGESTED ESSENTIAL OILS
None (see Further Advice)

SUGGESTED HERBS
Externally: calendula and St John's wort ointment (see Botanic Prescription under Cold Sores)

FURTHER ADVICE
Although oils such as chamomile and lavender are often recommended, they may further irritate a baby's delicate skin. Far better to apply a preventative proprietary zinc and castor oil cream. Should a rash develop, apply St John's wort and calendula ointment (also available from pharmacies). Let your baby's skin breathe by leaving off the nappy for at least one hour a day (with protective covering for the carpet or cot!).

PSORIASIS

SUGGESTED ESSENTIAL OILS

Specifics: bergamot (but see Caution, page 221), chamomile (German and Roman), lavender
General: Any oil according to aroma preference for uplifting spirits

Methods of Use

Warm compress, bath, ointment, general body massage to reduce stress (but only where skin is healthy). For psoriasis of the scalp, see Aromatic Prescriptions

Aromatic Prescriptions

1. Bath: dissolve 500g sea salt in the water. Add up to 8 drops appropriate essential oil. Take 3–4 times a week
2. Scalp lotion: 100ml distilled water, 3 teaspoons cider vinegar, 2 drops German chamomile, 2 drops lavender. Put vinegar in dark glass bottle, add essential oil and shake well. Top up with distilled water and shake again. Rub into the scalp 2–3 times daily

SUGGESTED HERBS

To relax and strengthen nervous system: chamomile, hops, linden blossom, oats, valerian, vervain
To promote skin health: dandelion, elm (decoctions of the dried inner bark), heartsease (wild pansy), nettle.
Externally: infused oil of St John's wort

Botanic Prescriptions

1. Decoction of dandelion root mixed 50/50 with nettle. Add 20 drops oats tincture per teacup
2. Infusion of linden blossom. Add 15 drops heartsease tincture per teacup

FURTHER ADVICE

Psoriasis is characterised by red raised patches topped by silvery scales. It can affect any part of the body, including the scalp. Studies have shown that 60 per cent of sufferers experience improvement by taking 6 × 500 mg evening primrose oil capsules daily. Sunlight and sea-water usually give temporary relief. Sea-water contains minerals virtually identical to those in blood plasma (responsible for feeding and strengthening all body cells). If possible, consult a holistic nutritionist and/or a medical herbalist. Homeopathy is also worth considering.

RINGWORM

SUGGESTED ESSENTIAL OILS

Eucalyptus, geranium, lavender, lemon, peppermint, pine

Methods of Use

Lukewarm or cold compress, aromatic ointment, bath

SUGGESTED HERBS

Externally: calendula ointment (see recipe under Athlete's Foot)
Internally: echinacea (to boost the immune system)

FURTHER ADVICE

This fungal infection manifests as a red, itchy rash in circular patches anywhere on the body. Expose skin often to fresh air and sunlight. Wash all clothing and linen in very hot or boiling water to avoid reinfection.

THE RESPIRATORY SYSTEM

Supplying the cells with life-giving oxygen is the shared responsibility of the respiratory and circulatory systems. And since the lungs share the role of eliminating waste with the skin, kidneys and colon, if a problem develops in any of these systems the body compensates by increasing the burden on the others.

Respiratory ailments affect the mucous membranes. These include the linings of the noses, sinuses, mouth, throat, windpipe and lungs. The fine coverings of the eyes and the linings of certain parts of the inner ear are also covered by mucus-producing membranes. When health is compromised, perhaps through poor diet, emotional disharmony or cigarette smoke, we become more susceptible to bacterial and viral infection. Should the cause of the problem be ignored, this can lead to congestion or chronic catarrh. The aim of natural treatment is to change the consistency of the mucus by using decongestant herbs and essences. Above all, treatment is geared to strengthening the immune system.

RESPIRATORY AILMENTS

It is particularly difficult to generalise about appropriate flower essences for respiratory ailments. Asthma sufferers, however, commonly require essences for addressing various states of anxiety: for example Aspen, Chamomile, Mimulus, Pine, Larch, Red Chestnut, Rescue Remedy and Valerian.

ASTHMA

SUGGESTED ESSENTIAL OILS
Eucalyptus, frankincense, lavender, marjoram, melissa (true), peppermint, pine, rose otto, rosemary, tea tree
Internally: garlic oil capsules

Methods of Use
Bath, regular massage (especially to chest, back, neck and shoulders), vaporiser, dry inhalation

Aromatic Prescription
Massage/bath/vaporiser: 2 drops rose otto, 2 drops marjoram, 1 drop frankincense

SUGGESTED HERBS
Angelica, chamomile, echinacea, evening primrose (leaves), feverfew, lavender, lemon balm, linden blossom, marjoram, peppermint, pine needle, rosemary

Botanic Prescription
1. Infusion: 1 part lemon balm, 2 parts marjoram. Add 10 drops echinacea tincture per teacup
2. Infusion: equal parts evening primrose and feverfew

FURTHER ADVICE
There is usually a family history of asthma, eczema and sometimes migraine. Allergies are often implicated, for example, air pollutants, dust mites, pollen, animal fur, moulds, dairy products. Fear and nervous tension may provoke an attack. Seek to reduce stress. You might like to take up singing as this greatly improves lung capacity. For chronic asthma (a potentially life-threatening condition) it is essential to seek constitutional treatment from a fully accredited holistic practitioner, *whilst remaining under medical supervision.*

CAUTION

Avoid saunas and steam inhalations as they may provoke an asthma attack. Before using any essential oil (or external application of a herbal preparation) always carry out a skin test (see page 88).

BRONCHITIS

SUGGESTED ESSENTIAL OILS
Angelica, cedarwood, eucalyptus, frankincense, lavender, lemon, marjoram (sweet), orange, peppermint, pine, rose otto, rosemary, sandalwood, tea tree
Internally: garlic oil capsules

Methods of Use
Steam inhalations, vaporiser, bath (not eucalyptus), chest and back rub (see Aromatic Prescription)

Aromatic Prescription
Relaxing bedtime back and chest rub: 50ml almond oil, 5 drops frankincense, 5 drops sandalwood, 5 drops lavender

SUGGESTED HERBS
Angelica, basil, echninacea, ginger, heartsease, lemon, marjoram, nasturtium, pine needle, sage, vervain, violet (sweet)

Botanic Prescription
Infusion: equal quantities of sage and marjoram. Add 15 drops echninacea tincture per teacup

FURTHER ADVICE
Symptoms are a chesty cough, high temperature, chest pain, aching muscles, irritation between the shoulder blades, depression. Ensure that you have plenty of bed rest. Also, take hot lemon and honey drinks with a pinch of dried ginger or cayenne pepper. Chronic bronchitis (often accompanied by emphysema) requires professional intervention. If this is the case, seek the cooperation of your doctor as well as embarking on constitutional treatment from a medical herbalist or homeopath.

CATARRH

SUGGESTED ESSENTIAL OILS
Cedarwood, eucalyptus, frankincense, ginger, lavender, lemon, marjoram, orange, peppermint, pine, rose otto, rosemary, sandalwood, tea tree

Methods of Use
Bath (not eucalyptus), steam inhalation, dry inhalation, chest rub (see Aromatic Prescriptions under Bronchitis)
Internally: garlic capsules

SUGGESTED HERBS
Chamomile, elderflower, feverfew, lemon balm, marjoram, peppermint, pine needle, sage, violet (sweet)

Botanic Prescriptions
1. Infusion: equal parts elderflower, lemon balm and chamomile
2. Infusion of peppermint. Add 10 drops of violet tincture per teacup

FURTHER ADVICE
Chronic catarrh is indicative of a faulty diet and/or allergy. Seek professional advice from an holistic nutritionist and/or medical herbalist or homeopath.

COLDS

SUGGESTED ESSENTIAL OILS
Angelica, cedarwood, coriander (seeds), eucalyptus, ginger, lavender, lemon, marjoram, orange, peppermint, pine, tea tree
Internally (as a preventative): garlic oil capsules

Methods of Use
Bath (not eucalyptus), steam inhalation, dry inhalation, vaporiser, chest rub (see Aromatic Prescriptions under Bronchitis)

SUGGESTED HERBS
Chamomile, elderflower, ginger, lemon, marjoram, mustard, peppermint, pine needle

Botanic Prescriptions
1. Hot decoction of ginger. Add 1 dessertspoon lemon juice per teacup. Sweeten with honey to taste.
2. Infusion: equal parts chamomile, peppermint and elderflower

FURTHER ADVICE
Two other highly beneficial treatments are the mustard foot bath (see page 113) and the Epsom salts bath (see page 142).

COUGHS

SUGGESTED ESSENTIAL OILS
Angelica, cedarwood, clary sage, eucalyptus, ginger, marjoram, pine, rose otto, rosemary, sandalwood, tea tree
Internally: garlic capsules (not for dry cough)

Methods of Use
Gargle (see Aromatic Prescription), dry inhalation (drops on handkerchief), bath, vaporiser, massage oil (rub on chest and gently over throat)

Aromatic Prescription
Gargle: 2 teaspoons cider vinegar, 1 drop sandalwood or eucalyptus, 1 drop lemon. Top up with 1 teacup warm water, then stir in 1 teaspoon honey. Use 2–3 times daily, but do not swallow

SUGGESTED HERBS
Angelica, honeysuckle, marjoram, peppermint, pine needle, sage, vervain, violet (sweet)

Botanic Prescription
Cough with phlegm: hot decoction of angelica (root or seed). Add 3 teaspoons lemon juice per teacup. Sweeten with honey to taste
Dry cough: infusion of vervain. Add 10 drops violet tincture per teacup. Sweeten with honey to taste

FURTHER ADVICE
If a cough is persistent or painful, or if there is brown or discoloured mucus, or blood, seek urgent medical attention.

EARACHE

SUGGESTED ESSENTIAL OILS
Chamomile (German and Roman), lavender, peppermint, rosemary

Method of Use
Warm 1 eggcup olive or almond oil and add 1 drop essential oil. Using a pipette (from pharmacists), put a few drops into the ear and seal in with a small ball of cotton wool

SUGGESTED HERBS
As for Colds. See also Coughs and Flu (page 113)

FURTHER ADVICE
Earache, often associated with a cold or flu, is usually caused by infection spreading from the eustachian tube in the ear. If persistent, see a doctor, especially if there is pus or a bloody discharge.

EYE INFECTIONS (STICKY, IRRITATED, STYES)

SUGGESTED ESSENTIAL OILS
Never apply oils to the eyes as they can cause pain and irritation. However, genuine rosewater from a reputable supplier can be used to bathe the eyes

Method of Use
Externally, as for herbal preparations

SUGGESTED HERBS
Agrimony, calendula, chamomile, rose petal, sage
Internally (to boost immunity): echinacea

Botanic Prescription
For dry irritated eyes, bathe with cold infusions of any of the recommended herbs, or apply a cold compress. For sticky eyes (and styes), bathe with warm infusions of the same herbs

FURTHER ADVICE
Styes are similar to boils (see page 127), but can be treated as suggested here. Conjunctivitis is a more serious contagious condition which may need medical attention (though herbs will hasten the healing process). Other eye infections can often be relieved with herbal lotions. However, chronic cases are indicative of a run-down state. Therefore, constitutional treatment under the guidance of a medical herbalist, holistic nutritionist or homeopath is essential.

FLU

SUGGESTED ESSENTIAL OILS
As for Colds

Methods of Use
Bath, steam inhalation, dry inhalation (drops on handkerchief), massage oil (rubbed on to chest and gently over throat)

Aromatic Prescription
Chest rub (see Aromatic Prescriptions under Bronchitis)

SUGGESTED HERBS
As for colds

FURTHER ADVICE
Try a mustard footbath. Put 1 level teaspoon English mustard powder in a bowl of hand-hot water, then soak your feet for 10 minutes. At the same time, enjoy a hot lemon, ginger and honey drink (see Botanic Prescription under Colds). Afterwards, go straight to bed and 'sweat it out'. Another helpful remedy is the Epsom salts bath (page 142).

HAYFEVER

SUGGESTED ESSENTIAL OILS
Chamomile (German and Roman), echinacea, eucalyptus, melissa (true), peppermint, pine, rose otto
Internally: garlic capsules

Methods of Use
Bath, dry inhalation (drops on handkerchief), massage (especially to chest and back), vaporiser

SUGGESTED HERBS
Elderflower, feverfew, lavender, lemon balm, peppermint, pine needle, rose petal

Botanic Prescription
Infusion: 1 part lavender, 4 parts rose petal. Add 10 drops elder flower tincture per teacup. Sweeten with honey to taste

FURTHER ADVICE
Take 1 teaspoon local honey from the comb, wax and all, every day for a year to help build your immunity to pollens in your immediate environment. If home treatment is only partially successful, seek advice from a medical herbalist, homeopath or holistic nutritionist (see also Asthma).

Sinusitis

SUGGESTED ESSENTIAL OILS
Eucalyptus, lavender, lemon, peppermint, pine, tea tree
Internally: garlic capsules (to boost immune system)

Methods of Use
Steam inhalation, dry inhalation (drops of essential oil on handkerchief), bath, vaporiser, massage (very light stroking downwards over eyes and cheekbones to encourage drainage of mucus)

SUGGESTED HERBS
Agrimony, echinacea, elderflower, feverfew, lavender, peppermint, pine needle, rosemary

Botanic Prescription
1. Decoction of fresh pine needles mixed 50/50 with infusion of peppermint. Add 10 drops echinacea tincture per teacup
2. Infusion: 1 part lavender, 1 part agrimony, 3 parts elderflower

FURTHER ADVICE
Sinusitis is an infection of the sinus cavities (the four air-containing cavities of the face), often associated with colds and flu. However, chronic sinusitis may be caused by food intolerance (possibly to dairy products or wheat), prolonged stress or air pollution. Try to reduce stress; it may be advisable to consult a medical herbalist, homeopath or holistic nutritionist.

Throat infections

SUGGESTED ESSENTIAL OILS
Sore throat: bergamot, clary sage, eucalyptus, geranium, ginger, lavender, lemon, peppermint, pine, sandalwood, tea tree
Laryngitis/hoarseness: clary sage, eucalyptus, frankincense, lavender, lemon, sandalwood

Methods of Use
Gargle (see Aromatic Prescription under Coughs), massage oil (apply to throat)

SUGGESTED HERBS
Gargle: Agrimony, echinacea, lemon, sage, violet (sweet)

Botanic Prescription
Gargle: infusion of sage. Add 2 teaspoons lemon juice or cider vinegar per teacup. Best used warm. Gently reheat the infusion (but not the lemon juice or vinegar) each time before use

FURTHER ADVICE
A sore throat is often the first sign of a cold, flu or some other viral infection. Laryngitis is inflammation of the larynx (voice box), producing huskiness and weakness of the voice and sometimes a harsh dry cough. Try to rest the voice.

THE CIRCULATORY SYSTEM

Every cell in the body needs a constant supply of blood to bring in oxygen and nutrients and to remove metabolic wastes. If the supply is insufficient, we experience a marked decrease in vitality. The heart itself does not extract vital oxygen from the main circulation, but is nourished by the blood which passes through the coronary arteries – the heart's main weak spot. Should they become narrowed through cardiovascular disease, the amount of blood able to pass through the heart is reduced. Coronary dysfunction is, in fact, the greatest single cause of death.

The management of serious heart and circulatory problems are beyond the scope of self-treatment. However, provided you remain under medical supervision there is a great deal you can do to ease the symptoms and perhaps even halt the progress of problems like high blood pressure and angina. This can be achieved by giving up smoking (or not starting in the first place), taking adequate exercise, eating sensibly and trying to reduce the stress in your life.

Circulatory problems often mean there is fluid retention. Massage (with or without essential oils) is supremely effective in helping the body to eliminate excess fluid and toxic wastes. Of course, not everyone is fortunate enough to be able to receive regular massage. None the less, herbal remedies can play a major role in the healing process.

CIRCULATORY PROBLEMS

The flower essences recommended for Anxiety (see page 119) may also be helpful for those suffering from high blood pressure and palpitations. Poor circulation and cold extremities, particularly if accompanied by impaired memory, indicate the flower essence Rosemary.

BLOOD PRESSURE, HIGH (HYPERTENSION)

SUGGESTED ESSENTIAL OILS
Chamomile (German and Roman), Clary sage, lavender, lemon, marjoram, melissa (true), ylang ylang
Internally: garlic capsules

Methods of Use
Bath, massage, personal perfume, vaporiser

Aromatic Prescription
Massage/bath/vaporiser: 3 drops marjoram, 2 drops Roman chamomile, 4 drops lemon

SUGGESTED HERBS
Lemon balm, linden blossom, olive (leaves), valerian

Botanic Prescription
1. Decoction of olive leaves mixed 50/50 with infusion of lemon balm
2. Infusion: Equal parts lemon balm and linden blossom

FURTHER ADVICE
Although often symptomless in the early stages, signs include morning headache, dizziness on sudden change of position, palpitations, shortness of breath and blurred vision. Prolonged stress, smoking, obesity, sedentary lifestyle, pregnancy and faulty diet are contributing factors. Holistic treatment is essential, including deep breathing and relaxation exercises, as well as sensible exercise. Regular aromatherapy massage is one of the best natural treatments. However, persistent high blood pressure must be investigated by a medical practitioner.

BLOOD PRESSURE, LOW (HYPOTENSION)

SUGGESTED ESSENTIAL OILS
Angelica, coriander, geranium,
ginger, lemon, marjoram, neroli,
pine, rosemary

Methods of Use
Bath, brisk massage

Aromatic Prescription
See recipe under Sluggish
Circulation below

SUGGESTED HERBS
Angelica, dandelion, ginger,
ginseng, rosemary

Botanic Prescriptions
1. Decoction of angelica root or
   seed. Add 10 drops ginseng
   tincture per teacup
2. Decoction of dandelion root
   mixed 50/50 with infusion of
   rosemary

FURTHER ADVICE
Low blood pressure only becomes a
problem when it is associated with
dizziness, fainting and debility. If so,
seek medical advice.

CIRCULATION, SLUGGISH

SUGGESTED ESSENTIAL OILS
Angelica, bergamot, coriander,
eucalyptus, geranium, ginger,
lavender, lemon, marjoram, melissa
(true), neroli, orange, peppermint,
pine, rose, rosemary
Internally: garlic capsules

Methods of Use
Bath (not eucalyptus), foot/hand
bath, brisk massage

Aromatic Prescriptions
1. Bath/massage: 2 drops geranium,
   1 drop ginger, 3 drops neroli
2. Bath/massage: 2 drops marjoram,
   2 drops pine, 2 drops rosemary

SUGGESTED HERBS
Angelica, basil, dandelion, ginger,
horse chestnut, lavender, lemon
balm, peppermint, rosemary, sage,
vervain

Botanic Prescriptions
1. Infusion of horse chestnut (use
   dried)
2. Infusion: 1 part lavender, 2 parts
   sage, 2 parts vervain
3. Decoction of ginger, sweetened
   with honey to taste

FURTHER ADVICE
Sluggish circulation manifests as
cold extremities, susceptibility to
chilblains and exceptional
intolerance to cold. Circulation is
improved by regular full body
massage, fresh air and exercise,
correct breathing and good
nutrition.

PALPITATIONS

SUGGESTED ESSENTIAL OILS
Lavender, melissa (true), neroli, orange, petitgrain, rose, ylang ylang

Methods of Use
Dry inhalation (drops on handkerchief), vaporiser, personal perfume, regular full body massage as a preventative measure

Aromatic Prescription
Massage/bath/vaporiser: 2 drops rose otto or 3 drops rose absolute, 4 drops orange, 2 drops ylang ylang

SUGGESTED HERBS
Chamomile, lemon (peel and leaves), lemon balm, linden blossom, orange (flowers and leaves), rose petal, valerian

Botanic Prescriptions
1. Infusion: equal quantities of linden blossom, lemon balm and rose petals
2. Infusion: decoction of lemon leaves or organic lemon peel mixed 50/50 with infusion of orange flowers

FURTHER ADVICE
Pounding of the heart other than after exercise, emotional shock or excitement needs further investigation. It may be the result of prolonged stress, allergy, hormonal fluctuation (e.g. menopause), chronic high blood pressure, or consuming nicotine or caffeine. It may also indicate a heart problem. Try to reduce stress, and have a medical check-up.

VARICOSE VEINS (also HAEMORRHOIDS)

SUGGESTED ESSENTIAL OILS
Frankincense, geranium, lavender, lemon, rose
Internally: garlic capsules

Methods of Use
Cold or tepid compress, aromatic ointment, *very gentle* application of appropriate massage oil

Aromatic Prescription
30g unperfumed base cream, 5 drops frankincense, 4 drops geranium or 2 drops rose otto, 5 drops lemon. Smooth into affected areas 2–3 times daily

SUGGESTED HERBS
Calendula, St John's wort. Also, St John's wort and calendula ointment (see under Cold Sores, page 127) Internally: horse chestnut, nettle, rosehip

Botanic Prescription
Infusion of horse chestnut (use dried) mixed 50/50 with infusion of nettle

FURTHER ADVICE
Take adequate exercise. Yoga, especially the inverted positions, is good. Alternatively, rest with your feet higher than your head for about 10 minutes every day. The specific remedy is rutin, found in buckwheat and available in tablet form from health food stores, which helps strengthen capillary walls and reduces swelling. It is also helpful for haemorrhoids (varicose veins of the rectum).

THE DIGESTIVE SYSTEM

Dietary habits apart, the functioning and health of the digestive system is closely related to our emotional state. Almost everyone has experienced a 'gut reaction' to a powerful emotion such as fear, anger or anxiety. This may have resulted in a momentary tightening of the abdomen, or a fluttering sensation in the solar plexus. Prolonged distress, however, can lead to disturbances ranging from diminished appetite, constipation and heartburn, to diarrhoea, nausea or, more seriously, a gastric ulcer. As with most conditions explored in this chapter, holistic treatment (which takes into account the emotional state of the sufferer) is essential. Bearing this in mind, the following charts suggest natural treatments for a number of common ailments affecting the digestive system.

PROBLEMS OF THE DIGESTIVE SYSTEM

The flower essences recommended for Stress and Anxiety (see pages 119 and 124 respectively), may also be helpful for digestive problems, particularly gastric ulcers.

CONSTIPATION

SUGGESTED ESSENTIAL OILS
Marjoram, orange, rose otto, rosemary. Also, oils for reducing stress if this is a contributing factor (see page 124)

Method of Use
Massage, particularly abdominal (clockwise circular strokes with the flat of the hand). If stressed, aromatic baths and full body massage with appropriate oils

SUGGESTED HERBS
Basil, dandelion, centaury, chamomile, chicory, apple (stewed fruit), violet (sweet)

Botanic Prescription
1. Decoction of dandelion. Add 20 drops of violet tincture per teacup
2. Decoction of chicory root mixed 50/50 with infusion of basil

FURTHER ADVICE
The main causes are lack of dietary fibre (especially fresh fruit and vegetables), inadequate fluid intake, sedentary lifestyle, nervous tension, depression and failure to respond to a 'call of nature'. Long-term use of chemical laxatives, and strong herbal laxatives like senna, inhibit the movement of food along the gut and actually worsen the problem. Drink 2–3 mugs of warm spring water immediately after breakfast to stimulate the bowels. Chronic constipation must be investigated by a medical practitioner, then treated under the guidance of an holistic therapist.

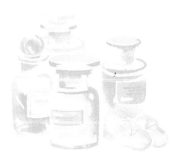

DIARRHOEA

SUGGESTED ESSENTIAL OILS
Chamomile (German and Roman), ginger, marjoram, sandalwood
Internally: garlic capsules

Method of Use
Warm compress over abdomen

SUGGESTED HERBS
Astringents: agrimony, meadowsweet, rosehip, sage, sweet chestnut (dried catkins), walnut (dried catkins)
For griping pain: angelica, ginger, peppermint
For stomach bugs: ginger

Botanic Prescriptions
1. Decoction of ginger mixed 50/50 with infusion of agrimony
2. Infusion of meadowsweet mixed 50/50 with infusion of rosehips
3. Decoction of sweet chestnut catkins mixed 50/50 with decoction of angelica seeds or root

FURTHER ADVICE
Diarrhoea is a symptom of an underlying problem such as stress, bacterial infection (e.g. holiday diarrhoea), gastric flu, the side-effects of certain drugs, food poisoning, and drastic and sudden changes in diet. As well as taking a herbal remedy, drink plenty of bottled or boiled water to prevent dehydration. Persistent diarrhoea should be investigated by a medical practitioner.

GASTRIC ULCER (INCLUDING DUODENAL AND PEPTIC ULCERS)

SUGGESTED ESSENTIAL OILS
To reduce stress: choose soothing, relaxing oils e.g. cedarwood, chamomile (German and Roman), frankincense, lavender, marjoram, neroli, rose otto, sandalwood, ylang ylang
To settle the stomach (inhalant): peppermint

Methods of Use
The aim of aromatherapy is to reduce stress rather than to treat the ulcer directly. Regular full body massage, aromatic bath, personal perfume. A few drops of peppermint oil can be dropped on a handkerchief and inhaled as required

SUGGESTED HERBS
Calendula, chamomile, peppermint, slippery elm

Botanic Prescriptions
To coat lining of stomach, alleviate pain and protect against over-acid secretions. Take 1 teaspoon slippery elm powder, make into a paste with a little cold water and add 1 teacup boiling water, stirring all the time. Sweeten with a little honey if desired. Eat a few teaspoons three times daily before meals

FURTHER ADVICE
Faulty diet, smoking and prolonged stress are contributing factors. Take regular and frequent light meals, avoiding foods which cause excessive acid secretion (e.g. bacon, egg white, tea, coffee, chocolate, alcohol). If the ulcer is caught in the early stages stress-reducing techniques and soothing herbs will make the stomach secrete mucus to heal the wound. Consult a medical practitioner for correct diagnosis.

GINGIVITIS

SUGGESTED ESSENTIAL OILS
Bergamot, eucalyptus, lemon, tea tree

Method of Use
Mouthwash: put 1–2 drops essential oil into a small glass or teacup of warm water and use 2–3 times a day

SUGGESTED HERBS
Mouthwash (infusion or diluted tincture): agrimony, calendula, echinacea, rose (leaves), sage

FURTHER ADVICE
Gingivitis is inflammation of the gums caused by poor oral hygiene and/or a diet high in sugar and processed foods. If left untreated, it may develop into severe gum disease (pyorrhoea) and tooth loss. Gentle, regular and effective brushing is essential. The best and cheapest cleanser and gum strengthener is salt water ($1/2$ teaspoon salt in a small cup of lukewarm water). Visit your dentist regularly (preferably one who practises holistic dentistry).

HALITOSIS (OFFENSIVE BREATH)

SUGGESTED ESSENTIAL OILS
Bergamot, peppermint

Method of Use
Mouthwash (as described for Gingivitis)

SUGGESTED HERBS
Chew a whole clove or the leaves of peppermint, parsley or fennel

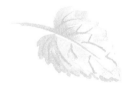

FURTHER ADVICE
Usually the result of eating foods like garlic and onions, it may also be caused by poor dental hygiene, periodontal disease, gastric disorders, constipation, catarrh, smoking, excessive alcohol, or possibly an underlying health problem. If the problem persists, have a medical check-up, perhaps followed by treatment under a medical herbalist or homeopath.

INDIGESTION (also HEARTBURN)

SUGGESTED ESSENTIAL OILS
Chamomile (German and Roman), clary sage, coriander, ginger, marjoram, peppermint

Methods of Use
Gentle clockwise abdominal massage, dry inhalation of peppermint (drops on a handkerchief)

SUGGESTED HERBS
Basil, centaury, chamomile, ginger, lemon balm, marjoram, peppermint, slippery elm

Botanic Prescriptions
1. Infusion: equal parts basil, marjoram and peppermint
2. Infusion: equal parts lemon balm and chamomile

FURTHER ADVICE
Common causes of indigestion are too much rich food and drink, irregular meals, eating too quickly, incompatible food combinations (e.g. bread with oranges) and nervous tension. Indigestion, particularly heartburn, is common during pregnancy and in cases of hiatus hernia. Persistent indigestion should be investigated by a health professional as it may indicate a stomach ulcer or gallstones. Food allergy may also be implicated.

IRRITABLE BOWEL SYNDROME

SUGGESTED ESSENTIAL OILS
Chamomile (German and Roman), lavender, marjoram, melissa (true), neroli, peppermint, rose otto
Internally: peppermint oil capsules (from health food stores)

Methods of Treatment
Warm compress over abdomen, very gentle clockwise abdominal massage. To reduce stress: aromatic baths and full body massage with any relaxing essences of your choice

SUGGESTED HERBS
Agrimony, chamomile, hops, lemon balm, marjoram, peppermint, slippery elm

Botanic Prescription
1. Slippery elm paste (see recipe under Gastric Ulcer)
2. Infusion: 2 parts agrimony, 1 part lemon balm, 1 part chamomile

FURTHER ADVICE
Symptoms include abdominal cramps, colic, bloating, flatulence and alternate bouts of diarrhoea. Prolonged stress, inadequate exercise and faulty nutrition are usually implicated. Try to reduce stress, and consult a medical herbalist or homeopath or a holistic nutritionist. Many sufferers have food intolerance, particularly to diary products. Other foods may also contribute to the problem.

MOUTH ULCERS

SUGGESTED ESSENTIAL OILS
Peppermint, tea tree

Method of Use
Mouthwash (see Aromatic Prescription)

Aromatic Prescription
Put 1 drop tea tree in a teacup of warm water and use 2–3 times daily

SUGGESTED HERBS
Calendula (tincture), sage

Botanic Prescription
Infusion of sage. Add 10 drops calendula tincture per teacup and use as a mouthwash 2–3 times daily

FURTHER ADVICE
Mouth ulcers can be caused by biting the inside of the mouth; irritation from a denture; or a run-down condition, perhaps through prolonged stress or antibiotic treatment. If necessary, seek to reduce stress through regular aromatherapy massage or relaxation techniques. If antibiotics are the cause, eat lots of live yoghurt to restore the natural intestinal flora destroyed by the drug. Otherwise, try to obtain lacto bacilus supplements (yoghurt culture) from health food stores.

NAUSEA (also MOTION SICKNESS)

SUGGESTED ESSENTIAL OILS
Angelica, coriander, ginger, lavender, peppermint

Method of Use
Dry inhalation (drops on a handkerchief). Choose the oil you find most pleasant and use singly (blends are not always tolerated)

SUGGESTED HERBS
Angelica, chamomile, ginger, meadowsweet, peppermint. Herbal travel sickness tablets containing ginger are available in health food stores

Botanic Prescription
Choose the plant remedy you find most palatable. Make an infusion/decoction (or use the diluted tincture) and take as often as required. For motion and pregnancy sickness suck crystallised ginger

FURTHER ADVICE
The causes of nausea include stress, constipation, faulty diet, overeating, mild food poisoning, indigestion, pregnancy, VDU stress and motion sickness (affecting the organ of balance in the inner ear). Fresh air tends to alleviate all nausea. Persistent nausea with no apparent cause should be investigated by a medical practitioner.

THE MUSCULAR AND SKELETAL SYSTEM

The most common problems associated with the muscular and skeletal system are arthritis and rheumatism. There are many forms, including bursitis, gout, sciatica, fibrositis (also known as muscular rheumatism), osteoarthritis and rheumatoid arthritis. All are painful and restrict movement. There may also be inflammation and swelling, calcification of the joints, and loss of synovial fluid which lubricates the joints. Rheumatism is a term that indicates any of the various diseases of the musculoskeletal system. However, there is a contradistinction between osteoarthritis and rheumatoid arthritis.

Osteoarthritis is a 'wear and tear' condition in which the cartilage protecting the ends of the bones flakes off, leaving rough edges and preventing the joints from functioning smoothly. It usually affects the weight-bearing joints, especially the knees, hips, back and neck. The condition may also be asymmetrical – for instance, while the left knee feels stiff and painful, the right one feels fine.

Rheumatoid arthritis is an auto-immune disease in which the body's defence system goes haywire and attacks its own tissues, a disease marked by exacerbations and remissions. The joints most commonly affected are the hands, wrists, ankles, and feet, often with a high temperature and swellings involving the same joint on both sides of the body.

The orthodox approach is to prescribe anti-inflammatory drugs and sometimes corticosteroids, all of which can have unpleasant side-effects. Surgery such as hip replacement may also play a part. Yet contrary to common medical belief these two potentially crippling diseases can be overcome. Indeed, there are many recorded cases of people who have used natural therapies such as acupuncture, massage, herbal medicine, homeopathy, reflexology and dietary reform to reduce pain greatly and increase mobility in the affected parts. However, natural healing takes time, patience and commitment, so comparatively few people give alternative therapy a fair chance.

The main aim of treatment is to detoxify the system and balance the acid/alkaline composition of the blood (arthritis and rheumatism are associated with over-acidity). Stress may be reduced and flexibility increased by methods such as mineral salt baths, massage, gentle stretching, deep relaxation exercises and a predominantly alkaline diet: cut out or reduce to a bare minimum acid-producing foods and beverages such as pork, tea, coffee and chocolate, and eat plenty of fruit, vegetables, sprouted seeds and grains.

However, no one diet is perfect for everyone – you might find that grapes or apples exacerbate your own symptoms. It is advisable therefore to consult a holistic nutritionist (see Useful Addresses on page 265) who will devise a personal dietary plan. Alternatively, if you can perfect the skill of dowsing (see page 74) this can be a marvellous way of ascertaining the right foods for your own unique mind/body complex.

THE EPSOM SALTS BATH

In all cases of musculoskeletal discomfort, an Epsom salts bath is one of the most effective pain relievers. It also greatly reduces stress and can even ward off colds and flu if taken at the onset of symptoms. Epsom salts (magnesium sulphate, a naturally occurring mineral) are inexpensive and can be obtained from pharmacists. The salts alleviate pain by promoting perspiration and drawing acidic wastes (mainly uric acid) from the muscles and joints through the pores of the skin. Add to the bathwater as much as 450g salts. Relax for about 15 minutes, but do not use soap as it interferes with the action of the salts. If possible, try to rest for at least two hours afterwards, and avoid becoming chilled. (See CAUTION for Epsom salts, opposite.)

MUSCULAR AND SKELETAL PROBLEMS

The flower remedy Willow is often indicated for people with arthritic and rheumatic complaints. Those prone to muscular aches and pains due to overexertion should consider Dandelion, Impatiens, Oak or Vervain. Ensure that the chosen remedy matches the psycho-spiritual pattern of the individual concerned.

ARTHRITIS AND RHEUMATISM

SUGGESTED ESSENTIAL OILS
Angelica, cedarwood (Atlas), chamomile (German and Roman), coriander, ginger, juniper berry, lavender, marjoram, pine, rosemary
Internally: garlic oil capsules

Methods of Treatment
Massage, compress (for painful joints), baths, aromatic ointment

Aromatic Prescriptions
1. Massage: 25ml extra virgin olive oil, 4 drops cedarwood, 4 drops juniper berry, 3 drops pine
2. Aromatic ointment: 50g unperfumed base cream, 5 drops coriander, 2 drops ginger, 8 drops lavender, 5 drops rosemary. Stir the essential oils into the cream. Apply 2–3 times daily, preferably after a bath

SUGGESTED HERBS
Heather (decoction added to bath), infused oil of St John's wort
Internally: chamomile, dandelion, elderflower, elderberry, ginger, heartsease, juniper berries (but see Cautions, page 173), lemon, marjoram, meadowsweet, nettle, pine needle, rosemary, sage. Also, evening primrose oil capsules (3 × 500 mg daily)

Botanic Prescriptions
1. Infusion: equal parts chamomile and meadowsweet. Add 1 dessertspoon lemon juice per teacup
2. Infusion: equal parts nettle, marjoram and heartsease (wild pansy)
3. Decoction of fresh pine needles mixed 50/50 with infusion of sage

FURTHER ADVICE
If there is no improvement after three months, seek the advice of a medical herbalist. Regular aromatherapy massage will help to ease pain and uplift the spirits. Other helpful therapies are acupuncture or homeopathy (not both together because they are known to cancel each other out). Regular gentle exercise will improve mobility in the joints and possibly halt the progress of the disease. Try to reduce stress and make appropriate dietary changes, preferably with the help of a holistic therapist.

CAUTION

Always move arthritic joints as much as possible after an Epsom salts bath to prevent congestion, which will cause further pain. Do not have one if you have high blood pressure or a heart condition. Elderly or frail people should use 225g salts to start with, gradually increasing as the bath becomes better tolerated.

CAUTION

Never apply massage over inflamed and swollen joints. This state comes and goes, particularly with rheumatoid arthritis. Massage over affected areas is fine in between flare-ups and will help ease the severity of future exacerbations.

MUSCULAR ACHES AND PAINS

SUGGESTED ESSENTIAL OILS
Chamomile (German and Roman), coriander, eucalyptus, ginger, juniper berry, lavender, lemon, marjoram, pine, rosemary

Methods of Use
Massage, bath, compress

Aromatic Prescription
1. Massage: 25ml St John's wort oil, 2 drops ginger
2. Massage: 25ml extra virgin olive oil, 7 drops juniper berry, 2 drops German chamomile (or 3 drops Roman)

SUGGESTED HERBS
All those suggested for Stress (page 124). Also, massage with infused oil of St John's wort

CAUTION
Never massage if the muscle is inflamed and swollen. Use cold compresses instead.

FURTHER ADVICE
If you are prone to muscular aches and pains, the condition may be related to an arthritic or rheumatic complaint, or it may be stress-related. If caused by a recent injury or fibrositis, the pain will be sharp or searing. Old injuries and chronic muscular tension manifest as a dull ache (see also First Aid on page 154).

THE URINARY SYSTEM

The kidneys form the body's main waste disposal system, with the skin, lungs and colon following close behind. They also control vital water balance in the body tissues, and are involved with cleaning and filtering the blood. Moreover, the kidneys regulate the relative salt balance in the body, excreting excessive amounts of potassium salts and sodium chloride. As if this were not enough, they also maintain the optimum acid/alkaline content of the blood. In a healthy body this ratio should be 80 per cent alkaline to 20 per cent acid. In fact, the acid/alkaline balance of the blood is also influenced by diet.

The most abundant waste product the kidneys have to deal with is urea, the end product of protein digestion. The kidneys also produce between 1 and 2 litres of urine a day. Microscopic droplets of this waste-laden fluid continuously feed into a tiny reservoir called the ureter in the centre of each kidney. Its exit, the urethra, reaches an opening in the front of the vagina in women and the tip of the penis in men. In women the urethra is shorter, which is why they are more susceptible to invasion by bacteria, resulting in problems such as cystitis.

Of course, serious kidney and urinary disorders are way beyond the scope of home treatment. However, there is much you can do to maintain the healthy functioning of your kidneys and urinary tract, and thus prevent the development of serious disorders. As well as putting into practice the basics of a healthy diet and lifestyle, kidneys need to be flushed out. It is important to drink 3–4 litres of fluid a day, but not entirely in the form of tea, coffee and alcohol. Try to include at least half a litre of plain water, preferably bottled or spring. Above all, never ignore the pressing demands of a full bladder. If urine is retained for too long, it is susceptible to chemical change which in turn can lead to infection.

With a few reservations, the only urinary infection which can be treated at home is cystitis. This is why it is the only condition for which a suggested treatment strategy is given. Although cystitis mostly occurs in women, men are by no means immune. Those who have undergone surgery involving the urethra or who suffer from an enlarged prostate gland are more likely to suffer.

URINARY INFECTION

If stress is contributing to frequent attacks of cystitis, the flower essences suggested for Stress and Anxiety are worth considering (pages 119 and 124). Apart from herbs and essential oils, one of the finest remedies for cystitis is cranberry juice (available from health food stores). It works by alkalising infected urine, thus helping to reduce its scalding effect. Take one wineglassful three times daily.

CYSTITIS

SUGGESTED ESSENTIAL OILS
Bergamot, cedarwood, chamomile (German and Roman), eucalyptus, frankincense, juniper, lavender, pine, sandalwood, tea tree

Methods of Use
Warm compress over lower back, bath. As a preventative measure, regular aromatherapy massage (paying particular attention to lower back)

SUGGESTED HERBAL REMEDIES
Chamomile, dandelion, eucalyptus (leaves), meadowsweet, nasturtium, pine needle

Botanic Prescription
Infusion: equal parts pine needles and eucalyptus leaves

FURTHER ADVICE
Symptoms are burning pains when passing urine, as well as pain in the groin before, during and just after urination. Commonly, it is related to bacterial infection, though paint fumes and industrial chemicals may initiate an attack, as can stress. Food intolerances may also be implicated. Prolonged sexual activity can sometimes trigger the problem. As a preventative, drink a glass of water immediately after sex and empty the bladder as soon as possible. As well as herbal remedies, flush out your kidneys by drinking copious amounts of warm water. If you are prone to cystitis, seek the advice of a holistic health practitioner.

CAUTION

If there is blood or pus in the urine, seek urgent medical attention.

THE FEMALE REPRODUCTIVE SYSTEM

Essential oils and herbs are especially helpful for easing problems associated with the female life-cycle. But before exploring treatment strategies, it would seem appropriate to begin this section with some startling information that no woman can afford to ignore.

In her book *Passage To Power – Natural Menopause Revolution*, leading health writer Leslie Kenton draws our attention to the devastating effects of xenoestrogens (oestrogen-mimicking chemicals) which have come to pollute our environment. Xenoestrogens are petroleum by-products used in the manufacture of plastics, electronic components, agrochemicals and many other industrial products. Gradually, over the years, we may accumulate these fat-soluble chemicals in the fat of our own bodies, which results in oestrogen dominance. This manifests as oestrogen or oestrogen-like chemicals in the presence of a relative insufficiency of progesterone in a woman's body.

Because progesterone is a precursor to many other steroid hormones, when the body's production of it is over-ruled by oestrogen other hormones are not produced adequately either. The absence of these steroids can result in problems such as weight gain, headaches, bad temper, chronic fatigue and loss of libido – all of which are part of the clinically recognised premenstrual syndrome or PMS. Oestrogen dominance can also result in irregular periods, low fertility, high blood pressure, endometriosis, cancer of the womb, fibrocystic breast disease, breast cancer, increased risk of stroke and heart disease – even osteoporosis (brittle bone disease), a condition normally attributed to *decreased* oestrogen levels after menopause. There is also strong evidence to suggest that environmental xenoestrogens are to blame for the increase in male osteoporosis, birth defects, prostate cancer and infertility.

'One of the greatest ironies at the turn of the millennium,' writes Kenton, 'is that women have been encouraged to use oestrogens. They have been sold both as a means of birth control and for counteracting the negative symptoms of menopause. Yet it turns out that excessive oestrogen may well be the greatest enemy any woman in the industrialised world ever faces.' Much of her book is therefore devoted to the use of 'natural' progesterone synthesised from the Mexican wild yam.

However, we should not lose sight of the fact that yam-derived progesterone (usually marketed in the form of a cream for rubbing into the skin), has been put through a number of chemical processes, resulting in a substance supposedly identical to that produced in the body. In view of what we have already learned about 'nature identical' drugs (see Chapter 2), this is an erroneous assumption. Indeed, according to Lynn McTaggart, editor of *What Doctors Don't Tell You* (February 1996, Vol. 6, No. 11), one manufacturer of natural rub-on progesterone states that the cream may cause 'spotting' in between periods and may even increase thyroid activity. This is surely indicative of a drug with potential side-effects.

Of particular interest to women, just as medicine now recognises that there are both beneficial and harmful cholesterol in relation to protecting the body from heart disease, so there are 'good' oestrogens and 'bad' oestrogens. Oestrogen-like compounds in certain foods and medicinal herbs actually help to protect women against cancer of the breast and reproductive system by binding with oestrogen receptor sites so that xenoestrogens are not so readily taken up. They also help to alleviate menopausal hot flushes, PMS, heavy or painful periods, and many other illnesses associated with the female reproductive system.

According to Herman Aldercreutz, nutritional chemist at the University of Helsinki, and others, the best protective oestrogenic foodstuffs are tofu (soya bean curd), miso (fermented soya paste), rye bread, green lentils, pomegranates and French beans. Other foods with hormone-balancing properties are sprouted seeds and grains (especially alfalfa), celery, yam, papaya, bananas, figs, dates, apples, grapes, cherries, citrus fruits, avocado, fennel, anise, liquorice, seaweed, garlic, beetroots, potatoes, parsley and raw unheated honey.

Of the medicinal herbs, hops and sage are especially rich in phyto-oestrogens (*phyto* means plant); whereas Oriental ginseng contains hormone-like saponins which encourage the body to produce the quantities of oestrogen and progesterone it needs. The Mediterranean herb chaste tree is highly beneficial for women, especially during menopause. It contains glycosides, flavonoids and micronutrients which act in concert to stimulate the synthesis of progesterone – although it also appears to have a regulatory effect on oestrogen.

But what about essential oils? It is not clear whether the essential oils of plants like hops, fennel and sage contain the same phyto-oestrogens found in the raw plant material. As far as I am aware, there have been no official studies on the subject. However, since phyto-sterols are fat-soluble, they may well be present in the distilled oil. Certainly, empirical evidence amongst aromatherapists and their clients confirms the efficacy of these and other hormone-balancing essences.

Then there is the question of HRT. While it would be wrong to rule out HRT completely, far fewer women than the proponents of the drug would have us believe actually need medication to control their body chemistry. Despite tireless campaigns by doctors and drug companies, half of all women prescribed HRT stop within six months, according to a recent survey by National Opinion Polls. So the 'feel good' drug is not living up to its expectations. Although women used to be given oestrogen-only versions of HRT, this was found to increase by twenty-fold the risk of endometrial cancer. To counteract this, women who still have a womb are now given the additional artificial hormone progestogen, which is supposed to mimic naturally occurring progesterone.

Some of the reported side-effects of progestogens (*Physicians Desk Reference*, 1995) include breast tenderness, fluid retention, skin rashes, anaphylasix (severe allergic reactions requiring life-saving shots of adrenalin), depression, nausea, insomnia and blood clots in the veins. When taken with oestrogens, the side-effects may include raised blood pressure, headaches, dizziness, nervousness, fatigue, increased body hair and thinning scalp hair, a cystitis-like syndrome, itchy skin and PMS-like symptoms.

As if these symptoms were not bad enough, despite claims that oestrogen/progestogen combined formulas of HRT are protective against breast cancer and cardiovascular disease, in fact the opposite is true (*Lancet* 1991: 338: 274–7). It may be true that combined formulas of HRT offer some protection against osteoporosis, but only when taken for upwards of seven years – far longer than most women stay on the drug. As soon as it is discontinued, bone mineral density declines rapidly, and other menopausal symptoms like hot flushes and night sweats may return with a vengeance (*New England Journal of Medicine*, 14 October 1993).

Since experts cannot agree about the safety of HRT (whether derived from natural sources or completely synthetic), my own approach is to advocate a life-enhancing programme combining excellent nutrition, weight-bearing exercise (allowing the body to bear its own weight) such as walking to help develop strong bones, and, if necessary, a combination of herbal remedies, flower essences and aromatherapy.

In so doing, even women who have undergone hysterectomy have found that they can live healthily without hormone supplementation. But should natural methods fail to control deeply distressing symptoms – which may occur in women who have undergone radical hysterectomy involving removal of the ovaries – then HRT may well be the only answer.

WOMEN'S HEALTH

When choosing flower essences, consider those recommended for Anxiety and Stress (see pages 119 and 124). An extremely helpful flower remedy for women going through menopause is Walnut, for it helps engender a positive acceptance of change. For PMS consider remedies such as Chamomile, Impatiens, Lavender, Olive, Scleranthus and Mustard.

AMENORRHOEA (MISSED, SCANTY OR IRREGULAR PERIODS)

SUGGESTED ESSENTIAL OILS
Clary sage, hops, juniper berry, marjoram, rose otto

Methods of Use
Bath, massage (especially to lower back and abdomen), warm compress (abdomen). Supplementary methods: vaporiser, dry inhalation (drops on a handkerchief)

Aromatic Prescription
Bath/massage/compress: 4 drops clary sage, 1 drop rose otto, 2 drops juniper berry

SUGGESTED HERBS
Calendula, chaste tree, hops, rose petal, sage

Botanic Prescription
1. Infusion of rose petals (or calendula or sage). Add 15 drops chaste tree tincture per teacup
2. Infusion: equal parts calendula and rose petals. Add 15 drops hops tincture per teacup

FURTHER ADVICE
Barring pregnancy or menopause, the condition may be caused by prolonged stress, emotional shock or excitement, long-distance air travel, obesity, anorexia nervosa, excessive exercise or hormonal fluctuation (e.g. discontinuing the pill, breastfeeding). It sometimes indicates a serious underlying health problem. Attention to diet and lifestyle is essential. If there is no improvement after a few months of self-treatment, especially if you are trying to conceive, do have a medical check up.

DYSMENORRHOEA (PAINFUL PERIODS)

SUGGESTED ESSENTIAL OILS
Angelica, calendula, chamomile (German and Roman), clary sage, frankincense, hops, juniper berry, lavender, marjoram, melissa (true), rose otto, rosemary

Methods of Use
Bath, warm compress (abdomen), massage (feather-light stroking downwards over abdomen to alleviate pain and congestion); regular full body massage as a preventative

Aromatic Prescriptions
During period (bath/compress): 4 drops marjoram, 2 drops lavender
Preventative (massage): 2 drops frankincense, 2 drops clary sage, 1 drop rose otto or 2 drops rosemary

SUGGESTED HERBS
Angelica, calendula, chamomile, chaste tree, hops, lemon balm, marjoram, rose petal, St John's wort, valerian

Botanic Prescription
Infusion: equal parts lemon balm and marjoram. Add 10 drops valerian tincture or St John's wort tincture per teacup

FURTHER ADVICE
Severe pain may be symptomatic of a gynaecological disorder. If there is no improvement after three months of self-treatment, do seek medical advice, perhaps followed up with constitutional treatment under the guidance of a medical herbalist or homeopath.

MENOPAUSAL SYMPTOMS

SUGGESTED ESSENTIAL OILS

For hot flushes and night sweats: clary sage

General (balancing to mind and body): bergamot, chamomile (Roman), clary sage, frankincense, geranium, lavender, melissa (true), neroli, rose otto, sandalwood, ylang ylang

Methods of Use

Hot flushes and night sweats: bath, massage

General: bath, massage, vaporiser, personal perfume

Aromatic Prescription

Bath/massage/vaporiser: 1 drop rose otto or 2 drops geranium, 2 drops frankincense, 3 drops clary sage

SUGGESTED HERBS

Specific for hot flushes, night sweats: sage. Menstrual flooding: chaste tree, sage. Hormone-balancers: calendula, chaste tree, evening primrose oil (see Further Advice), ginseng, hops. For vaginal dryness: chaste tree. Anti-depressants: lemon balm, oats, rose petal, St John's wort

Botanic Prescriptions

1. Infusion of sage. Add 15 drops chaste tree tincture per teacup
2. Infusion: equal parts hops and lemon balm. Add 15 drops ginseng tincture per teacup

FURTHER ADVICE

Take steps to reduce stress. To help prevent the development of osteoporosis, take adequate weight-bearing exercise such as walking. Eat plenty of hormone-balancing foods (see pages 146–7). Evening primrose oil is highly beneficial: it helps turn essential fatty acids into prostaglandins, which help balance hormones naturally. Take 2 × 500 mg evening primrose oil daily. Where oestrogen deficiency really is a problem (i.e. after hysterectomy), you may benefit from a herbal 'HRT' formula (see Useful Addresses on page 264).

MENORRHAGIA (HEAVY PERIODS)

SUGGESTED ESSENTIAL OILS

Chamomile (German and Roman), geranium, lemon, rose otto. Also, jasmine absolute as a supplementary treatment (see Methods of Use)

Methods of Use

Bath, massage (gentle massage into abdomen and lower back). Jasmine absolute (to supplement massage and aromatic baths with other oils): personal perfume, dry inhalation (drops on handkerchief)

Aromatic Prescription

Bath/massage: 2 drops Roman Chamomile, 2 drop geranium, 3 drops lemon

SUGGESTED HERBS

Agrimony, lemon (peel), oak (bark), rose petal, sage, sweet chestnut (leaves), walnut (catkins)

Botanic Prescription

1. Infusion of sage mixed 50/50 with decoction of lemon peel (organic)
2. Decoction of oak bark
3. Infusion: 2 parts agrimony, 2 parts rose petal

FURTHER ADVICE

Heavy periods may be symptomatic of menopause, or possibly fibroids, polyps or a more serious disorder such as endometriosis. If the problem continues for more than a few cycles seek medical advice, perhaps followed up with holistic treatment from a medical herbalist or homeopath.

MILK FLOW (TO PROMOTE)

SUGGESTED ESSENTIAL OILS
Fennel (sweet), lemongrass (not profiled in the Directory of Healing Plants)

Methods of Use
Breast massage, warm compress

SUGGESTED HERBS
Basil, chaste tree, nettle, vervain

Botanic Prescription
Infusion: equal parts basil and nettle

FURTHER SUGGESTIONS
Try to reduce stress and improve your diet. Drink plenty of bottled water. Start breastfeeding as soon as possible after birth to stimulate milk production. Wash off all traces of essential oil prior to feeding. Seek the advice of your midwife as well.

MILK FLOW (TO DECREASE)

SUGGESTED ESSENTIAL OILS
Peppermint. Essential oil of sage will also decrease milk production, but is not recommended for home use (see Cautions, page 202). Supplementary measure: jasmine absolute (see Methods of Use)

Methods of Use
Cold (or tepid) compress, massage oil (apply 2–3 times daily, but do not actually massage the breasts as this may stimulate flow). Jasmine absolute (to supplement peppermint compresses/massage oil): personal perfume, dry inhalation (drops on a handkerchief)

SUGGESTED HERBS
Sage

Botanic Prescription
Infusion of sage. Take 3–4 times daily until desired result is achieved

FURTHER ADVICE
It may be necessary to reduce fluid intake, but seek the advice of your midwife first.

PMS (PREMENSTRUAL SYNDROME)

SUGGESTED ESSENTIAL OILS
Chamomile (German and Roman), citrus essences, clary sage, geranium, hops (but not if depressed), frankincense, juniper berry, lavender, marjoram, melissa (true), neroli, rose otto, sandalwood, ylang ylang

Methods of Use
Baths, massage (preferably full body, otherwise head, neck, shoulders or just back), vaporiser, dry inhalation (drops on handkerchief), personal perfume

Aromatic Prescription
Bath/massage/vaporiser: 2 drops Roman chamomile, 1 drop rose otto or 2 drops geranium, 3 drops clary sage

SUGGESTED HERBS
Diuretic: dandelion root. Hormone balancers: calendula, chaste tree, evening primrose oil (capsules). For anxiety and nervous tension: chamomile, hops, oats, vervain (see also page 209). Anti-depressants: ginseng, lemon balm, St John's wort (see also page 172)

Botanic Prescriptions
1. Decoction of dandelion root. Add 10 drops chaste tree tincture per teacup
2. Infusion: equal parts calendula and lemon balm. Add 10 drops St John's wort tincture per teacup

FURTHER SUGGESTIONS
The symptoms of PMS may include fluid retention, breast tenderness, headaches, nausea, anxiety, depression, irritability, sleep disturbances, food cravings and more. Try to reduce stress and ensure that you take adequate outdoor exercise. A professional aromatherapy massage now and again will help to balance the nervous system, and thus reduce or alleviate many symptoms. Take 4 × 500 mg evening primrose oil capsules daily. Include plenty of hormone-balancing foods in your diet (see pages 146–7). Snack on these throughout the day in order to stabilise blood sugar levels and balance mood.

PREGNANCY SICKNESS ('MORNING SICKNESS')

SUGGESTED ESSENTIAL OILS
Ginger, lavender, peppermint

Methods of Use
Vaporiser, dry inhalation (drops on handkerchief)

SUGGESTED HERBS
Chamomile, meadowsweet, peppermint. Also crystallised stem ginger (see Further Advice)

FURTHER ADVICE
Nausea or vomiting are common in the first few months. Although it is most frequent in the morning when the stomach is empty, it can happen at other times until the body has adjusted to the massive hormone changes. Low blood sugar and possibly low blood pressure may also be implicated. Before getting up, eat an arrowroot biscuit or a piece of unbuttered wholemeal toast, perhaps spread with a little ginger conserve. It is best to avoid medication in pregnancy, though the gentle remedies here can be used if necessary. Inhalation of a single recommended essential oil (according to aroma preference) can settle the stomach. Infusions of nervine herbs (one suggested herb at a time according to taste) can also be taken. Or chew a little crystallised stem ginger if liked.

CAUTION

Do not apply essential oils to the skin during the first trimester of pregnancy. The recommended oils are for inhalation only

SORE OR CRACKED NIPPLES

SUGGESTED ESSENTIAL OILS
Chamomile (German and Roman), rose otto

Method of Use
Massage, ointment (see Aromatic Prescription)

Aromatic Prescription
30g unperfumed base cream, 6 drops German chamomile. Stir in the oil and apply to nipples after each feed

SUGGESTED HERBS
Calendula and St John's wort ointment (see Botanic Recipe Prescription under Cold Sores, page 127)

FURTHER ADVICE
This problem is common in the first weeks before the nipples have 'hardened' to the effects of continual sucking. To allow time for healing, wear nipple shields (from pharmacies). These will enable the baby to suck without causing you discomfort. Wash off all traces of cream or ointment before each feed.

VAGINAL THRUSH (CANDIDA)

SUGGESTED ESSENTIAL OILS
Lavender, tea tree
Internally: garlic capsules

Methods of Use
Bath, sitz bath (add 4 drops essential oil to a bowl of warm water and sit for 5–10 minutes)

SUGGESTED HERBS
Bath, sitz bath: agrimony, calendula, lavender, oak (decoction of bark), walnut (decoction of fresh leaves)
Internally: calendula, echinacea, rosemary, sage

Botanic Prescriptions
Internally:
1. Infusion of calendula. Add 10 drops echinacea tincture per teacup
2. Infusion: equal parts sage and rosemary

FURTHER ADVICE
Thrush is a fungal infection producing a thick white discharge accompanied by intense itching. Antibiotics are often implicated: they destroy helpful colonies of bacteria and encourage resident thrush colonies to multiply. Other possible causes are the pill, high sugar/high yeast diet, sexual contact with an infected partner (men carry candida but do not always show symptoms) and synthetic fibres (especially tights). Drastically reduce sugar, yeast and alcohol consumption. Take lactobacillus acidophilis tablets (yoghurt culture), which are available from health food stores to restore normal intestinal flora. If symptoms persist, seek the advice of a holistic nutritionist and/or medical herbalist.

NATURAL FIRST AID

The following chart will help you to select essential oils and herbal preparations for minor burns, cuts and abrasions, insect stings, sprains and strains. Serious burns and wounds, however, need urgent medical attention. Indeed, orthodox medicine is extremely good at treating such injuries. But how can we tell when a burn or wound warrants medical attention?

If a wound or sting becomes infected, with yellow or green pus accompanied by much swelling and pain, antibiotic drugs may be essential. Superficial or first-degree burns and scalds can be treated at home for they involve only the outer skin layer. They are marked by redness, warmth and tenderness, sometimes blistering.

Second-degree burns are characterised by blistering, pain and swelling. The burn may also be weepy. Third-degree burns are characterised by immediate lack of pain (because the nerve endings have been destroyed), whiteness and/or charring. Home treatment in either situation should be limited to applying a clean dry dressing, then seek urgent medical attention. Never in any circumstances attempt to burst blisters or peel damaged skin as this will only encourage infection.

ADDITIONS TO THE FIRST AID KIT

As well as the basic equipment common to any first aid kit, such as sterile dressings, waterproof plasters, scissors, bandage, tweezers and so on, it is prudent to include a bottle of Bach Rescue Remedy. Calendula ointment (with or without the addition of St John's wort) is also highly recommended. Both versions are widely available from chemists and health food stores, or you could make your own (see page 127).

The best (and least expensive) essential oils for first aid treatments are lavender and tea tree. As an alternative to tea tree, you may prefer eucalyptus oil. You will also need some bicarbonate of soda for treating bee and ant stings, and cider vinegar for treating sunburn, wasp stings, mosquito and horsefly bites.

Although not featured in the Directory of Healing Plants, distilled witch-hazel is another wonderful remedy for the natural first aid kit, valued for its astringent and blood-clotting properties. It can be applied to minor burns, cuts, sprains and bruises.

Therapeutic Charts for Natural First Aid follows on page 154

FIRST AID

For external first aid applications, where herbal tinctures and aromatic compresses are suggested in the following charts use twice the usual recommended quantities given in Chapter 6.

BURNS AND SCALDS (MINOR)

SUGGESTED ESSENTIAL OILS
Eucalyptus, geranium, frankincense, lavender, tea tree

Methods of Use for Oils and Herbs
Cool by plunging into cold water, or spray with a cold shower, or keep under running cold water, for 10 minutes. If a chemical burn, remove any splashed clothing and flush the affected area with running water. Then apply neat essential oil, or calendula ointment, or infused oil of St John's wort, or witch-hazel. Larger burns and scalds can be treated with cold aromatic compresses (or a cold compress containing diluted calendula tincture)

SUGGESTED HERBS
Infused oil of St John's wort, distilled witch-hazel, calendula ointment, calendula tincture

FURTHER ADVICE
Never apply ointments or vegetable oils, including essential oils diluted in vegetable oil, without first cooling the skin with plenty of water. Fatty substances will 'fry' on hot skin, increasing the possibility of infection.

IMPORTANT

Serious burns need urgent medical attention.

CUTS AND GRAZES

SUGGESTED ESSENTIAL OILS
Eucalyptus, frankincense, lavender, lemon, pine, tea tree

Methods of Use for Oils and Herbs
First clean by swabbing with wet cotton wool or holding the injured part under running water. Apply neat lavender or tea tree, or an aromatic antiseptic ointment (see page 97). For larger wounds, apply cold aromatic compresses (or a cold compress containing tincture of calendula or St John's wort). Cover with a bandage or plaster if necessary.

SUGGESTED HERBS
Diluted tincture of calendula, distilled witch-hazel. If the cut is quite deep, use diluted tincture of St John's wort

FURTHER ADVICE
If soil particles are clinging to the wound, remove with spotlessly clean tweezers (wipe tweezers first with neat essential oil)

IMPORTANT

If there is any risk of infection such as tetanus, seek urgent medical attention.

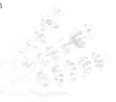

INSECT BITES AND STINGS

SUGGESTED ESSENTIAL

Eucalyptus, lavender, tea tree
Insect repellent: cedarwood, eucalyptus, lavender, patchouli, rosemary, tea tree

Methods of Use for Oils and Herbs

Bee stings: hold tweezers as near to the skin as possible (avoiding venom sac), grasp stinger and remove it. To neutralise the acidic venom, apply bicarbonate of soda (an alkali) made into a paste with a little water. Bicarbonate of soda also neutralises acidic ant venom
Wasp stings: wasp venom is alkaline, so an acidic remedy is necessary. Dab with cider vinegar or lemon juice (also for mosquito and horsefly bites).
Most other insect bites and stings: can be treated with neat essential oil, diluted herbal tincture or herbal ointment.

SUGGESTED HERBS

Calendula and/or St John's wort tincture, calendula and/or St John's wort ointment

FURTHER ADVICE

Bee and wasp stings: after the initial vinegar or bicarb treatment apply neat essential oil, herbal ointment or diluted herbal tincture, any of which will help prevent infection. To repel insects: apply a massage oil containing a 3 per cent concentration of suitable essential oil. For the home or workplace, the same oil(s) can be used in the vaporiser.

IMPORTANT

Bee and wasp stings affect some people seriously. If this is the case, summon urgent medical attention.

SPRAINS AND BRUISES

SUGGESTED ESSENTIAL OILS

Chamomile (German and Roman), eucalyptus, geranium, lavender, marjoram, pine, rosemary

Methods of Use for Oils and Herbs

For sprains and bruises: start with a cold or icy aromatic or herbal compress (witch-hazel is excellent), then apply an aromatic or herbal ointment
For sprains: after the compress, apply gentle massage above towards the heart and below the injury (not directly on it) to drain off excess fluids. Then apply an aromatic or herbal ointment.

SUGGESTED HERBS

Calendula (tincture or ointment), elder (decoction of leaves), distilled witch-hazel

FURTHER ADVICE

A sprain occurs at a joint such as a wrist or ankle when the ligaments and tissues around the joint are suddenly wrenched or torn. Symptoms are pain and tenderness around the joint, often followed by swelling and bruising. Rest the injured part and raise it to prevent accumulation of excess fluids (support with cushions or pillows).

STRAIN (MUSCULAR)

SUGGESTED ESSENTIAL OILS
As for Sprains and Bruises

Methods of Use
Begin with a cold or tepid essential oil compress. Once the swelling has subsided take a hot aromatic bath (up to 8 drops essential oil and 4 tablespoons sea salt), followed by massage with an infused oil or an aromatherapy blend.

SUGGESTED HERBS
Infused oil of calendula, or a 50/50 blend of infused oil of calendula and St John's wort

FURTHER ADVICE
A strain occurs when a muscle or group of muscles is overstretched and possibly torn by violent or sudden movement, for example back strain as a result of heavy lifting.

Rest is essential. If you have strained the muscle of an arm or leg, raise the injured part above the level of your heart to prevent the accumulation of excess fluids (support with cushions or pillows).

SUNBURN

SUGGESTED ESSENTIAL OILS
Chamomile (German and Roman), geranium, lavender, rosemary, tea tree

Methods of Use for Oils and Herbs
Take 2–3 cool (preferably cold) aromatic baths throughout the day, adding up to 8 tablespoons cider vinegar and 8 drops essential oil.

Afterwards, pat the skin dry and apply an appropriate aromatherapy massage oil, or infused oil of calendula, or calendula ointment. For very sore patches it is less painful to use oil than ointment: paint it on with a small, soft bristle brush. Aloe vera juice (from health food shops) will prevent sunburnt skin from peeling. It also takes out the heat and sting, stops blistering and converts minor sunburn into a tan. Put some into a cosmetic spray bottle and mist the skin several times daily.

SUGGESTED HERBS
Calendula: infused oil, ointment. Also aloe vera juice

PART THREE

DIRECTORY OF HEALING PLANTS

Agrimony: It is an herb under the sign of Jupiter. ... The decoction of the herb made with wine is good against the biting and stinging of serpents. ...

Beech Tree: It is a plant of Saturn. ... The water found on the hollow places of decaying beeches will cure both man and beast of any scurf, scab or running tetters, if they be washed therewith. . . .

Violets: They are a fine pleasing plant of Venus. ... The green leaves are used with other herbs for inflammations and swellings ... and for the piles also, being fried with yolks of eggs and applied thereto. ...

NICHOLAS CULPEPER,
The English Physician, or Herball, 1653

CHAPTER NINE

INTRODUCTION TO THE DIRECTORY

THE DIRECTORY IS DIVIDED into two parts: Major and Minor. The first is a repertory of plants which are commonly employed in at least two systems of botanic medicine, such as herbalism and aromatherapy. The second is a slightly abbreviated version featuring a number of plants which may be extensively employed in one area of healing, but which play a lesser or non-existent role in other systems.

The plants are arranged in alphabetical order according to their Latin or botanical names. This is because the common names of plants differ from one region to another whereas the botanical names are recognised throughout the world.

Each profile includes a botanical description to aid identification. Where botanical terms such as *achene* and *lanceolate* are used, their meanings are given in the Glossary of Botanical Terms on pages 254–5.

The Principal Constituents section may be of no more than passing interest to many people, though it may prove useful to students of botanic medicine and others with an interest in biochemistry or pharmacognosy. Far more information is available for some plants than for others: this reflects the amount of research carried out and not necessarily the importance of the plant.

The main uses in herbalism, aromatherapy, flower therapy and homeopathy are described where applicable. Where medical terms such as *antispasmodic* and *vulnerary* are used, their meanings are given in the Glossary of Medical Terms on pages 256–8.

The Major Directory includes three additional sections: History, Culinary Uses, and Cultivation and Collection. The historical note gives the origin of the botanical and common names (if known), along with certain mythological or folklore associations. The other two categories are self-explanatory, though readers are assumed to have a basic knowledge of cookery and gardening. However, detailed advice on collecting, drying and preparing your own herbal remedies can be found in Chapter 6.

Any precautions to be observed in relation to the use of a particular essential oil or herb are given in the CAUTIONS note at the end of the relevant plant profile.

Illustrations for all the plants profiled can be found in Chapter 10 with the exception of one or two which have very restricted uses.

A WORD ABOUT HOMEOPATHY

Homeopathic uses are given simply to illustrate the plant's multifaceted potential. It is beyond the scope of this book to delve into the complexities of

---

CAUTION

If you are unsure about the identity of a potential culinary or medicinal herb, it is essential to seek the advice of a knowledgeable person.

---

practical homeopathy (which also includes substances of animal and mineral origin). If you wish to use homeopathic medicine it is advisable to consulta fully accredited practitioner who will tailor the treatment to your own specific needs. This is very important, for there are hazards with self-prescribing.

Even though homeopathic medicines are pharmacologically inactive (and therefore non-toxic), unlike flower essences they can be alarming in their action. For example, overuse or misuse of a remedy may result in an exacerbation of the very symptoms for which it is being prescribed – a phenomenon known as 'proving'. Moreover, when dealing with a chronic complaint it is not unusual for completely different physical and emotional symptoms to arise, possibly stemming from years of suppressive allopathic (conventional) treatments.

The skill of the homeopath lies in his or her ability to ensure that the correct potency (and frequency of use) is prescribed for the individual concerned, thus greatly reducing the possibility of sudden and severe reactions. If the latter sounds unlikely, consider the words of the renowned homeopath James Tyler Kent (1826–1916), 'I would rather share a room with a nest of vipers than be subjected to the administrations of an inexperienced homeopath!'

> For advice on preparing and administering herbs, essential oils and flower remedies, see Chapter 6.

CHAPTER TEN

MAJOR DIRECTORY

❀ ❀ ❀

CONTENTS

The plants in this directory are organised alphabetically by their Latin, or botanical name. For ease of reference, common names for plants are referred to in the index and below.

AESCULUS HIPPOCASTANUM
CHESTNUT, HORSE

Family: Hippocastanaceae (Horse Chestnut Family) **Synonyms:** *Hippocastanum vulgare*, White Chestnut
Parts Used: bark, fully ripe chestnuts. Two Bach flower essences are prepared from the same tree: White Chestnut
(flowers), Chestnut Bud (buds and twigs)

DESCRIPTION AND HABITAT
(See illustration, page 177)
A tall deciduous tree reaching up to 30m, with a broad, dense crown and smooth, later grey-brown and scaly, bark. The sticky, brown buds open into large palmate leaves with five to seven leaflets. On the smaller branches are curious horseshoe markings, the scars of the previous year's leaf-stalks. The flowers are white, blotched red at the base, and borne in dense, erect panicles. The fruits are round, green and prickly, splitting in late autumn to release one or two hard, shiny brown 'conkers'. The tree is a native of northern Greece and Albania, and has long been cultivated in other parts of the world for its ornamental value. Wild trees are found in damp mountain woodland; naturalised trees can often be found growing on waste ground and in copses.

HISTORY
The tree's generic name *Aesculus* derives from the Latin word *esca*, meaning food. *Hippocastanum* is simply the Latin word for horse chestnut. The origin of the name may well be the horseshoe markings on the smaller branches. In Turkey horse chestnuts were formerly fed to horses and cattle suffering from coughs.

PRINCIPAL CONSTITUENTS
The seeds (horse chestnuts): saponins, tannin, flavones, starch, fatty oil and the glycocides aesculin and fraxin. The bark contains no saponins and is higher in tannins.

HERBAL MEDICINE
Horse chestnut has astringent, fever-reducing and anti-thrombotic properties. An infusion of dried chestnuts aids the treatment of phlebitis (inflammation in the veins), varicose veins and haemorrhoids. Herbalists also prescribe the remedy for enlargement of the prostate gland. Externally, decoctions of the bark or fruit may be used as a lotion (or incorporated into an ointment) for the same conditions, and also for leg ulcers, cuts and grazes, ringworm and sunburn.

FLOWER THERAPY
The flower remedy Chestnut Bud is prepared from the sticky leaf buds. Collect the buds and short twigs during spring and potentise using the Boiling Method. The remedy is for those who never seem to learn from past experiences (see page 68). For the White Chestnut flower remedy, collect the blooms in early summer and potentise using the Sun Method. This remedy is indicated for persistent worrying thoughts and mental arguments (see page 73).

HOMEOPATHY
The homeopathic remedy mirrors its herbal uses. It is also indicated for constipation combined with a feeling of prolapse in the rectum.

CULTIVATION AND COLLECTION
The trees can be propagated from seed, but they take a long time to develop. Young trees can be obtained from tree and shrub specialists. Plant during the autumn in any fertile soil in a partially shaded position. The tree requires a great deal of space! The chestnuts are gathered as they fall from the trees during late autumn. The bark is collected in the spring. Dry the bark or fruit in the sun, or employ slight artificial heat.

ANGELICA ARCHANGELICA

ANGELICA

Family: Umbelliferae/Apiaceae (Carrot Family) **Synonym:** *Angelica officinalis*
Parts Used: essential oil, flowers (flower therapy), leaves, roots, seeds, stems

DESCRIPTION AND HABITAT
(See illustration, page 177)
A tall, robust aromatic herb growing up to 3m tall with a dark, turnip-like rhizome, stout roots and large, serrated leaves. If prevented from flowering it is a short-lived perennial, but if allowed to bloom it is biennial. In the second year it develops a thick, furrowed, hollow stem. The greenish flowers are in large umbels, the fruit ('seed') pale yellow, oval, flattened and ribbed. All parts of the plant emit a musky aroma. Native to Syria, it has spread throughout Europe along rivers and other moist places.

HISTORY
The name 'angelica' derives from the Greek *angelos*, a heavenly messenger. The plant was believed to impart divine protection from witches and demonic possession.

PRINCIPAL CONSTITUENTS
Essential oil (including phellandrene, pinene, limonene, linalool etc.), tannins, bitters, angelica acid, furocoumarins, resin, starch, sugar.

HERBAL MEDICINE
The plant is a circulatory stimulant, expectorant and digestive. Decoctions of crushed seed or root restore appetite after prolonged illness, help flatulence, respiratory ailments, cystitis, migraine, painful periods, absence of periods outside pregnancy and are reputedly helpful for the recovering alcoholic. The aroma of the crushed leaves may alleviate travel sickness.

AROMATHERAPY
The oil is captured by steam distillation of the roots or seed; the latter is safest for home use (see Cautions). It has the viscosity of alcohol and is virtually colourless. The aroma is earthy-herbaceous with a piquant top note. Its odour effect is warming and stimulating; a reputed aphrodisiac. If used in excess the aroma is soporific. Angelica is helpful for rheumatic aches and pains, menstrual cramp, respiratory disorders, indigestion, fatigue, migraine and stress-related disorders. It blends well with citrus essences, clary sage and patchouli.

FLOWER THERAPY
Collect the blooms in late summer and potentise using the Sun Method. Use for promoting a sense of protection and inner guidance at times of immense difficulty, especially bereavement.

HOMEOPATH
Homeopathic doses of angelica are said to help the recovering alcoholic.

CULINARY USES
Stalks can be candied for use in cakes. Leaf shoots can be added to salads, the stems and roots steamed as vegetables – or cooked with rhubarb and apples, and the seeds used to flavour bread and pastries. The essential oil is used in some gins and vermouths.

CULTIVATION AND COLLECTION
Sow freshly ripened seed in rich, damp soil in early spring in a part-shaded site. Dig up the roots in their first autumn and before they become woody; dry using gentle heat. Collect the leaves in early summer, before flowering. Gather newly ripened seed in late summer.

CAUTION

Harvest only cultivated plants or purchase from a reputable supplier, for it can be confused with poisonous plants of the same family. Both the herbal remedy and the essential oil can stimulate menstruation, so avoid during pregnancy. Never apply essential oil of angelica root (seed is fine) to skin before exposure to natural or simulated sunlight, as it can cause pigmentation. The oil is highly odoriferous, so use in very low concentration. Angelica may irritate sensitive skin.

CALENDULA OFFICINALIS

CALENDULA

Family: Compositae/Asteraceae (Daisy Family) **Synonym:** Pot Marigold
Parts Used: flowers, leaves

DESCRIPTION AND HABITAT
(See illustration, page 177)
An annual aromatic herb growing to 45cm tall. The pale green leaves are lanceolate and alternate. All parts of the plant are roughly hairy. Calendula is grown for its bright orange or yellow daisy-like flowers, which bloom from early summer until late autumn. The blooms emanate a bitter-sweet aroma, unpleasant to some people. The fruit ('seed') is a rough, curved achene. Although native to southern Europe, the plant is grown in gardens everywhere.

HISTORY
The botanical name *Calendula*, a diminutive of the Latin word *Calendae* (meaning first day of the month), refers to the plant's habit of flowering all year round in its native habitat. In former times, Christians called the flower 'Marygolde' and dedicated it to the Virgin Mary. The word 'gold' refers to the aura seen around the virgin's head.

PRINCIPAL CONSTITUENTS
Essential oil, sterols, pigments (carotenoids), bitter compounds, saponins, flavonoids, mucilage, resin.

HERBAL MEDICINE
The plant has anti-inflammatory, astringent, cicatrisant, vulnerary, antifungal, cholagogic and emmenagogic properties. Infusions of the flowers can heal gastric and duodenal ulcers. The remedy is also helpful for digestive disorders, delayed periods, painful periods and menopausal distress. Externally it is used for stubborn wounds, bed sores, nappy rash, sore or cracked nipples, persistent ulcers, varicose veins, bruises, athlete's foot, ringworm and eczema, and as a mouthwash for infected gums.

AROMATHERAPY
A solvent-extracted absolute is available, though it is hard to find. Aromatherapists prefer the infused oil, which is employed primarily for its skin-healing properties. Low concentrations of appropriate essential oils are often used to enhance its healing effects. The bitter-sweet aroma is compatible with citrus essences, chamomile (German and Roman), clary sage, geranium, lavender, neroli, petitgrain, rose and ylang ylang.

FLOWER THERAPY
The flowers are gathered during high summer and potentised using the Sun Method. Helpful for those with a tendency to use cutting or sharp words, Calendula facilitates the development of empathy and compassion.

HOMEOPATHY
The tincture and ointment are applied for the same conditions as in herbal medicine. Internally, the potentised remedy is prescribed for extremely nervous individuals, particularly if there is also suppressed menstruation, nausea, chronic catarrh, unhealthy skin, eye injury or poor circulation.

CULINARY USES
The leaves and petals can be added to salads. The petals alone enhance the flavour and appearance of rice, fish and cheese dishes.

CULTIVATION AND COLLECTION
Sow the seed in a sunny position in spring. The plants will grow in any well-drained soil. Once established, they will seed themselves freely. Flowers and leaves are collected throughout the summer months. Either the flowering tops or just the petals can be collected during late summer and dried in a warm, shady place.

CAUTION

Avoid internal use of the herb in pregnancy as it may stimulate the uterus.

CHAMAEMELUM NOBILE

CHAMOMILE, ROMAN

Family: Compositae/Asteraceae (Daisy Family) **Synonyms:** *Anthemis nobilis*, Camomile
Parts Used: essential oil, flowers, leaves

DESCRIPTION AND HABITAT
(See illustration, page 177)
An almost hairless perennial herb up to 30cm tall, with mat-like trailing stems. The leaves are grey-green and finely divided into many feathery segments. The solitary flowerheads are daisy-like, with white outer petals and a yellow conical centre. The cultivated double form is the preferred variety for medicinal uses. The whole plant has a sweet, apple-like aroma. It is native to southern and western Europe, and naturalised in North America. In the wild, chamomile can be found in grassy places, particularly on sandy soil.

HISTORY
The generic name, *Chamaemelum*, derives from the Greek word *khamaimelon*, meaning 'earth apple', alluding to the plant's apple-like scent. The Ancient Egyptians used the herb in the 'House of Life' where ailing people were sent to be restored; such buildings were attached to major temples.

PRINCIPAL CONSTITUENTS
Essential oil (mainly comprising esters, pinene, fanesol, nerolidol, chamazulene, pinocarvone, cineol), mucilage, coumarin, flavone glycosides.

HERBAL MEDICINE
Chamomile has anti-inflammatory, antiseptic, carminative, sedative, stomachic and diaphoretic properties. Infusions of the herb are prescribed for feverish conditions, nausea, flatulence, painful indigestion, irritable bowel syndrome, gastric ulcers, painful menstruation, rheumatism, headaches, asthma, hayfever, anxiety and insomnia. Herbalists recommend the remedy for anxiety and sleeplessness in children, and for colicky infants. Used externally as a cooled infusion, chamomile is helpful for inflamed and sore eyes. It can also be used as a hair rinse for imparting golden highlights to light brown or fair hair.

AROMATHERAPY
The essential oil, a pale yellow liquid, is captured by steam distillation of the flowerhead. The sweet, dry aroma has an apple-like nuance with a warming, calming effect. It makes a good skin care oil suitable for most skin types and is helpful for acne, allergies, burns, eczema, inflamed skin conditions, earache, wounds, period pain, PMS, headache, insomnia, nervous tension and other stress-related disorders. It blends well with citrus oils, clary sage, lavender, geranium, neroli, rose and ylang ylang.

FLOWER THERAPY
Collect the flowerheads in late summer and potentise using the Sun Method. Chamomile is indicated for all stress-related problems, especially when accompanied by insomnia, moodiness, irritability, anger, nightmares and hypersensitivity. Although the Californian FES remedy is prepared from the related *Anthemis cotula*, from the author's experience *Chamaemelum nobile* is of equal value.

HOMEOPATHY
The preparation is potentised from the related *Chamomilla recutita* and used for the same conditions as *C. nobile* (as cited under Herbal Medicine), especially if anger, irritability and oversensitivity are present.

CULTIVATION AND COLLECTION
Chamomile can be raised from seed, though it is easier to obtain young plants from a garden centre. It needs a light, well-drained soil in full sun. Plant out in mid-spring. Gather the flowers (and young leaves if desired) in late summer and use fresh or dried.

CAUTION

The herbal remedy is generally safe for home use. The essential oil, however, must be avoided during the first trimester of pregnancy because it may stimulate menstruation. The oil is highly odoriferous, so use in the lowest recommended quantities.

CHRYSANTHEMUM PARTHENIUM

FEVERFEW

Family: Compositae/Asteraceae (Daisy Family)
Parts Used: flowers, leaves

DESCRIPTION AND HABITAT
(See illustration, page 177)
A perennial aromatic herb, bushy in habit and growing up to about 60cm. The finely divided leaves give the plant a feathery appearance. The small, daisy-like flowers have yellow centres and white ray petals and are borne in clusters from midsummer to autumn. The whole plant emits a pungent, bitter aroma disliked by bees. Feverfew is native to south-east Europe and Asia but naturalised throughout the world. It grows on waste ground, walls and roadsides and is also a common garden plant.

HISTORY
The common name is a corruption of Latin *febrifugia*, a reference to the plant's former use to reduce fever. According to Gerard, it is also 'good for such as be melancholic and pensive'. Culpeper described it as 'very effectual for all pains in the head coming of a cold cause'.

PRINCIPAL CONSTITUENTS
Sesquiterpene lactones, essential oil (containing chamomile camphor), bitter compounds, tannins, mucilage.

HERBAL MEDICINE
Feverfew is anti-inflammatory, vasodilatory, sedative, digestive and a uterine stimulant. Infusions of the flowers and leaves have proved effectual for migraine and other headaches, dizziness, asthma, catarrh, sinusitis, insomnia, arthritis and delayed, scanty or painful periods. It can also help mild depression. Externally, a strong infusion soothes swellings and open wounds.

FLOWER THERAPY
At the time of writing the remedy (prepared by the Sun Method) is being fully researched. It is proving beneficial for cyclic headaches such as those experienced during or immediately before menstruation.

HOMEOPATHY
The homeopathic remedy (*Pyrethrum parthenium*) mirrors the herbal uses but includes convulsions, twitching and delirium.

CULTIVATION AND COLLECTION
Scatter the seed over the surface of a well-prepared seed bed where the plants are to grow, and then water in. Feverfew thrives in poor soil in a sunny position, seeding itself readily in walls and between cracks in paving. The fresh leaves are collected in the summer. For drying, collect just before the flowers open between midsummer and mid-autumn.

CAUTION

Internal doses should be avoided during pregnancy as feverfew is a uterine stimulant. The fresh leaves (though not the dried herb) may cause mouth ulcers in sensitive people, but not if the herb is put between two slices of bread and eaten as a sandwich. The usual dosage for migraine sufferers is just one or two leaves daily.

CITRUS LIMON

LEMON

Family: Rutaceae (Rue Family) **Synonym:** *C. limonum*
Parts Used: essential oil, fruit, leaves, pips

DESCRIPTION AND HABITAT
(See illustration, page 178)
A small evergreen tree growing up to 5m tall, producing small, fragrant white flowers tinged with pink, followed by bright yellow fruit. The lemon is native to Asia, but has become naturalised in the Mediterranean region. It is also cultivated extensively in Italy, Cyprus, Israel, California and elsewhere.

HISTORY
The Ancient Egyptians used crushed lemon pips as an antidote to scorpion venom. The lemon therefore came to be included in mixtures to counter the effects of toxic substances including excessive doses of opium. It was also seen to protect against the ill effects of putrid meat and fish. According to the Roman writer Virgil, it is efficacious for steadying the pulse rate of 'trembling old men'.

PRINCIPAL CONSTITUENTS
Skin of the fruit: essential oil (including limonene, terpinene, pinene, myrcene, citral, linalol, geraniol, citronellal), hesperidin. Juice: citric acid (vitamin C).

HERBAL MEDICINE
As well as its anti-scurvy properties (due to high levels of vitamin C), lemon is antiseptic, diuretic, hypotensive, diaphoretic and bactericidal. Taken as a hot drink with honey, it helps feverish conditions such as colds and flu. The juice diluted in a little water makes an excellent gargle for sore throats. The fruit is helpful in acidic conditions like arthritis and rheumatism, for it becomes alkaline during digestion. The fresh juice applied externally will neutralise the poison of wasp stings. A squeeze of lemon juice can also rid shellfish of 92 per cent of their bacteria. The crushed pips mixed with honey will eliminate threadworms. Lemon is also helpful for high blood pressure and palpitations. In France, the leaves are used as a soothing, uplifting tea for stress and anxiety.

AROMATHERAPY
The oil is captured by cold expression of the peel of the fruit (a distilled oil is also available, but has an inferior aroma). The pale yellow liquid has a fresh, sharp aroma just like the fresh fruit, and the effect is uplifting and cooling. Lemon is helpful for acne, boils, chilblains, warts (applied neat), arthritis, rheumatism, high blood pressure, poor circulation, asthma, bronchitis, catarrh, colds and flu. It blends well with other citrus oils, chamomile (Roman and German), frankincense, juniper berry, lavender, neroli, petitgrain, rose, sandalwood and ylang ylang.

FLOWER THERAPY
The flowers are gathered in high summer and potentised by the Sun Method. The remedy is believed to enhance the intellect, and is therefore helpful for those engaged in study.

CULINARY USES
The fruit, juice and peel have many culinary uses, particularly in drinks, salad dressings and sauces, and as a constituent and flavouring in sweet and savoury dishes.

CULTIVATION AND COLLECTION
Although lemons can be grown under glass in northern Europe (young trees can be obtained from specialist nurseries), trees growing in their natural habitat are considered superior for medicinal purposes.

CAUTION

It is essential to obtain unwaxed, organic lemons from a health food store or good supermarket, because the ordinary kind are riddled with pesticide residues. The essential oil is phototoxic and must not be applied to skin before exposure to natural or simulated sunlight, as it may cause pigmentation. The oil has a short shelf-life and should be used within 6–9 months of purchase. It may irritate sensitive skin.

CORIANDRUM SATIVUM

CORIANDER

Family: Umbelliferae/Apiaceae (Carrot Family)
Parts Used: dried fruits ('seeds'), essential oil, flowers, fresh root

DESCRIPTION AND HABITAT
(See illustration, page 178)
A hairless aromatic annual up to 60cm tall. The slender stem bears flat, parsley-like lower leaves and finely divided upper leaves. The small flat umbels of white to pale lilac flowers appear from midsummer to early autumn, followed by the small ovoid fruits which drop as soon as they are ripe. The leaves emit a peculiarly musky scent, whereas the ripe fruits are piquant and spicy. Coriander is native to the Mediterranean region and India, but is cultivated throughout the world.

HISTORY
The generic name *Coriandrum* probably derives from the Greek *koris*, meaning 'bug', for the aroma of the fresh leaves is said to be reminiscent of the smell of bed bugs! In his treatise on herbal medicine entitled *The Art of Simpling* (1657), English herbalist William Coles tells us that the spicy aroma of crushed coriander seed enhances clarity of thought.

PRINCIPAL CONSTITUENTS
Fruits: essential oil (containing linalol, borneol, geraniol, carvone, anethole, pinene), fatty oil, tannins, pectin, sugars. Leaves: bitters, tannins, vitamin C.

HERBAL MEDICINE
The dried fruits are used by themselves (or in tea mixtures with other aromatic seeds such as caraway and fennel) primarily for indigestion, colicky pain and flatulence.

AROMATHERAPY
The essential oil is extracted by steam distillation of the crushed ripe fruits. The oil is colourless to pale yellow with the viscosity of alcohol, and possesses a spicy, faintly musky aroma. Its odour effect is warming, uplifting and mentally stimulating; a reputed aphrodisiac. It is helpful for rheumatism, muscular aches and pains, poor circulation, digestive problems, colds and flu, mental fatigue and nervous exhaustion. Coriander blends well with other spices, citrus essences, frankincense, jasmine, juniper berry, petitgrain, neroli, pine and sandalwood.

CULINARY USES
The fruits ('seeds') and fresh root can be added to curries. A few fresh leaves will impart a unique musky-pungent taste to a green salad, which is relished by some and detested by others!

CULTIVATION AND COLLECTION
Sow the seed in shallow rows during late spring in a dry, light soil in a sunny, sheltered position. The leaves can be picked throughout the growing season. The fruits ripen suddenly in late summer and fall without warning. Alternatively, cut the flower stems just as the aroma of the seeds starts to become pleasantly spicy; finish ripening in paper bags in a warm, dry place. Dig up the roots during autumn and use fresh.

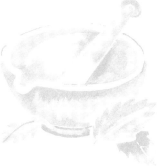

ESCHSCHOLZIA CALIFORNICA

CALIFORNIAN POPPY

Family: Papaveraceae (Poppy Family)
Parts Used: flowers, leaves

DESCRIPTION AND HABITAT
(See illustration, page 178)
The Californian poppy has finely cut blue-green leaves and masses of bright orange-yellow, saucer-shaped flowers, which are carried in profusion from the beginning of summer through to early autumn. There are also several hybrids whose colours include scarlet, orange, white, yellow, crimson and rose-carmine. The orange-yellow variety is preferred for healing purposes. A native of the west of North America, it thrives best in poor, sandy soils and sunny sites. The plant was introduced into Europe in the nineteenth century as an ornamental and medical plant.

HISTORY
The plant (pronounced esh-*sholt*-se-a) is named after Dr J.F. von Eschscholtz, a naturalist and physician who was attached to a Russian exploring expedition to north-west America a century ago. It has since become the state flower of California, and thus associated with fame, fortune and glamour. Interestingly, the flower was particularly abundant around Hollywood, the place once known to the native Americans as the 'land of dreams and illusion'. Hollywood, of course, is the home of the film industry and dubbed 'Tinsel Town' – the place of dreams and fantasy in the making!

PRINCIPAL CONSTITUENTS
Alkaloids similar to opium poppy; flavone glycosides.

HERBAL MEDICINE
Californian poppy is sedative, hypnotic, anodyne and antispasmodic. It is used as a non-addictive and weaker alternative to the opium poppy. Infusions of the flowers and leaves are helpful for tension headaches, migraine, anxiety, insomnia, palpitations, stress-related muscular aches and pains, and high blood pressure. Herbalists consider it safe enough for excitability and sleeplessness in children. As well as making good use of its sedative properties, the native Americans used the remedy for colicky pains and toothache.

FLOWER THERAPY
Gather the flowers during high summer and potentise using the Sun Method. Useful for those with escapist or addictive tendencies, constantly seeking outside themselves for enlightenment. It is as well to remember the old saying: 'All that glistens is not gold.'

HOMEOPATHY
Homeopaths employ the tincture in material doses for nervous conditions, such as those mentioned under Herbal Medicine.

CULTIVATION AND COLLECTION
The plants thrive in the poorest of soils and in full sun (the flowers remain closed if grown in the shade). Sow the seeds, just covering them, directly in the ground during early spring. Collect the flowers and leaves during the summer months. Use fresh or dried.

CAUTION

The Californian poppy is generally regarded safe for home use. It must not be confused with the opium poppy (Papaver somniferum), which is extremely poisonous and should never be used for self-medication.

FILIPENDULA ULMARIA

MEADOWSWEET

Family: Rosaceae (Rose Family)
Parts Used: flowers, leaves

DESCRIPTION AND HABITAT
(See illustration, page 178)

A perennial herb with reddish, upright stems up to 1.2m. The leaves are pinnate with toothed edges, dark green above, and white and downy on the underside. The small, creamy white flowers are borne in clusters at the stem tips, giving the appearance of feathery plumes. They have a pleasing, almond-like fragrance. The scent of the leaves is quite different from that of the flowers. Meadowsweet is native to northern Asia and Europe, where it can be found growing in damp meadows and on river banks.

HISTORY

The common name is derived from the Anglo-Saxon word *medu* (mead), because the plant was once used to flavour the drink made from fermented honey. It was in the flowerheads that salicylic acid was first discovered in 1839, and from this substance aspirin was later synthesised.

PRINCIPAL CONSTITUENTS

Salicylates, tannins, mucilage, flavonoids, heliotropine, yellow pigment, vanillin, essential oil, vitamin C, sugar.

HERBAL MEDICINE

Meadowsweet is antipyretic, anti-inflammatory, antispasmodic, astringent, diuretic and antirheumatic. Infusions of the flowers and leaves are helpful for flu, headaches, rheumatic and arthritic pain. It is also one of the most effective herbs for children's diarrhoea, gastritis and peptic ulcers. Meadowsweet is often described as a 'herbal aspirin', but without the side-effects. The tannin and mucilage content act to buffer the adverse effects of isolated salicylate, which can cause gastric bleeding.

AROMATHERAPY

The essential oil of meadowsweet is not generally available. However, the infused oil (see page 96) can be used as a massage oil for rheumatic aches and pains, or solely for its sweet, uplifting aroma. It blends well with citrus essences, cedarwood, chamomile (German and Roman), clary sage, geranium, jasmine, lavender, neroli, rose, sandalwood and ylang ylang.

FLOWER THERAPY

The flowers are collected during late summer and potentised using the Sun Method. Meadowsweet is for anxious individuals who experience a feeling of tightness in the head and neck. The remedy engenders a deep sense of release.

HOMEOPATHY

The homeopathic remedy is called *Spiraea ulmaria*, the old Latin name for meadowsweet. It is prescribed for burning and pressure in the oesophagus (food pipe), which makes swallowing difficult; also for vertigo, headache or a feeling of blood rushing to the head. The remedy was formerly used for epilepsy and hydrophobia.

CULTIVATION AND COLLECTION

The plant is rarely cultivated, though it can be raised from seed (obtained from a wildflower seed specialist). Sow the seeds in spring in a rich, moist soil. There is usually no need to thin the seedlings out, as meadowsweet grows best *en masse*. A shaded or semi-shaded site is essential.

HELIANTHUS ANNUS

SUNFLOWER

Family: Compositae/Asteraceae (Daisy Family)
Parts Used: fixed oil, flowers, roots, seeds

DESCRIPTION AND HABITAT
(See illustration, page 179)
A tall, erect annual reaching up to 3m or more, with a single stout, rough, hairy stem. The leaves are large, heart-shaped, rough in texture and deeply veined, growing alternately up the stem. Each stem bears one large golden yellow flower about 30cm across. The large grey seeds are protected by a hard, black and white seed coat. Sunflowers are native to South America, but are widely cultivated throughout the world.

HISTORY
The genus name, *Helianthus*, derives from the Greek *helios*, meaning sun, and *anthos*, meaning a flower. For the golden-ray florets resemble the sun, and always turn towards the direction of its rays. In its native Peru, the Inca people associated the sunflower with their sun god, Atahualpa. Head-dresses and other regalia were fashioned in the form of the flower. Its image was also carved into solid gold and used to decorate temples.

PRINCIPAL CONSTITUENTS
Flowerheads: flavo-glycosides, anthocyano-glycosides, xanthophyll, sapogenin. Seeds: fixed oil with fatty acids, carotenoids, lecithin.

HERBAL MEDICINE
The plant is not much used in modern herbalism. The flowers, leaves and seeds are believed to be febrifuge and antispasmodic. Infusions (also the diluted tincture) were formerly used to treat malaria, whooping cough, bronchitis and tuberculosis. Decoctions of the root were employed for their laxative effect. Sunflower seeds are highly nutritious: as well as containing calcium, magnesium, potassium and other trace minerals, they are a good source of protein and vitamins B, D and E. The cold-pressed oil can be used as a rub for aching muscles and joints.

AROMATHERAPY
The cold-pressed or unrefined oil has a slightly sweet, nutty aroma and a fine texture. It makes an excellent base for just about any essential oil.

FLOWER THERAPY
Take a single flowerhead and potentise using the Sun Method. An extra-large glass bowl will be required! The flower essence is for those who have low self-esteem or, on the contrary, are prone to vanity and self-aggrandisement. It brings out the sun-like qualities of the expressive self, but in a balanced way.

CULINARY USES
Sunflower oil is popular in cooking. The cold-pressed version has a delicious nutty taste and is excellent in a salad dressing. The seeds can be eaten raw, though they taste better when lightly toasted. Sprinkle over salads, baked potatoes, steamed vegetables and other savoury dishes.

CULTIVATION AND COLLECTION
Sunflowers grow well in rich, fertile soil in a sunny position. Propagation is by seed sown under glass in spring; the seedlings should be planted out in early summer. The huge flowers bloom during late summer, and the seeds are ripe when the flowerheads begin to droop. The heads are then cut and left to dry, and when the seeds are fully dried they will fall out easily. The leaves are gathered throughout the growing season and used fresh. Dig up the roots in the autumn and dry in a warm, dark place.

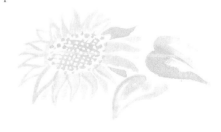

HUMULUS LUPULUS

HOPS

Family: Cannabaceae (Hemp Family)
Parts Used: essential oil, flowers

DESCRIPTION AND HABITAT
(See illustration, page 179)
A vigorous perennial climber growing up to 8m. The twining stems bear three- to five-lobed, heart-shaped leaves with serrated edges, in opposite pairs. The male flowers hang in loose bunches while the females are cone-like catkins known as strobiles; the genders are on separate plants. Native throughout Europe, it is found in hedgerows, copses and thickets in deep, rich soil.

HISTORY
The common name comes from Anglo-Saxon *hoppan*, meaning to 'climb'. However the origin of the generic name *Humulus* is uncertain, although some authorities suggest *humela*, an old German word for the plant. The Romans used the young shoot tips in salads and cooked like asparagus. Hops have produced the characteristic bitter taste of beer since the Middle Ages or earlier.

PRINCIPAL CONSTITUENTS
Lupulin, bitters, resin, tannin, oestrogenic substances. Also an essential oil which includes humulene, myrcene (only in the fresh oil), caryophyllene, farnescene.

HERBAL MEDICINE
Hops are primarily sedative, hypnotic, antiseptic and astringent. The remedy is used for insomnia, restlessness and headache. It is also helpful for gastrointestinal spasm, and therefore irritable bowel syndrome. Before the days of mechanisation, female hop pickers could suffer disrupted menstruation due to the aroma and/or absorption of the essential oil through their hands. This is due to the oestrogen content, which can also quell sexual desire in men.

AROMATHERAPY
The oil is captured by steam distillation of newly dried strobiles. It is a yellowish liquid with a sweet, warm, spicy aroma whose effect is soothing and soporific. It is helpful for spasmodic coughs, nervous indigestion, headaches, menstrual irregularity, menstrual cramps, menopausal symptoms, insomnia and nervous tension. The oil blends well with citrus essences, juniper berry, and pine.

FLOWER THERAPY
The stobiles are collected in late summer and potentised using the Sun Method. Hops helps to ease distress associated with transition, especially the psycho-spiritual turmoil commonly experienced during adolescence and menopause.

HOMEOPATHY
The remedy is used for nervous problems like insomnia, muscle twitching, tremors, dizziness and delirium.

CULTIVATION AND COLLECTION
It is best to gather wild hops. Use a knife to collect the females only, in late summer when the bracts are dry and papery.

CAUTION

The pollen from the strobiles may cause contact dermatitis. Similarly the fresh essential oil may cause skin reactions, probably because of its myrcene content. But as the oil ages it becomes benign to skin. Nevertheless, always use it in the lowest concentrations. Since the plant and its oil are sedative, hops should be avoided by those suffering from depression and lethargy.

HYPERICUM PERFORATUM

St John's Wort

Family: Hypericaceae (St John's Wort Family) **Synonyms:** Hypericum, Perforate St John's Wort
Parts Used: flowers, leaves, stems

DESCRIPTION AND HABITAT
(See illustration, page 179)
An upright perennial with a stout, creeping rhizome which bears clumps of erect stems, branches near the top and reaching up to 60cm tall. The woody-based stems have two lengthways ridges along each side. The opposite, small, ovate, pale green leaves bear small translucent dots (oil glands) which are clearly seen when held up to the light. The vibrant yellow, star-shaped flowers are black-dotted, especially at the edges. St John's wort, native to Europe and western Asia, can be found on grassy banks and in meadows and hedgerows.

HISTORY
The name *Hypericum* is derived from Greek *hyper*, meaning 'above', and *eikon*, meaning 'picture': in medieval times it was hung over picture frames to ward off evil spirits. The glands in the leaves, which look like tiny punctures, explain the specific name, *perforatum*. They were thought to look like wounds, and in the Middle Ages the plant was used by the Knights of St John of Jerusalem to heal the wounds of Crusaders.

PRINCIPAL CONSTITUENTS
Glycosides (including a red pigment, hypericin), flavonoids, tannins, pectin, essential oil, resin.

HERBAL MEDICINE
St John's wort is anti-inflammatory, vulnerary, diuretic, astringent, expectorant and sedative. Internally, it is helpful for arthritic and rheumatic complaints, nerve pain, bedwetting, diarrhoea, coughs, bronchitis, anxiety and nervous tension, depression and menopausal distress. Current research indicates its efficacy in seasonal affective disorder (SAD). The infused oil (see page 96) can be used as a rub to ease the pain of fibrositis and sciatica. It also promotes the healing of wounds, bruises, minor burns and eases the pain and inflammation of varicose veins.

AROMATHERAPY
The infused oil is used for the same conditions cited in herbalism. Low concentrations of appropriate essential oils are often added to enhance the therapeutic effects. The sweetish, astringent aroma combines well with angelica, citrus essences, coriander, geranium, ginger, juniper, lavender and rosemary.

FLOWER THERAPY
The flowers are collected in midsummer (ideally on St John's Day in the northern hemisphere) and potentised by the Sun Method. St John's wort is for oversensitive individuals (especially children) prone to disturbing dreams, night terrors and paranoiac feelings. The remedy engenders a sense of protection.

HOMEOPATHY
The remedy is seen as invaluable for nerve injuries, especially of the spine, fingers, toes and nails. It is also regarded as an anti-tetanus remedy to be taken as soon as possible after injury. Emotional symptoms may include depression and a morbid fear of falling from heights.

CULTIVATION AND COLLECTION
The plant can be propagated by division of the root stock in autumn or spring. Alternatively, sow the seed in the ground in early spring, preferably in a lime-rich soil in a sunny situation. The entire plant above ground is collected just before all the blooms are fully open.

CAUTION

In hypersensitive individuals, excessive use internally or externally causes a skin allergy which becomes aggravated by exposure to sunlight.

JUNIPERUS COMMUNIS

JUNIPER

Family: Cupressaceae (Cypress Family)
Parts Used: berries, essential oil

DESCRIPTION AND HABITAT
(See illustration, page 180)
A small, coniferous evergreen tree or shrub, reaching up to 4m. It has reddish stems and bluish green prickly needles. Small yellow flowers bloom in early summer. The berries take three years to ripen and are first green, then bluish and finally black. The whole plant emanates a pine-like aroma. Juniper is native to North Africa, Europe (including Britain), northern Asia, Korea and Japan. It can be found growing wild on chalk, limestone or peaty soils.

HISTORY
In former times the odour of juniper branches, hung on the door of the house, were reputed to keep snakes away. They were also burnt in public squares, streets and houses during epidemics of plague and cholera, and in the hospitals of Paris during the smallpox epidemic of 1870. Since biblical days juniper has been considered a magical plant with the power to drive away evil spirits.

PRINCIPAL CONSTITUENTS
Essential oil (including pinene, myrcene, borneol, camphene, limonene, terpenic alcohol), sugars, flavonoids, glycosides, resin, tannins, organic acids.

HERBAL MEDICINE
A decoction of juniper berries is considered a specific for complaints of the urinary tract (e.g. cystitis) due to its potent diuretic and antiseptic actions. It increases the volume of urine, to which it gives an odour of violets. Juniper is also prescribed for arthritis (it promotes the elimination of uric acid), bronchial catarrh, intermittent fevers, general debility, flatulence and infected skin problems.

AROMATHERAPY
The highest quality essential oil is obtained by steam distillation of the berries. It is a virtually colourless liquid. The aroma is fresh and woody with a peppery overtone. Its odour effect is uplifting and yet also warming and calming; a reputed aphrodisiac. Juniper is helpful for skin and hair care (oily), acne, weeping eczema, haemorrhoids, wounds, arthritic and rheumatic complaints, muscular aches and pains, loss of periods outside pregnancy, painful periods, cystitis, PMS, nervous tension and stress-related disorders. It blends well with bergamot, cedarwood, frankincense, geranium, lavender, neroli, petitgrain, rosemary and sandalwood.

HOMEOPATHY
The remedy is used in material doses (infusion or tincture) for disorders of the urinary tract.

CULINARY USES
Juniper berries are used commercially to flavour gin and liqueurs. In the kitchen the crushed berries add a piquant flavour to roasts, casseroles and especially baked or stuffed red cabbage.

CULTIVATION AND COLLECTION
The berries should be gathered when ripe in the autumn for sowing in early spring. The seed is slow to germinate, so it is easier to obtain a good specimen from a garden centre or tree nursery. Juniper is a hardy, slow-growing tree and will thrive in soil which is either acid (peaty) or alkaline (chalk or limestone). It prefers an open site. The berries can be used fresh or dried.

CAUTION

Do not use juniper during pregnancy or where there is kidney disease. When choosing the essential oil, ensure that the bottle is labelled 'Juniper Berry' and not 'Juniper'. The latter is an inferior oil distilled from fermented berries and/or the leaves and twigs.

LAVANDULA ANGUSTIFOLIA

LAVENDER

Family: Lamiaceae/Labiatae (Mint Family) *Synonyms:* L. officinalis, L. vera
Parts Used: essential oil, flowers, leaves

DESCRIPTION AND HABITAT
(See illustration, page 180)
An evergreen aromatic shrub growing up to 60cm tall, with lanceolate bluish green leaves. The bluish mauve flowers are carried in spikes at the end of thin stems. Lavender is native to the mountainous regions of southern Europe, but is widely cultivated elsewhere, especially England.

HISTORY
The name *Lavandula* is derived from the Latin *lavare*, to wash. Throughout history lavender has been used for its scent as a strewing herb, and for placing among linen and clothes. The plant was dedicated to Hecate, the goddess of witches, and was said to afford protection against the forces of darkness. It was one of the plants taken to America by the Pilgrim Fathers.

PRINCIPAL CONSTITUENTS
Essential oil (including linalol, linalyl acetate, lavandulol, lavandulyl acetate, terpineol, limonene, caryophyllene), tannins, coumarins, flavonoids.

HERBAL MEDICINE
Lavender is carminative, antirheumatic, cholagogic, diuretic, antimicrobial, antispasmodic, antidepressant, sedative, hypotensive, nervine, cicatrisant, vulnerary and rubefacient. Weak infusions are helpful for disorders of nervous origin, such as insomnia, poor digestion, migraines and irritability; and for respiratory disorders such as acute laryngitis, bronchitis, coughs and hayfever. Externally, the cooled infusion is used to treat vaginal infections, cuts and sores, minor burns and insect stings. The infused oil can be used as a liniment to help ease rheumatic aches and pains.

AROMATHERAPY
The essential oil is obtained by steam distillation of the flowering tops. It is a colourless to pale yellow liquid, with a sweet floral-herbaceous aroma. The odour effect is uplifting, calming and refreshing. Lavender is helpful for skin care (most skin types), acne, allergies, athlete's foot, boils, bruises, eczema, dandruff, dermatitis, burns, chilblains, psoriasis, ringworm, and insect bites and stings; also as an insect repellent and for asthma, earache, coughs, colds and flu, catarrh, laryngitis, headache, insomnia, migraine, nervous tension, PMS and stress-related disorders. It blends well with citrus essences, cedarwood, clary sage, coriander, frankincense, geranium, juniper berry, neroli, rose, petitgrain and pine.

FLOWER THERAPY
The flowers are collected during high summer and potentised using the Sun Method. The remedy is for those who feel strained, tense, anxious and physically depleted. Lavender enables such individuals to balance sensitivity with the needs of the body.

CULTIVATION AND COLLECTION
Lavender is usually propagated by cuttings taken in autumn, kept in sandy compost under cover during winter and planted out the following spring. It will thrive in any well-drained soil in a sunny position, but must be protected from hard frosts. Collect the flowers during high summer, cutting the whole stalk. Once dried, the flowers can be rubbed off the stalks and stored in jars.

MELISSA OFFICINALIS

LEMON BALM

Family: Lamiaceae/Labiatae (Mint Family) *Synonyms:* Balm, Bee Balm
Parts Used: flowers (flower therapy), leaves

DESCRIPTION AND HABITAT

(See illustration, page 180)

A bushy perennial with a height and spread of about 60cm, producing bright green lemon-scented leaves in opposite pairs. The small, two-lipped flowers, which grow in whorls in the upper leaf axils, change colour as they mature from pale yellow to white or pale blue. Lemon balm is native to the Middle East and the Mediterranean and has become widely naturalised in Europe.

HISTORY

The name *Melissa* is derived from the Greek word for the honeybee, for the herb produces abundant nectar. The common name is an abbreviation of balsam, after its sweet-smelling aroma when fresh. Like many other Mediterranean herbs, it was introduced to Britain by the Romans.

PRINCIPAL CONSTITUENTS

Essential oil (including citral, citronellol, eugenol, geraniol, linalyl acetate), bitter principles, tannins, resin.

HERBAL MEDICINE

Lemon balm is carminative, antispasmodic, hypotensive, stomachic, diaphoretic and sedative. It is used in infusions for digestive disorders, nausea, flatulence, nervous anxiety, headache and insomnia. The plant also has a tonic effect on the heart and circulatory system and can lower high blood pressure. It is helpful in feverish conditions like colds and flu.

AROMATHERAPY

The essential oil is obtained by steam distillation of the leaves and flowering tops. It is a pale yellow liquid with a light, fresh and distinctly lemony scent. The odour effect is uplifting and calming. Lemon balm is helpful for allergies (skin and respiratory), cold sores, eczema, asthma, bronchitis, indigestion, nausea, irregular menstruation, insomnia, migraine, anxiety, nervous exhaustion and other stress-related disorders. It blends well with citrus essences, chamomile (German and Roman), geranium, lavender, petitgrain, neroli, and rose.

FLOWER THERAPY

The flowers are collected during the height of summer and potentised by the Sun Method. Used for loss of vitality and a sense of spiritual stagnation, particularly when associated with over-concern for others. The remedy engenders inner strength and courage.

CULINARY USES

Lemon balm is used to flavour fish and poultry dishes, jams and desserts. The fresh leaves can be eaten with salads and every kind of vegetable. It can also be made into a refreshing tisane.

CULTIVATION AND COLLECTION

The plant is easily propagated by dividing the rootstock in the autumn when the stems have died back, or in the spring before new growth occurs. It also seeds itself freely. The fresh leaves should be collected when young. If you cut all the leaves in one go in spring (for drying) you will have another harvest six weeks later, but with smaller leaves.

CAUTION

Despite its strong aroma, lemon balm produces a tiny amount of essential oil (labelled 'Melissa, True'). The genuine oil it is as costly as rose otto. Many of the so-called melissa oils are blends of cheaper lemon-scented essences such as lemon, lemongrass and citronella, sometimes with the addition of synthetic chemicals, so it is important to buy from a reputable supplier. Although melissa is popular with aromatherapy doctors in Germany, it is a relative newcomer to aromatherapy and has not been thoroughly tested on humans. Available data indicates that the oil can irritate sensitive skin. Always use it in the lowest recommended concentrations.

MENTHA PIPERITA

PEPPERMINT

Family: Lamiaceae/Labiatae (Mint Family)
Parts Used: essential oil, flowering tops, flowers (flower therapy), leaves, stems

DESCRIPTION AND HABITAT
(See illustration, page 180)
A perennial herb growing up to 1m tall and spreading prolifically by rhizomes. The opposite, bright green leaves are oval and serrated, with pointed tips. The pink or lilac flowers are arranged in long, stout terminal spikes. The whole plant emanates a fresh, piercing, distinctly minty aroma. Peppermint is a hybrid between water mint (M. *aquatica*) and spearmint (M. *spicata*), both of which are native to the Mediterranean. The plant has naturalised throughout Europe and America.

PRINCIPAL CONSTITUENTS
Essential oil (including menthol, carvone, cineol, limonene, menthone, pinene, thymol), flavonoids, carotenoids, choline, azulenes, rosmarinic acid, tannins, bitter compounds.

HERBAL MEDICINE
Peppermint is stomachic, carminative, cholagogic, antispasmodic, anti-inflammatory, expectorant and antiseptic. Infusions are prescribed for indigestion, gall bladder problems, diarrhoea, flatulence and abdominal spasms. Peppermint also aids the healing of gastric ulcers. Inhalations of the herb are helpful for bronchial catarrh. Externally, the tincture can be incorporated into an ointment base and applied as a linament to ease muscular aches and pains. It has mild local anaesthetic properties.

AROMATHERAPY
The essential oil is obtained by steam distillation of the flowering tops. It is a pale yellow liquid with a fresh, piercing, minty aroma. Its odour effect is enlivening, cooling and head-clearing. Peppermint is helpful for bruises, sprains, swellings, ringworm, scabies, toothache, neuralgia, muscular aches and pains, indigestion, halitosis, irritable bowel syndrome (taken internally as peppermint capsules), mouth ulcers, mouth thrush, nausea, feverish conditions, colds and flu, headache, mental fatigue and migraine. It blends well with clary sage, eucalyptus, lavender, lemon and rosemary. The oil is highly odoriferous, so use sparingly.

FLOWER THERAPY
The flowers are gathered during late summer and potentised using the Sun Method. Peppermint is used for mental dullness and lethargy. The remedy facilitates clarity of thought.

HOMEOPATHY
The homeopathic remedy mirrors the herbal uses, though it is also indicated for vaginal pruritis and dry cough.

CULINARY USES
Peppermint is used to flavour a wide range of foods, including sauces, ices, fruit salad, confectionery (e.g. mint creams), new potatoes and peas. The fresh or dried herbs can be taken hot or iced as an uplifting tisane.

CULTIVATION AND COLLECTION
The easiest way to propagate the plant is by division of the roots or rhizomes. Plant in a rich, moist soil in a sheltered position. Pick the fresh leaves as required. For drying, cut stems and leaves before flowering.

CAUTION

The essential oil should always be used in the lowest recommended concentrations as it may irritate sensitive skin. Since the oil promotes menstruation, it is best to avoid during the first trimester of pregnancy.

MAJOR DIRECTORY PLANTS

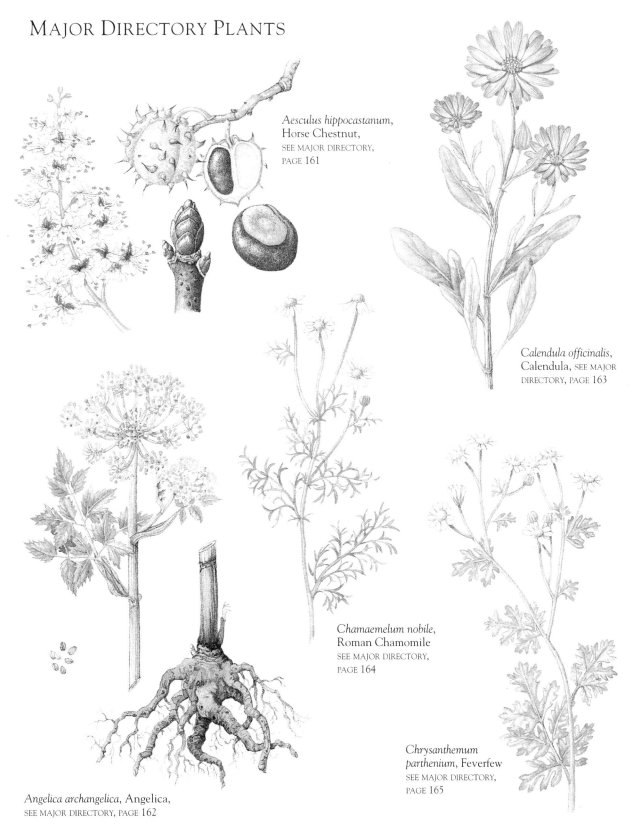

Aesculus hippocastanum,
Horse Chestnut,
SEE MAJOR DIRECTORY,
PAGE 161

Calendula officinalis,
Calendula, SEE MAJOR
DIRECTORY, PAGE 163

Chamaemelum nobile,
Roman Chamomile
SEE MAJOR DIRECTORY,
PAGE 164

*Chrysanthemum
parthenium,* Feverfew
SEE MAJOR DIRECTORY,
PAGE 165

Angelica archangelica, Angelica,
SEE MAJOR DIRECTORY, PAGE 162

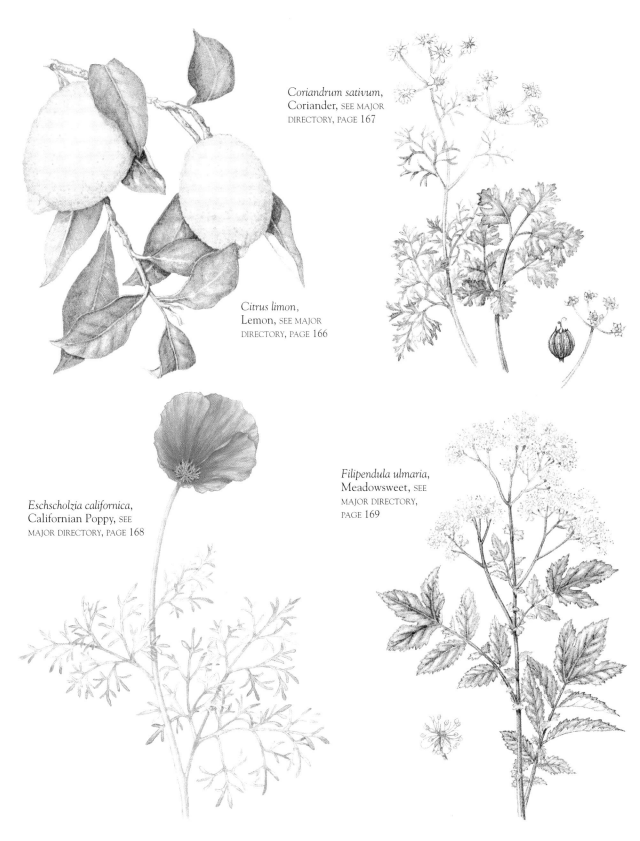

Coriandrum sativum,
Coriander, SEE MAJOR
DIRECTORY, PAGE 167

Citrus limon,
Lemon, SEE MAJOR
DIRECTORY, PAGE 166

Eschscholzia californica,
Californian Poppy, SEE
MAJOR DIRECTORY, PAGE 168

Filipendula ulmaria,
Meadowsweet, SEE
MAJOR DIRECTORY,
PAGE 169

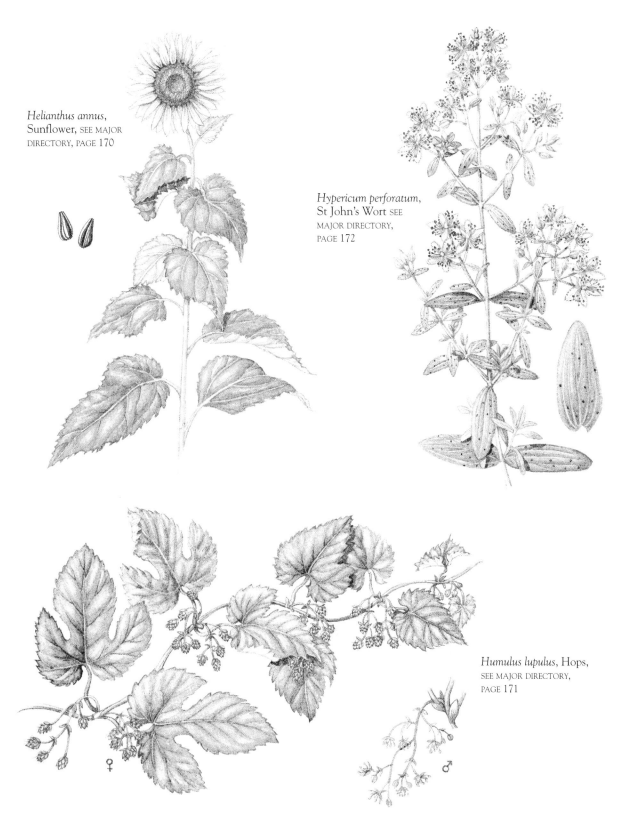

Helianthus annus,
Sunflower, SEE MAJOR
DIRECTORY, PAGE 170

Hypericum perforatum,
St John's Wort SEE
MAJOR DIRECTORY,
PAGE 172

Humulus lupulus, Hops,
SEE MAJOR DIRECTORY,
PAGE 171

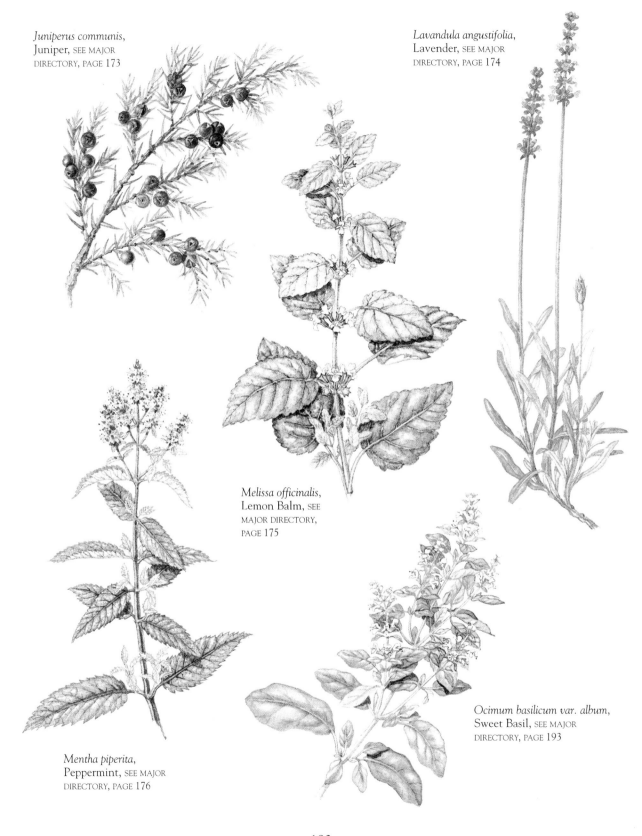

Juniperus communis,
Juniper, SEE MAJOR
DIRECTORY, PAGE 173

Lavandula angustifolia,
Lavender, SEE MAJOR
DIRECTORY, PAGE 174

Melissa officinalis,
Lemon Balm, SEE
MAJOR DIRECTORY,
PAGE 175

Mentha piperita,
Peppermint, SEE MAJOR
DIRECTORY, PAGE 176

Ocimum basilicum var. album,
Sweet Basil, SEE MAJOR
DIRECTORY, PAGE 193

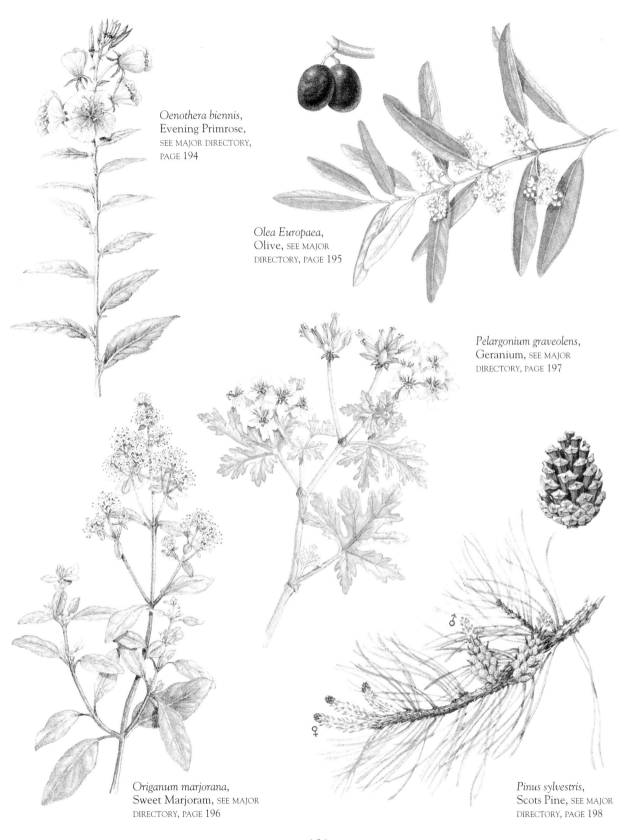

Oenothera biennis,
Evening Primrose,
SEE MAJOR DIRECTORY,
PAGE 194

Olea Europaea,
Olive, SEE MAJOR
DIRECTORY, PAGE 195

Pelargonium graveolens,
Geranium, SEE MAJOR
DIRECTORY, PAGE 197

Origanum marjorana,
Sweet Marjoram, SEE MAJOR
DIRECTORY, PAGE 196

Pinus sylvestris,
Scots Pine, SEE MAJOR
DIRECTORY, PAGE 198

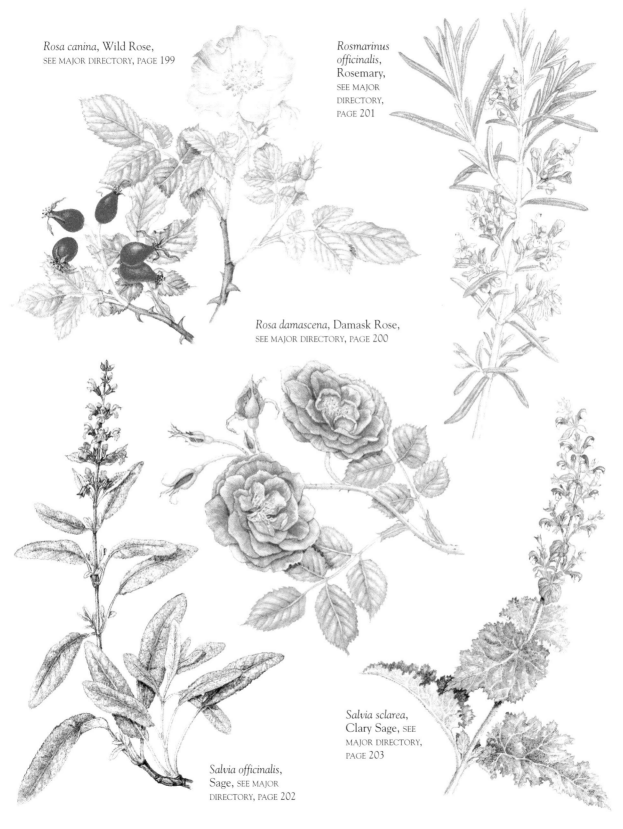

Rosa canina, Wild Rose,
SEE MAJOR DIRECTORY, PAGE 199

Rosmarinus officinalis, Rosemary, SEE MAJOR DIRECTORY, PAGE 201

Rosa damascena, Damask Rose, SEE MAJOR DIRECTORY, PAGE 200

Salvia sclarea, Clary Sage, SEE MAJOR DIRECTORY, PAGE 203

Salvia officinalis, Sage, SEE MAJOR DIRECTORY, PAGE 202

Sambucus nigra, Elder, SEE MAJOR
DIRECTORY, PAGE 204

Taraxacum officinale,
Dandelion, SEE
MAJOR DIRECTORY,
PAGE 205

Tilia cordata, Linden,
SEE MAJOR DIRECTORY,
PAGE 206

Tropaeolum majus,
Nasturtium, SEE MAJOR
DIRECTORY, PAGE 207

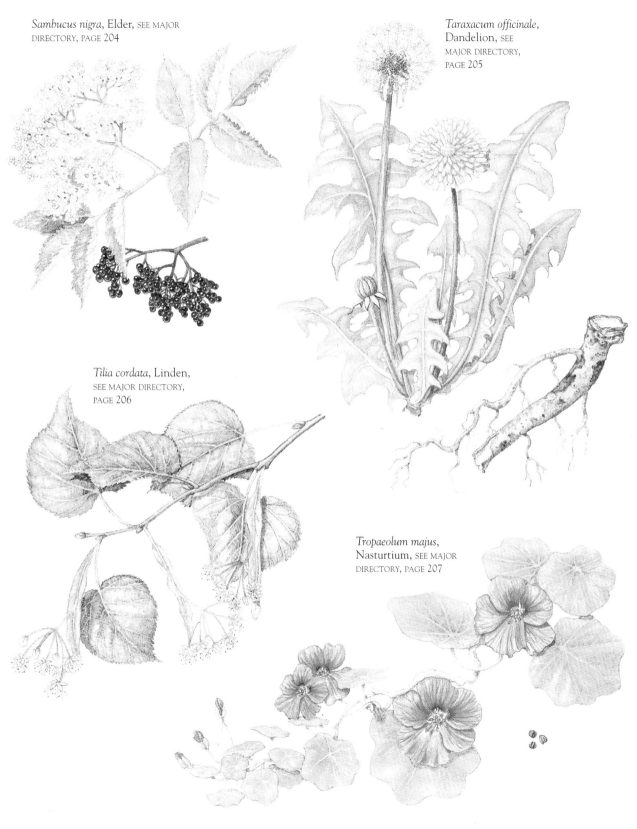

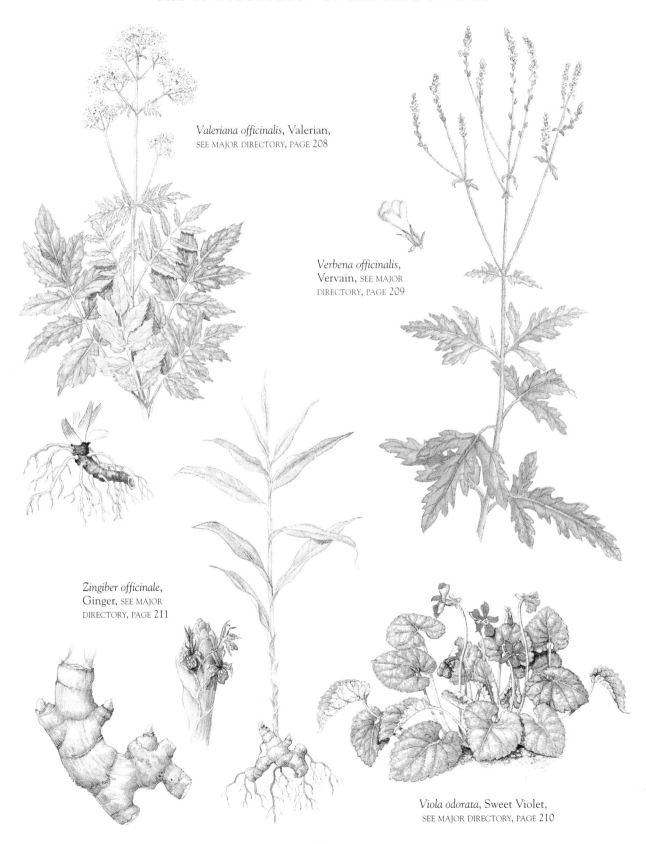

Valeriana officinalis, Valerian,
SEE MAJOR DIRECTORY, PAGE 208

Verbena officinalis,
Vervain, SEE MAJOR
DIRECTORY, PAGE 209

Zingiber officinale,
Ginger, SEE MAJOR
DIRECTORY, PAGE 211

Viola odorata, Sweet Violet,
SEE MAJOR DIRECTORY, PAGE 210

MINOR DIRECTORY PLANTS

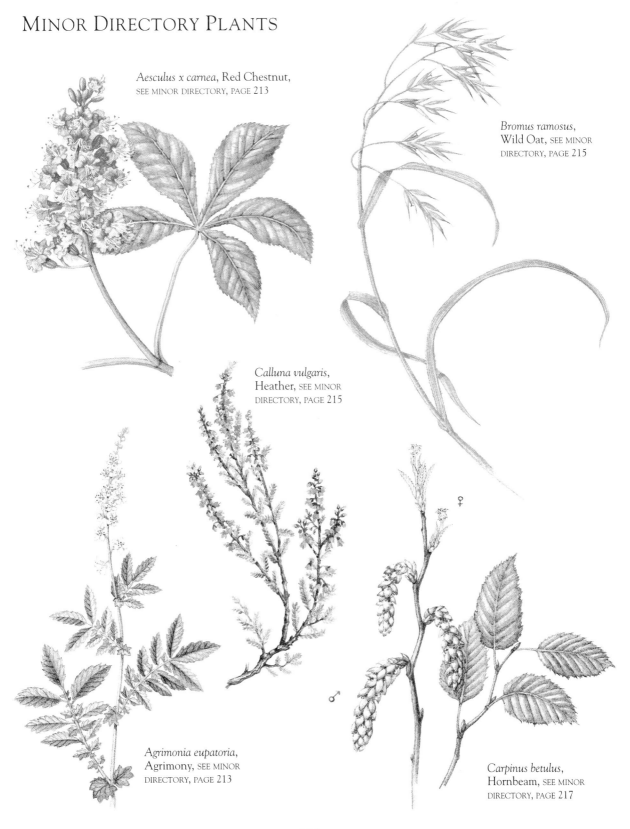

Aesculus x carnea, Red Chestnut, SEE MINOR DIRECTORY, PAGE 213

Bromus ramosus, Wild Oat, SEE MINOR DIRECTORY, PAGE 215

Calluna vulgaris, Heather, SEE MINOR DIRECTORY, PAGE 215

Agrimonia eupatoria, Agrimony, SEE MINOR DIRECTORY, PAGE 213

Carpinus betulus, Hornbeam, SEE MINOR DIRECTORY, PAGE 217

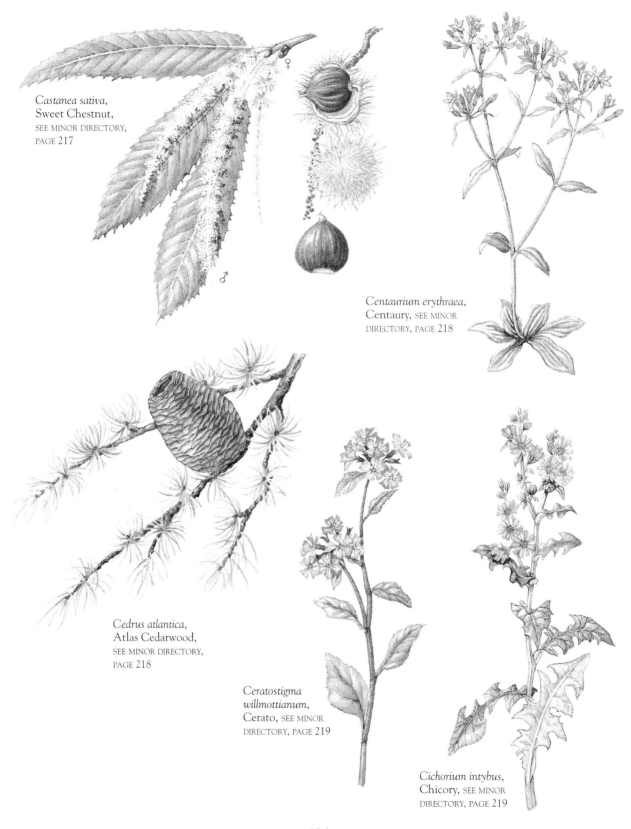

Castanea sativa,
Sweet Chestnut,
SEE MINOR DIRECTORY,
PAGE 217

Centaurium erythraea,
Centaury, SEE MINOR
DIRECTORY, PAGE 218

Cedrus atlantica,
Atlas Cedarwood,
SEE MINOR DIRECTORY,
PAGE 218

*Ceratostigma
willmottianum,*
Cerato, SEE MINOR
DIRECTORY, PAGE 219

Cichorium intybus,
Chicory, SEE MINOR
DIRECTORY, PAGE 219

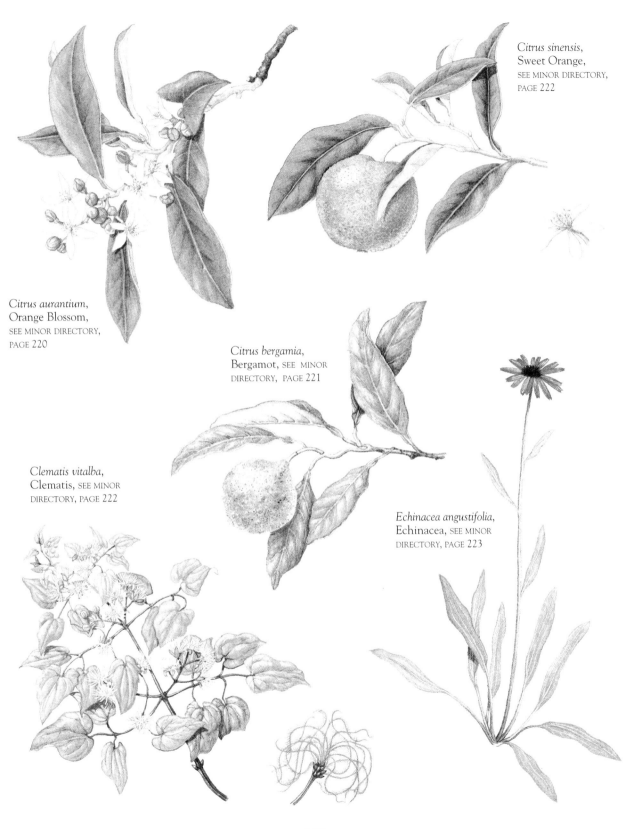

Citrus sinensis,
Sweet Orange,
SEE MINOR DIRECTORY,
PAGE 222

Citrus aurantium,
Orange Blossom,
SEE MINOR DIRECTORY,
PAGE 220

Citrus bergamia,
Bergamot, SEE MINOR
DIRECTORY, PAGE 221

Clematis vitalba,
Clematis, SEE MINOR
DIRECTORY, PAGE 222

Echinacea angustifolia,
Echinacea, SEE MINOR
DIRECTORY, PAGE 223

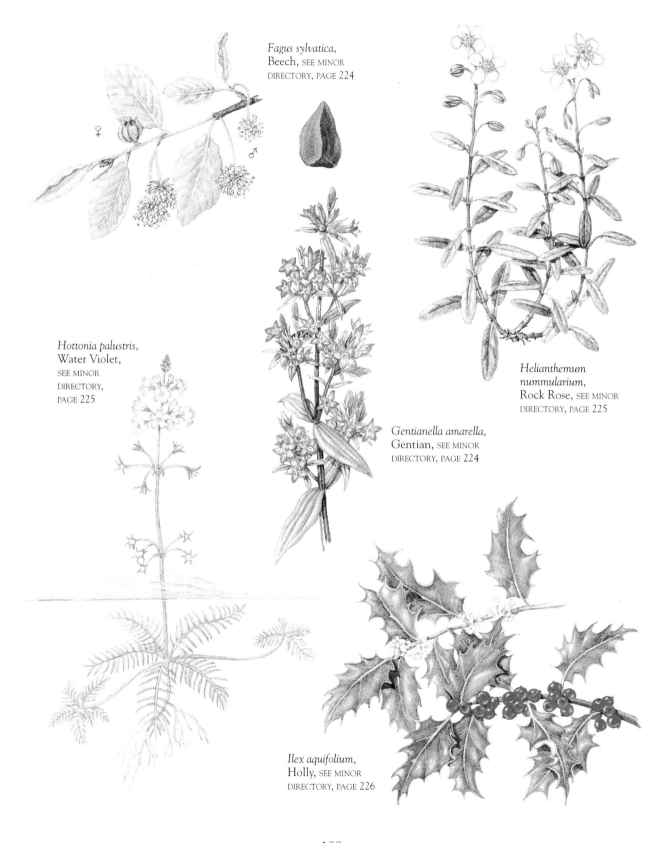

Fagus sylvatica,
Beech, SEE MINOR
DIRECTORY, PAGE 224

Hottonia palustris,
Water Violet,
SEE MINOR
DIRECTORY,
PAGE 225

*Helianthemum
nummularium,*
Rock Rose, SEE MINOR
DIRECTORY, PAGE 225

Gentianella amarella,
Gentian, SEE MINOR
DIRECTORY, PAGE 224

Ilex aquifolium,
Holly, SEE MINOR
DIRECTORY, PAGE 226

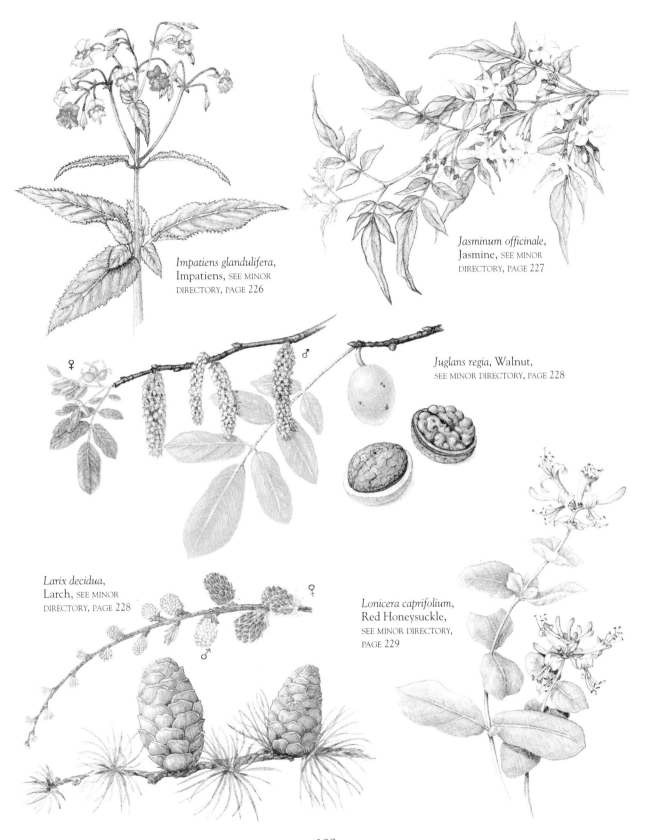

Impatiens glandulifera,
Impatiens, SEE MINOR
DIRECTORY, PAGE 226

Jasminum officinale,
Jasmine, SEE MINOR
DIRECTORY, PAGE 227

Juglans regia, Walnut,
SEE MINOR DIRECTORY, PAGE 228

Larix decidua,
Larch, SEE MINOR
DIRECTORY, PAGE 228

Lonicera caprifolium,
Red Honeysuckle,
SEE MINOR DIRECTORY,
PAGE 229

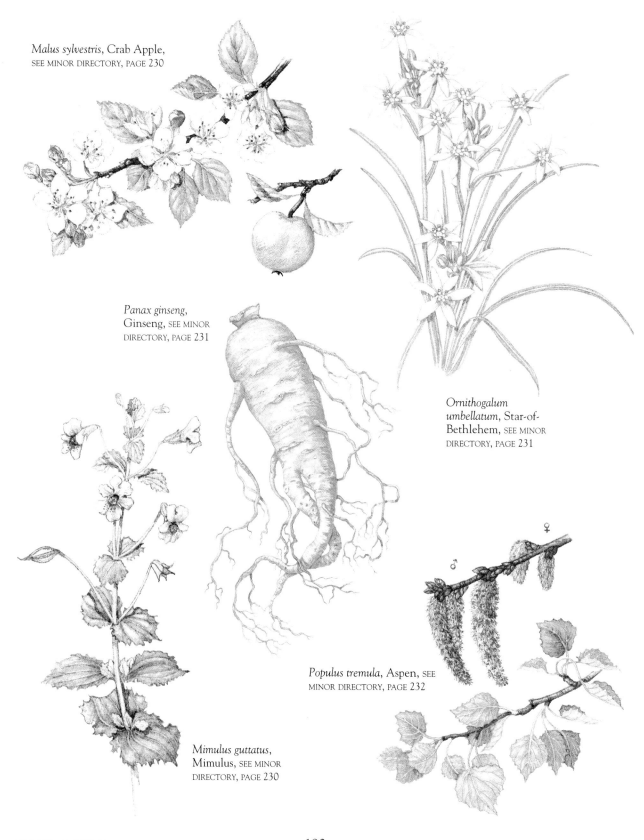

Malus sylvestris, Crab Apple, SEE MINOR DIRECTORY, PAGE 230

Panax ginseng, Ginseng, SEE MINOR DIRECTORY, PAGE 231

Ornithogalum umbellatum, Star-of-Bethlehem, SEE MINOR DIRECTORY, PAGE 231

Mimulus guttatus, Mimulus, SEE MINOR DIRECTORY, PAGE 230

Populus tremula, Aspen, SEE MINOR DIRECTORY, PAGE 232

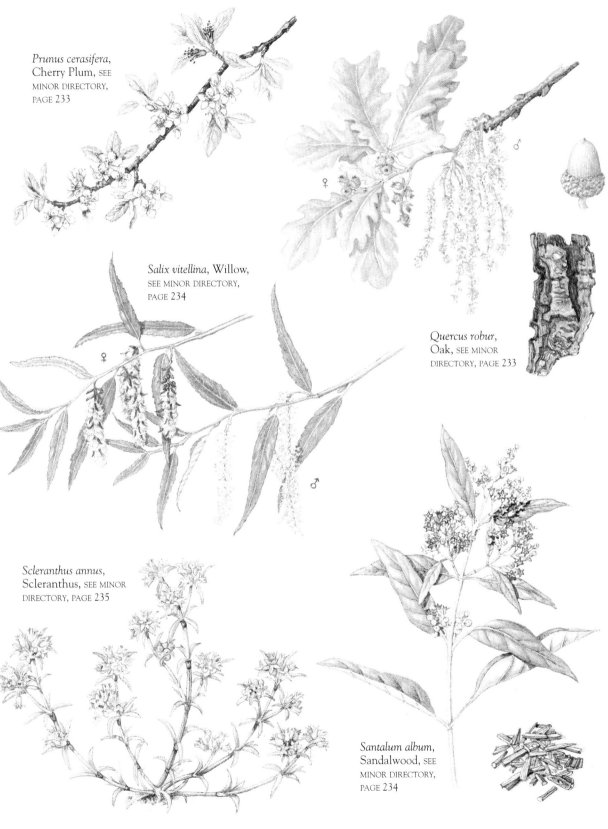

Prunus cerasifera,
Cherry Plum, SEE
MINOR DIRECTORY,
PAGE 233

Salix vitellina, Willow,
SEE MINOR DIRECTORY,
PAGE 234

Quercus robur,
Oak, SEE MINOR
DIRECTORY, PAGE 233

Scleranthus annus,
Scleranthus, SEE MINOR
DIRECTORY, PAGE 235

Santalum album,
Sandalwood, SEE
MINOR DIRECTORY,
PAGE 234

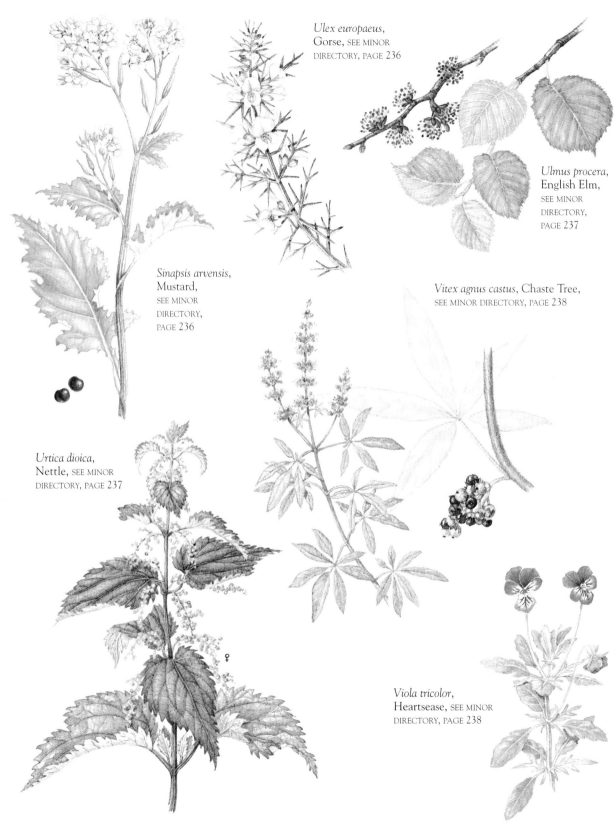

Ulex europaeus,
Gorse, SEE MINOR
DIRECTORY, PAGE 236

Ulmus procera,
English Elm,
SEE MINOR
DIRECTORY,
PAGE 237

Sinapsis arvensis,
Mustard,
SEE MINOR
DIRECTORY,
PAGE 236

Vitex agnus castus, Chaste Tree,
SEE MINOR DIRECTORY, PAGE 238

Urtica dioica,
Nettle, SEE MINOR
DIRECTORY, PAGE 237

Viola tricolor,
Heartsease, SEE MINOR
DIRECTORY, PAGE 238

OCIMUM BASILICUM VAR. ALBUM

BASIL, SWEET

Family: Labiatae/Lamiaceae (Mint Family)
Parts Used: essential oil, flowering tops, flowers (flower therapy), leaves

DESCRIPTION AND HABITAT

(See illustration, page 180)
An annual or short-lived perennial herb with strongly scented leaves reminiscent of a blend of fennel and cloves, growing up to 60cm tall. The slightly toothed leaves are opposite, short-stalked and oval with a slightly puckered surface. The white or pinkish flowers are usually arranged in whorls in the upper leaf axils. All parts of the plant are hairy and aromatic. Basil is native to southern Asia and the Middle East but has long been grown in Europe as an ornamental, culinary and medicinal herb.

HISTORY

The name 'basil' derives from the Greek word *basilikos*, meaning 'royal', because the herb was regarded as fit for a king's table. It is also said that scorpions are attracted to the aroma. In India basil is sacred to Vishnu, the Hindu god of justice and universal order.

PRINCIPAL CONSTITUENTS

Essential oil (comprising thymol, origanene, carvacrol, basil camphor), tannins, glycosides, saponin.

HERBAL MEDICINE

Basil has stomachic, carminative, expectorant, antispasmodic, mildly sedative and galactagogic properties. Infusions of the herb are indicated for gastric upset, stomach pains, flatulence, constipation and coughs. Externally, infusions of basil can be applied as a cool compress for slow-healing wounds, and in gargles.

AROMATHERAPY

The essential oil is steam-distilled from the flowering tops and leaves. It is pale yellow with the viscosity of alcohol and possesses a light, fresh, sweet-spicy scent with balsamic undertones. The odour effect is at first enlivening, giving way to a warm, comforting sensation. Basil is helpful for problems such as muscular aches and pains, respiratory disorders, delayed or scanty menstruation, colds and flu, mental fatigue, anxiety and depression (but see Cautions). It blends well with bergamot, clary sage, frankincense, geranium and neroli.

FLOWER THERAPY

The flowers are collected during late summer and potentised using the Sun Method. Basil is helpful for those who tend to separate spirituality and sexuality, believing that the two cannot be integrated.

HOMEOPATHY

Potentised from a related species, *Ocimum camum*, indicated for problems such as uterine prolapse, engorged breasts, pain while breastfeeding, fevers, painful joints, vomiting and diarrhoea.

CULINARY USES

A popular herb, preferably used fresh, to flavour soups, salads, tomato dishes, meat and fish. Wine made from the leaves is a reputed aphrodisiac.

CULTIVATION AND COLLECTION

Sow the seed indoors in late spring and plant outside in early summer, or after all danger of frost is past. Basil prefers a sunny, sheltered position in well-drained soil. Plants can also be grown in large pots on a sunny balcony or patio. Collect the leaves throughout the growing season and use fresh, or collect the flowering tops during high summer and dry in the shade.

CAUTION

The herb is perfectly safe for culinary use, but the essential oil (or strong infusions of the herb) are potentially hazardous. Avoid both oil and herb during pregnancy as they may stimulate menstruation. The oil can be highly irritant to sensitive skin, so use in the lowest recommended concentrations, or solely as a vaporising oil.

OENOTHERA BIENNIS

EVENING PRIMROSE

Family: Onagraceae (Willowherb Family)
Parts Used: leaves, flower stems, fixed oil (from seed), flowers (flower therapy)

DESCRIPTION AND HABITAT
(See illustration, page 181)
A biennial up to 1m tall with a branched, reddish stem. The large, cup-shaped, pale yellow flowers appear from midsummer. They open mainly in the evening, emanate a subtle fragrance and are followed by tubular, pointed seed pods. Native to North America, the plant is now naturalised in most of Europe. It is widespread on poor soils, especially embankments and sand dunes.

HISTORY
The origin of the botanical name *Oenothera* is thought to derive from Greek *oinos*, meaning 'wine', and *thera*, meaning 'hunt'. The plant was believed to increase the desire for wine, yet was also thought to dispel the effects of over-indulgence. The native Americans used to eat the leaves and roots as vegetables.

PRINCIPAL CONSTITUENTS
Fixed oil: essential fatty acids, especially gammalinoleic acid (GLA).

HERBAL MEDICINE
The leaves and outer flower stems are mildly sedative, mucilaginous and antispasmodic. Infusions were once used to treat asthma, whooping cough, diarrhoea, nervous indigestion and colic. The cooled infusion makes a soothing skin lotion for itchy skin rashes. The fixed oil (from the seed) has been subject to much scientific investigation and has proved beneficial for many conditions including eczema, psoriasis, various allergies, acne, alcohol withdrawal symptoms, multiple sclerosis (MS), PMS, rheumatoid arthritis and high blood pressure, also as a preventative of coronary artery disease. Its principal ingredient, GLA, is a precursor of a hormone-like substance called PGEI which has many desirable effects on the mind/body complex. The oil is usually taken in capsule form as a nutritional supplement.

HOMEOPATHY
The remedy (prepared from the fresh flowers, leaves and stems) is indicated for diarrhoea, especially if there is also dizziness, light-headedness, prickling of the skin, palpitations or fever.

FLOWER THERAPY
The variety used for the Californian (FES) flower essence is the closely related *O. hookeri*. The flowers are collected during summer and potentised using the Sun Method. The remedy is for those who feel rejected and unwanted, resulting in avoidance of commitment in relationships.

CULTIVATION AND COLLECTION
In early autumn, sprinkle the tiny seeds over the surface of a well-prepared seed bed where the plants are to grow, and water them in using a watering can with a fine spray. Do not thin the young plants for they grow best *en masse*. Evening primrose thrives in any well-drained soil in a sunny position and seeds itself readily. Collect the leaves and stems in summer and use fresh.

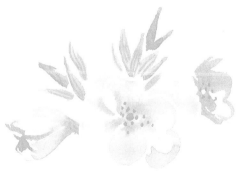

OLEA EUROPAEA

OLIVE

Family: Oleaceae (Olive Family)
Parts Used: fixed oil (from the fruit), flowers (flower therapy), fruit, leaves

DESCRIPTION AND HABITAT
(See illustration, page 181)
A slow-growing evergreen tree growing up to 6m tall, with numerous thin branches. The leathery, lanceolate leaves, carried in opposite pairs, are pale green above and silvery on the underside. The flowers, which appear in clusters of twenty or thirty, are very small with four creamy white petals. These are followed by the well-known olives, which contain a hard stone surrounded by edible, oily flesh. They are at first green, ripening to purple-black. The olive tree is native to the hot Mediterranean lands, but is cultivated in many parts of the world with a similar climate. It can be found growing wild in exposed dry places.

HISTORY
The olive has long been associated with peace and reconciliation. Noah's dove returned to the ark bringing an olive branch in its beak, and so the tree is also symbolic of hope and renewal. The Greeks – to whom their patron goddess Pallas Athene had brought the olive at the same time as the fig – made it their symbol of wisdom and so honoured it that only chaste men and virgins were allowed to grow it. The ancients made great use of olive oil in their food and in skin care.

PRINCIPAL CONSTITUENTS
Leaves: bitters, alkaloids. Oil: notably glycerides of oleic acid.

HERBAL MEDICINE
For constipation take a tablespoon of olive oil first thing in the morning, or stir it into soup eaten in the evening (taken in this way it is easily tolerated). Externally, the oil is useful for dehydrated, sore or inflamed skin, for the prevention of stretch marks during pregnancy and for reducing the itchiness of pruritis. The oil is also a natural sun filter, screening out, on average, up to 20 per cent of the sun's rays. It also makes an excellent massage oil for rheumatic aches and pains (with or without the addition of essential oil). The leaves possess substances which lower both high blood pressure and high blood sugar levels. The leaves are also astringent and febrifuge, and so the cooled decoction can be applied in cold compresses for fevers and for healing wounds.

AROMATHERAPY
Unrefined olive oil (labelled 'extra virgin') can be used as a base for essential oils. However, you may prefer to dilute it 50/50 (or more) with a less odorous oil, such as sweet almond. The pungent aroma of olive oil blends well with herbaceous and citrus essences, for example bergamot, lavender, lemon, marjoram, orange, and rosemary.

FLOWER THERAPY
Gather the flowering clusters from *wild* trees (such as those found in Crete) and potentise using the Sun method. It is for those who are so totally exhausted that their daily life is without pleasure (see page 71).

CULINARY USES
Use the unrefined extra virgin grade, which is obtained from the first cold pressing of the fruit. It can be used in cooking and as a salad dressing. Black or green olives are an indispensable ingredient in many Mediterranean dishes.

CULTIVATION AND COLLECTION
Olives can only be grown in hot, dry climates. The fruit is collected when still green, or once it has ripened to purple-black. The leaves are used fresh or dried.

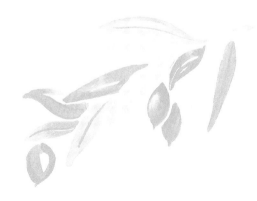

ORIGANUM MARJORANA

MARJORAM, SWEET

Family: Lamiaceae/Labiatae (Mint Family) **Synonym:** Knotted Marjoram
Parts Used: flowering tops, flowers (flower therapy), leaves

DESCRIPTION AND HABITAT
(See illustration, page 181)
A low-growing, bushy herb with branched stems. The greyish leaves are opposite, oval and short-stalked. The small, white or purplish two-lipped flowers are arranged in roundish clusters ('knots') in the leaf axils. The fruit consists of four smooth nutlets, which ripen only in warm regions. All parts of the plant are aromatic. Sweet marjoram is native to the Mediterranean, West Africa and south-west Asia.

HISTORY
The name *Origanum* is derived from the Greek *oros ganos*, which means 'joy of the mountains'. The Romans introduced the plant to Britain, mainly as a preserving and disinfectant herb.

PRINCIPAL CONSTITUENTS
Essential oil (including terpinenes, terpineol, sabinenes, linalol, carvacrol, linalyl acetate, geranyl acetate, citral, eugenol), tannins, bitter compounds, carotenes and vitamin C.

HERBAL MEDICINE
The herb has stomachic, carminative, choleretic, antispasmodic and weak sedative properties. Infusions are used for various gastrointestinal disorders and to aid digestion. It is also helpful for colds, flu, headaches and nervous tension. Incorporated into ointments and bath preparations, the herb can be used to ease rheumatic and muscular aches and pains.

AROMATHERAPY
The essential oil is captured by steam distillation of the dried flowering herb. It is a light amber liquid with a warm, woody, camphoraceous aroma. The odour effect is warming and calming; a reputed anaphrodisiac (quells sexual desire). It is helpful for chilblains, bruises, arthritis, muscular aches and pains, rheumatism, sprains and strains, respiratory ailments, colic, constipation, delayed menstruation, painful periods, PMS, insomnia, migraine, nervous tension and stress-related disorders. Marjoram blends well with bergamot, eucalyptus, juniper berry, lavender, rosemary and tea tree.

FLOWER THERAPY
Collect the flowers during early summer and potentise using the Sun Method. Marjoram is used for calming and soothing the nerves. It is also for those who harbour fear or a mistrust of life. The remedy engenders receptivity to the healing forces of nature.

HOMEOPATHY
The remedy is rarely used in modern homeopathy. However, according to Boericke in *Homoeopathic Materia Medica* of 1910, it is for powerful lascivious impulses in females, such as erotic dreams, masturbation and a desire for active exercise!

CULINARY USES
The herb will endure prolonged heat and is used to flavour stews, casseroles and roasts. The French use the dried herb to enhance the flavour of delicate vegetables such as cucumber and salsify, and also carrots. It blends well with basil for enhancing the flavour of tomato dishes.

CULTIVATION AND COLLECTION
Although the plant is hardy in its native habitat, it is susceptible to frosts so may have to be treated as a half-hardy annual. The seed is sown indoors in early spring, or outside in early summer. Sweet marjoram thrives in well-drained soil in a sunny position.

CAUTION

The essential oil is best avoided during pregnancy due to its ability to promote menstruation. However, the plant is safe if taken in normal amounts as a culinary herb.

PELARGONIUM GRAVEOLENS

GERANIUM

Family: Geraniaceae (Geranium Family) **Synonyms:** Pelargonium, Rose Geranium
Parts Used: essential oil, flowers (flower therapy), leaves

DESCRIPTION AND HABITAT
(See illustration, page 181)
A perennial shrub 1m high, with a spreading, branching habit. The leaves are palmate, deeply lobed and toothed. The small, rose-pink flowers have a dark purple spot on the upper two petals and appear in clusters in midsummer. The whole plant emanates a piercing floral scent, especially if a leaf is bruised. A native of South Africa, it is cultivated throughout the world for ornamental purposes. *P. graveolens* is among the few species cultivated for essential oil production, the highest-quality oil coming from the Indian Ocean island of Reunion.

HISTORY
The name derives from Greek *pelargos*, meaning 'stork', whose head and bill the seed head resembles; *graveolens* means 'aromatic' or 'strong-smelling'. Pelargoniums were introduced into Europe in the early 1600s as ornamentals, and in 1819 the French chemist Recluz first distilled the leaves for the essential oil.

PRINCIPAL CONSTITUENTS
Essential oil (including citronellol, geraniol, linalol, menthone, phellandrene, limonene)

HERBAL MEDICINE
The rose geranium is rarely used, though the distantly related wild species herb Robert (*Geranium robertianum*) and the American cranesbill (*G. maculatum*) have been employed since antiquity. They are primarily astringent, antihaemorrhagic, anti-inflammatory and vulnerary. Decoctions of the root are used for inflammations, heavy periods, dysentery and haemorrhoids.

AROMATHERAPY
The essential oil is extracted by steam distillation of the leaves, stalk and flowers. It is a greenish liquid with a piercing, sweet, rosy aroma, often with an unexpected hint of mint whose effect is refreshing and uplifting. It is helpful for skin care (for most skin types), burns, eczema, headlice, ringworm, neuralgia, haemorrhoids, poor circulation, engorgement of the breasts, menopausal problems, PMS, nervous tension and stress-related disorders. Geranium blends well with citrus essences, clary sage, coriander, jasmine, juniper, lavender, neroli, patchouli, petitgrain, rosemary and sandalwood.

FLOWER THERAPY
Gather the flowers in midsummer and potentise using the Sun Method. The remedy is for those who feel the need to engender a sense of joy and frivolity.

HOMEOPATHY
The species used is *Geranium maculatum* or cranesbill. The remedy mirrors the herbal uses; other symptoms for which it is used include dizziness with double vision, dryness of the mouth, burning at the tip of the tongue, and inability to empty the bowels despite a constant desire to do so.

CULINARY USES
Infusions of rose geranium leaves can be used to flavour ice cream and fruit salads.

CULTIVATION
It is easiest to obtain young plants from a garden centre. They grow well either in pots or the ground, in full sun in well-drained soil. The plant is tender and should be brought indoors before the first frosts. To increase stock, take cuttings in summer; they root very easily.

CAUTION
The oil is highly odoriferous and should be used in low concentration.

PINUS SYLVESTRIS

PINE, SCOTS

Family: Pinaceae (Pine Family) **Synonyms:** Scotch Pine, Scotch Fir
Parts Used: flowers (flower therapy), fresh needles, green cones (essential oil), leaf buds of young shoots

DESCRIPTION AND HABITAT

(See illustration, page 181)
A tall, evergreen conifer rising over 35m. The crown is at first conical, later becoming distinctively flattened. The bark is reddish brown and flaky towards the top of the trunk; grey or brown, roughly furrowed and cracking lower down. The leaves are bluish green needles. Male and female flowers occur on the same tree: males are a cluster of small yellow balls at the base of the new shoot, whereas females are red, cone-shaped and appear at the end of the new growth. When the female cones are ripe, after two or three years, the scales open to release the winged seeds. All parts of the tree contain resin from which turpentine is derived. Scots pine is native to northern and western Europe (including Britain) and parts of Russia, especially mountainous areas.

HISTORY

The species name, *sylvestris*, means 'of the woods'. The Ancient Egyptians prescribed the resin for respiratory diseases. Hippocrates used it for pneumonia. The Arabs extolled its virtues as a specific for 'ulcers of the lungs' (tuberculosis).

PRINCIPAL CONSTITUENTS

Essential oil (including bornyl acetate, citral, cadinene, dipentene, phelladrene, pinene, sylvestrene), vitamin C (in fresh material), tannin, resin, fatty acids.

HERBAL MEDICINE

Pine is expectorant, antiseptic, diuretic, stimulant and tonic. Decoctions of the needles, buds or cones (or a combination) help bronchial complaints, cystitis, rheumatism and arthritis. A double-strength decoction added to the bath eases muscular aches and pains, fatigue and nervous exhaustion. It can also be used as a steam inhalant for colds and sinusitis, as a gargle for laryngitis and as a hot compress for rheumatic and arthritic pain.

AROMATHERAPY

The essential oil is extracted by steam distillation of the needles. An inferior oil is extracted from the cones, twigs and wood chippings, but is not recommended for aromatherapy. The oil is a colourless to pale yellow liquid, its aroma strong, dry and balsamic with a camphoraceous undertone – the effect is refreshing, cooling and enlivening. Pine is helpful for cuts and abrasions, wounds, headlice, excessive perspiration, scabies, muscular aches and pains, arthritis, rheumatism, poor circulation, respiratory ailments, cystitis, colds and flu, neuralgia, fatigue and stress-related disorders. It blends well with bergamot, cedarwood, eucalyptus, frankincense, juniper, lavender, lemon, rosemary and tea tree.

FLOWER THERAPY

Collect the male and female flowers along with a few twigs in late spring, and potentise by using the Boiling Method. Pine is for those who harbour guilt, even when they are not to blame (see page 71).

HOMEOPATHY

Generally, the homeopathic remedy mirrors the herbal uses. It is also prescribed for children who have emaciated legs and weak ankles and are late walking. There may also be a sensation that the chest is thin and about to give way. Emotional symptoms include anxiety, despondency and an inability to think clearly, with perhaps a tendency to undertake tasks which remain uncompleted.

CULTIVATION AND COLLECTION

Sowing seed is the only means of propagation. It is collected from the ripe, woody cones and sown outdoors in late spring. The trees need acidic conditions and thrive in peaty soils provided the roots are not waterlogged. They also thrive in lighter, rocky soil on an exposed site.

CAUTION

The oil should be avoided by those with sensitive skin. Since it is very potent, always use in the lowest recommended concentrations.

ROSA CANINA

ROSE, WILD

Family: Rosaceae (Rose Family) *Synonym:* Dog Rose
Parts Used: flowers, hips, leaves

DESCRIPTION AND HABITAT
(See illustration, page 182)
A deciduous shrub reaching up to 3m, with graceful, arching stems covered in large, hooked thorns shaped like a dog's tooth. The leaves are composed of two to three pairs of leaflets with serrated edges. The white or pink five-petalled, sweetly scented flowers appear in abundance in midsummer, followed by bright red hips which ripen in early winter. The wild rose is common in woodlands and hedgerows on most soils throughout Europe.

HISTORY
Some sources suggest that *Rosa* is derived from ancient Celtic *rhod*, to denote a plant of little worth. Another suggestion is that the roots were used to cure the effects of being bitten by a rabid dog. The shrub is said to be extremely long-lived: one growing in a convent garden at Hildesheim in Germany is said to have been planted by a son of Charlemagne in AD 850.

PRINCIPAL CONSTITUENTS
Hips: vitamin C (up to 1 per cent), carotenes, vitamin B complex, sugars, pectin, tannins, maltic and citric acids, fixed oil.

HERBAL MEDICINE
Rose leaves are mildly laxative and diuretic. The cooled infusion can be applied as a wash to promote the healing of wounds, and as an astringent for oily skin. The petals are anti-inflammatory, astringent and decongestant. Infusions are employed for diarrhoea, coughs, colds and flu, and heavy, painful or irregular periods. Rose is used for inflamed skin: infusions of petals can be taken internally and/or applied as a wash. The hips are widely used for their tonic, astringent, mild diuretic and mild laxative effects. When fresh, they are an excellent source of vitamin C. Fresh or dried, they are beneficial for convalescents, against exhaustion and colds. Traditionally, rosehip tea is taken in spring to cleanse the blood. It is also a gentle tonic for the kidneys and gall bladder. A decoction from the hips makes a gargle for bleeding gums.

FLOWER THERAPY
The Bach remedy Wild Rose is prepared by the Boiling Method. Collect the flowerheads with a short length of stalk and a few leaves in midsummer. It is used for apathy and joylessness (see page 73).

CULINARY USES
A syrup can be made from the fresh hips to pour over sweet dishes like ice-cream or fruit salads. The sweetened puree may be spread on bread like jam or added to cereals. Two excellent country wines are made from the hips and petals.

CULTIVATION AND COLLECTION
Propagate by hardwood cuttings taken in autumn. Alternatively sow seed in spring, gathered from the previous autumn's hips: it will grow in any well-drained soil in full sun or partial shade. Collect leaves and flowers in midsummer, when the flowers are still in bud, and the hips once softened by the first frosts of autumn.

CAUTION

Rosehips are full of downy seeds which tickle the skin (and the throat if swallowed), so must be scraped out before using. The herb (not the flower remedy) has a stimulating effect upon the uterus and should be avoided during pregnancy.

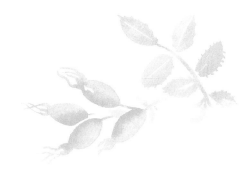

ROSA SPP: DAMASK ROSE R. DAMASCENA, CABBAGE ROSE R. CENTIFOLIA

ROSE

Family: Rosaceae (Rose Family) *Parts Used:* essential oil, flowers, hips, leaves, rosewater

DESCRIPTION AND HABITAT

(See illustration, page 182)

Most of the numerous roses in cultivation have medical and culinary uses. Those featured here are valued for their high-quality essential oil and rosewater. *R. damascena* is, like all roses, a deciduous shrub; it has prickly stems growing to about 1.5m tall, and whitish, hairy leaves. The 36-petalled pink flowers are richly fragrant. *R. centifolia* reaches 2.5m and has almost thornless stems. The many-petalled large and pink flowers are followed by bright red hips. The damask rose is native to Syria, but cultivated mostly in Bulgaria and Turkey for its essential oil. The birthplace of the cabbage rose is said to be ancient Persia; it is now cultivated mainly in Morocco, Tunisia, Italy, France and China for its essential oil.

HISTORY

Roses have been loved by all peoples and cultures. The Greek poetess Sappho crowned it 'The Queen of Flowers'. Rosewater was the favourite scent of the Persians and Arabs. Up to the Middle Ages roses were regarded as a panacea, and still play an important role in Eastern medicine. Traditionally the rose is symbolic of love and beauty.

PRINCIPAL CONSTITUENTS

Tannins, glycosides, pigments, essential oil (including citronellol, geraniol, nerol, phenyl ethanol, farnesol).

HERBAL MEDICINE

The flowers, leaves and hips have similar properties to those of the wild rose (see page 199). Rosewater is used by herbalists and aromatherapists to cleanse and tone all skin types, and can be incorporated into home-made skin-softening creams. It can also be used to bathe sore eyes.

AROMATHERAPY

There are two types of oil commonly available: rose otto, obtained by steam distillation of the fresh flowers, and rose absolute, obtained by solvent extraction of the fresh flowers (see also rose phytol, page 38). The distilled otto is preferred for aromatherapy (rosewater is a by-product of distillation); rose otto is virtually colourless and semi-solid at cool temperatures. The aroma is sweet and mellow with a hint of cloves and vanilla. Rose absolute is a dark yellow liquid with a rich sweet aroma, but it lacks the spicy/vanilla nuance of rose otto. The odour effect of both oils is warming and intoxicating, and reputedly aphrodisiac. Rose is helpful for skin care, eczema, palpitations, respiratory ailments, liver congestion, nausea, heavy periods, irregular periods, depression, insomnia, headache, PMS, nervous tension and other stress-related ailments. Both the otto and absolute blends well with cedarwood, citrus and floral oils, coriander, chamomile (German and Roman), clary sage, frankincense, jasmine, petitgrain, sandalwood and ylang ylang. Rose otto is highly odoriferous, so use sparingly.

HOMEOPATHY

R. damascena is used for hayfever, especially if the condition is accompanied by impaired hearing.

FLOWER THERAPY

Generally, red roses increase self-confidence and the ability to give and receive love; white roses engender inspiration and joy; pink roses heal a broken heart; while yellow roses transmute jealousy and resentment into positive self-acceptance.

CULINARY USES

Crystallised rose petals can be used as edible decorations. Rosewater sweetened with honey is delicious in fruit salads, and is used to flavour many Middle Eastern dishes.

CULTIVATION AND COLLECTION

Propagation is as for wild rose (page 199), except that most cultivated roses prefer an open, sunny site and a humus-rich soil. Collect fully open flowers in midsummer. The leaves are collected in spring, the hips when softened by the first frosts of autumn.

CAUTION

Rose exerts a stimulating effect upon the uterus, so both herb and oil should be avoided during pregnancy.

ROSMARINUS OFFICINALIS

ROSEMARY

Family: Lamiaceae/Labiatae (Mint Family)
Parts Used: essential oil, flowers (flower therapy), leaves, stems

DESCRIPTION AND HABITAT
(See illustration, page 182)
An evergreen, woody shrub with many upright branched stems, reaching 1.5m and more. The opposite leaves are simple, leathery, linear, dark green above and white-felted on the underside. The bluish, two-lipped flowers resemble tiny irises. All parts are strongly aromatic. Rosemary is native to the Mediterranean but cultivated throughout the world.

HISTORY
The name is derived from Latin *rosmarinus* or *ros maris*, 'dew of the sea', because it grew close to the sea. Since classical times it has had associations with the mind and improving the memory. Garlands of rosemary were worn by Ancient Greek students taking exams. Rosemary has therefore come to symbolise remembrance and fidelity.

PRINCIPAL CONSTITUENTS
Essential oil (including pinenes, camphene, limonene, cineol, borneol with camphor, linalol, terpineol, bornyl acetate), flavonoids, tannins, resin, organic acids, saponin, bitters.

HERBAL MEDICINE
Rosemary is rubifacient, cardiotonic, antirheumatic, diuretic, stomachic, nervine, a circulatory stimulant, cholagogic, tonic, antispasmodic and antiseptic. Infusions are helpful for jaundice, debility, headaches, flatulence, gallstones, low blood pressure, painful periods, poor circulation and mental fatigue. Applied as a compress, it promotes the healing of wounds.

AROMATHERAPY
The oil is obtained by steam distillation of the flowering tops. It is a colourless to pale yellow liquid with a camphoraceous, woody-balsamic aroma. The odour effect is refreshing and head-clearing, yet warming and invigorating; a reputed aphrodisiac. Rosemary is helpful for skin and hair care (oily) and the promotion of healthy hair growth; it is also effective in dealing with headlice, scabies, respiratory ailments, muscular aches and pains, rheumatism, poor circulation, painful menstruation, colds and flu, headaches, mental fatigue, depression and nervous exhaustion, as well as being an insect repellent. It blends well with basil, cedarwood, citrus essences, coriander, frankincense, lavender, peppermint, petitgrain and pine.

FLOWER THERAPY
Collect the flowers in early summer and potentise by the Sun Method. Rosemary is for those who tend to be forgetful and absent-minded. Their feet and hands may often be cold. The flower essence imparts a sense of revitalisation.

HOMEOPATHY
The remedy is used for uterine bleeding, especially if accompanied by a heavy sensation in the head, icy extremities and deficient memory.

CULINARY USES
The pungent-tasting herb is used to flavour roasts, casseroles and baked fish, and blends well with garlic.

CULTIVATION AND COLLECTION
Rosemary can be propagated from semi-ripe cuttings in late summer. Alternatively, it can be obtained from most nurseries. Grow it in a sheltered, sunny location in well-drained soil, and protect from frosts. Sprigs for home use can be picked all year round. It can also be dried and stored in the usual way.

CAUTION

Avoid rosemary during pregnancy, as it has a stimulating effect upon the uterus. There is a chance that it may trigger an epileptic attack in those who have this condition. Rosemary oil may irritate sensitive skin, so use only in low to medium concentrations.

SALVIA OFFICINALIS

SAGE

Family: Lamiaceae/Labiatae (Mint Family) **Synonyms:** Common Sage, Garden Sage, Red Sage
Parts Used: essential oil, flowers (flower therapy), leaves, stems

DESCRIPTION AND HABITAT
(See illustration, page 182)
An evergreen shrub growing up to 75cm tall. The greyish green leaves are opposite, oblong to oval or lanceolate, with a wrinkled appearance and texture. The stems are woody at the base, becoming soft towards the tips. The two-lipped flowers are bluish violet, reddish violet or white, arranged in clusters near the stem tips. All parts of the plant are strongly aromatic. Sage is native to northern coastal areas of the Mediterranean, but widely cultivated throughout the world.

HISTORY
The generic name, *Salvia*, derives from the Latin word *salvere*, meaning 'to be in good spirits'. The old French word *saulje* (also from *salvere* through *salvia*) has given us the modern English name. Sage was traditionally used as an aid to conception. To the Romans it was *herba sacra* or 'sacred herb'. In the Middle Ages there was an Arabic saying: 'Why should a man die when there is sage in his garden?'

PRINCIPAL CONSTITUENTS
Essential oil (including thujone, cineol, borneol, caryophyllene, linalool, camphors, salvene), oestrogenic substances, salvin, organic acids, flavonoids, tannins, bitter compounds.

HERBAL MEDICINE
Sage has many actions, including antiseptic, antifungal, astringent, diuretic, carminative and antispasmodic. It is fortifying to the nervous system, and has the ability to reduce sweating. It can also reduce the flow of breast milk. Infusions are helpful for colds and flu, nervous exhaustion, menopausal symptoms (e.g. hot flushes and night sweats), vaginal thrush and irregular periods. It is also highly beneficial as a gargle for sore throats, laryngitis and tonsillitis.

As a mouthwash it can be used for gum infections and mouth ulcers, or simply to keep teeth white.

AROMATHERAPY
Best avoided (see CAUTION)

FLOWER THERAPY
The flowers are collected during early summer and potentised using the Sun Method. Sage is for those seeking to find purpose and meaning in life. The remedy facilitates awareness of the inner voice of wisdom.

HOMEOPATHY
Like the material remedy, the homeopathic potency is a specific for night sweats.

CULINARY USES
The combination of sage and onion for stuffing poultry is well known. The finely chopped leaves can also be added to salads, pickles and cheese.

CULTIVATION AND COLLECTION
Sage can be grown from seed, although it is easily propagated by cuttings taken in spring from well-established plants, and planted well spaced directly into their permanent positions. Sage should be harvested before the flower spikes are produced. It takes longer to dry than other herbs, and will discolour if dried too quickly over a high heat.

CAUTION

The essential oil is unsuitable for aromatherapy due to high levels of the potentially toxic thujone. Clary sage is a safe alternative.

SALVIA SCLAREA

CLARY SAGE

Family: Labiatae/Lamiaceae (Mint Family)
Parts Used: essential oil, flowering stems, leaves

DESCRIPTION AND HABITAT
(See illustration, page 182)
A biennial herb with an erect, sparsely branched stem up to 1m high. The large leaves are broadly egg-shaped, wrinkled and serrated. The white, violet or pink two-lipped flowers are arranged in whorls at the end of the stem. All parts of the plant are strongly aromatic and hairy. Clary is native to the Mediterranean but has long been cultivated elsewhere as an ornamental plant.

HISTORY
The generic name, *Salvia*, derives from the Latin *salvus* (safe) referring to the plant's medicinal properties; *sclarea* is from *clarus* (clear) after the ancient use of the mucilaginous seeds to clear the eyesight.

PRINCIPAL CONSTITUENTS
Essential oil (including linalyl acetate, linalol, pinene, myrcene, phellandrene), tannins, bitter compounds.

HERBAL MEDICINE
The plant has tonic, astringent, cooling, carminative, antispasmodic and emmenagogic properties. Infusions of the leaves are helpful for digestive upsets, flatulence, diarrhoea, fevers and menstrual disorders such as painful or scanty periods.

AROMATHERAPY
The essential oil is captured by stream distillation of the flowering tops and leaves. The oil is a pale yellowish-green liquid with a sweet, musky-herbaceous aroma whose effect is uplifting, cooling and relaxing – a reputed aphrodisiac. It is helpful for high blood pressure, PMS, muscular aches and pains, respiratory problems, headaches, irregular periods, painful periods, depression and nervous tension. The oil is also used to ease childbirth (massaged into the lower back and/or vaporised). Clary sage blends well with bergamot, frankincense, jasmine, juniper berry, lavender, neroli, petitgrain and pine.

CULINARY USES
The essential oil is used commercially to flavour wine, vermouths and liqueurs. The leaves are occasionally used as a culinary herb to flavour soups and casseroles.

CULTIVATION AND COLLECTION
It grows best in fertile, well-drained soil in full sun. Sow the seeds during late spring in shallow drills. Once the seedlings are large enough to handle, plant them in a sunny position. Clary blooms in the second year. Collect the flowering tops and/or leaves during mid- to late summer and use fresh or dried.

CAUTION

Both the herb and essential oil stimulate the uterus and should be avoided during pregnancy.

SAMBUCUS NIGRA

ELDER

Family: Caprifoliaceae (Honeysuckle Family)
Parts Used: bark, flowers, fruits, leaves

DESCRIPTION AND HABITAT
(See illustration, page 183)
A deciduous shrub or small tree up to 8m tall with arched branches and greyish-brown, furrowed, corky bark. The dark green, unpleasant smelling lanceolate leaves are grouped in fives. The small creamy white flowers are arranged in flat-topped umbels, and when newly open and warmed by the sun emanate a pleasant musky fragrance. The fruits are purple-black berries on red stalks. Elder, native to Europe, western Asia and North Africa, is common in hedgerows and copses, on the edges of woods and near dwellings.

HISTORY
The common name probably derives from the Anglo-Saxon *ellaern* or *aeid*, meaning 'fire', for the stems were used for kindling. They were also used to make musical pipes, including the *sanbuk*, hence its botanical name *Sambucus*. Elder was planted near dwellings for it was believed to protect against black magic.

PRINCIPAL CONSTITUENTS
Flowers: a trace of essential oil (containing palmitic, linoleic and linolenic acids), triterpenes, flavonoids, pectin, mucilage, sugar. Berries: sugar, fruit acids, vitamin C, bioflavonoids. Leaves: cyanogenic glycosides, tannins, resins, fats, sugars, fatty acids. Bark: resin, viburnic acid, tannins, pectin, various alkaline salts.

HERBAL MEDICINE
The flowers are diaphoretic and anticatarrhal. Infusions are helpful for colds and flu, sinusitis, hayfever, migraine and insomnia, and as a gargle for sore throats. The cooled infusion makes a good skin tonic for most skin types and can also be used as an eyewash for conjunctivitis. The berries are diaphoretic, diuretic and laxative. Decoctions of fresh berries, sweetened with honey, are helpful for coughs, colds, constipation and rheumatism. Externally, the leaves are emollient and vulnerary; internally, they are purgative, expectorant, diruetic and diaphoretic (see Cautions). Infusions of the fresh leaves can be used as a compress or incorporated into an ointment and applied to bruises, sprains and chilblains.

FLOWER THERAPY
Collect the flowers during midsummer and potentise using the Sun Method. The remedy is for those who feel they are being psychically 'invaded'.

HOMEOPATHY
The remedy is primarily indicated for respiratory ailments, accompanied by constant fretfulness and timidity. Disturbing images may also arise when the eyes are shut.

CULINARY USES
The flowers and fruit make two very different wines. Elderflowers can also be made into fritters, or used to flavour gooseberries, baked pears and rhubarb.

CULTIVATION AND COLLECTION
The plant can be propagated from hardwood cuttings in late autumn. Alternatively, raise from seed sown thickly outside in late winter. A year later transplant to a permanent site in full sun or partial shade, damp if possible. The flowers are collected in spring and early summer and used fresh or dried. The leaves are collected throughout the growing season and used fresh. Pick the fully ripened berries in late summer and use fresh or dried.

> ## CAUTION
> *Preparations of the leaves and bark are strongly purgative and should never be used internally for self-medication.*

TARAXACUM OFFICINALE

DANDELION

Family: Compositae/Asteraceae (Daisy Family)
Parts Used: flowers, latex, leaves, roots

DESCRIPTION AND HABITAT
(See illustration, page 183)
A perennial herb up to 60cm tall with a long taproot. It has a basal rosette of hairless, dark green leaves with toothed edges. The familiar bright yellow flowers are followed by the 'clock' – a ball of wispy, plumed seeds that can travel up to 8 kilometres on the wind. All parts of the plant secrete a latex or milky juice. Dandelion is a native of Europe and Asia and a common weed of grassland, gardens and waste places. It has been introduced in many countries, including North America and Australia.

HISTORY
The common name is a corruption, through the French *dent de lion* (lion's tooth), of the medieval Latin *dens leonis*, after the jagged edge on the leaves. *Taraxacum* derives from the Greek *taraxos* and *achos*, meaning, respectively, 'disorder' and 'remedy'. In Tudor times the plant was nick-named piss-a-bed, referring to its diuretic ability.

PRINCIPAL CONSTITUENTS
Root: bitter principle (taraxacin), triterpenes, sterols, inulin, sugars, pectin, glycosides, choline, phenolic acids, tannins, potassium, latex. Leaves: lutein, carotenoids, bitter principles, vitamins (A, B, C, D), potassium, iron. Flowers: carotenoids, triterpenes.

HERBAL MEDICINE
Dandelion is stomachic, laxative, diuretic, cholagogic and nutritive. Infusions of the root can be used for painful indigestion, constipation, liver disorders, rheumatism, arthritis and fluid retention (including premenstrual bloating). Conventional diuretics leach potassium from the body, but dandelion maintains the natural mineral balance. Boiled with honey, the flowers make a soothing cough syrup. Applications of the latex pressed from the stalks are said to remove warts.

FLOWER THERAPY
The flowers are collected in midsummer and potentised using the Sun Method. The remedy is for those who suffer physical and emotional tension manifesting in the muscles, often as a result of prolonged distress (particularly grief) or overstriving.

HOMEOPATHY
The homeopathic remedy mirrors the herbal uses. It is also indicated for muscular pain of the neck and shoulders, aching limbs and neuralgia (nerve pain) of the knee.

CULINARY USES
The young leaves are good in salads, or they can be cooked like spinach. Dandelion 'coffee' can be made from the roots, dried, roasted and ground. The flowers make an excellent country wine.

COLLECTION AND CULTIVATION
The roots are best dug up in late summer. Split them longitudinally before drying in a warm, dark place. The leaves and flowers are best collected between mid-spring and late summer. Being a prolific weed, dandelion is not usually cultivated. On the contrary, most gardeners would like to know how to eradicate it!

TILIA CORDATA

LINDEN

Family: Tiliaceae (Lime Family) **Synonyms:** Small-Leaved Lime
Parts Used: flowers (linden/lime blossom)

DESCRIPTION AND HABITAT
(See illustration, page 183)
A tall deciduous tree reaching up to 30m, with a domed crown and downward-curving branches. The twigs grow in a zig-zag fashion, with prominent swollen buds set alternately at each bend. The bark is smooth and grey, becoming darker and fissured as the tree ages. The heart-shaped leaves are dark green above and paler beneath. The fruits are nut-like, the size of a pea, containing one to three seeds. The fragrant, creamy white flowers are borne in loose clusters during early summer. Linden is a woodland tree native to Europe, Siberia and Asia, though it is cultivated in other parts of the world as an ornamental.

HISTORY
The species name *cordata* refers to the heart-shaped leaves. The common names, 'lime' or 'linden', are derived from the Anglo-Saxon *lind*, a derivative of an Indo-European word meaning pliable: the inner bark fibres were once used for producing ropes and matting.

PRINCIPAL CONSTITUENTS
Essential oil (mainly farnesol), mucilage, flavonoid glycosides, courmarin, tannins, saponins, sugars.

HERBAL MEDICINE
Linden blossom is diaphoretic, antispasmodic, diuretic, hypotensive and mildly sedative. Infusions are used for calming the nerves, and for alleviating headaches, digestive upsets and respiratory catarrh. The remedy is also considered a specific for lowering raised blood pressure and easing palpitations. It is helpful for feverish conditions such as colds and flu.

AROMATHERAPY
A costly absolute can be obtained from the flowers and is used in the creation of high-class perfumes. It is a yellow semi-solid mass with a sweet, hay-like aroma. Unfortunately it is extremely difficult to find an unadulterated product, so it is rarely used in aromatherapy. However, the modified versions can be used solely for pleasure, as a personal perfume or heady room scent.

FLOWER THERAPY
Collect the flowers during midsummer and potentise using the Sun Method. Linden is used for developing receptivity to love. The remedy brings out nurturing qualities, engenders a sense of quietude and strengthens the relationship between mother and child.

HOMEOPATHY
The homeopathic remedy is prepared from the closely related *T. europa* or common lime. It is used for problems such as neuralgia, vaginal discharge, pelvic inflammation, intense itching and muscular weakness of the eyes.

CULINARY USES
The tisane can be enjoyed hot or iced, sweetened with honey.

CULTIVATION AND COLLECTION
Lime trees can be grown from seed if you are very patient, though it is best to obtain a young plant from a tree nursery. Plant in a sunny or semi-shaded position in moist loam soil. Collect the flower clusters during summer, and spread them out to dry in the dark. They require careful handling and should not be heaped up or pressed down.

TROPAEOLUM MAJUS

NASTURTIUM

Family: Tropaeolaceae (Watercress Family)
Parts Used: flowers, leaves, seeds

DESCRIPTION AND HABITAT
(See illustration, page 183)
A perennial or annual herb with a climbing or twining stem and bright green, umbrella-like leaves. The flowers are brilliant red, orange, yellow and occasionally mahogany red. Although only faintly aromatic, they produce abundant nectar and are much visited by bees. The fruit is a three-celled capsule. At dusk on hot summer days sparks are emitted from the heart of the flower. This strange phenomenon is connected with the plant's high phosphoric acid content. Nasturtium is native to South America, but widely cultivated throughout the world.

HISTORY
The name *Tropaeolum* is from the Greek *tropaion*, meaning 'trophy' – the flowers were thought to resemble helmets and shields, which were displayed as trophies of war. The common name derives from the Latin *nasus tortus*, meaning 'nose torture', because of its peppery aroma. Nasturtiums were introduced into Spain from Peru in the sixteenth century. Gerard mentions receiving seeds from France in 1597.

PRINCIPAL CONSTITUENTS
Vitamins A, C and E, nicotinamide, iron, sulphur, phosphoric acid, a glycoside, essential oil, fatty oil, proteins, trace minerals.

HERBAL MEDICINE
Nasturium is a natural antibiotic. Infusions of the leaves or seeds are helpful for chronic bronchitis and bronchial catarrh. Nasturtium is also a digestive tonic and a circulatory stimulant, making it a useful remedy in convalescence and general debility. It is also helpful for nervous depression and constipation, and for clearing spotty skin. Nasturtium can help certain forms of anaemia due to its high iron and vitamin C content (vitamin C aids the absorption of iron). Some herbalists use the plant for urinary infections such as cystitis. The diluted tincture makes an excellent hair tonic with a reputation for preventing baldness (doubtless because of its appreciable sulphur content).

FLOWER THERAPY
The flowers are collected during high summer and potentised using the Sun Method. Nasturtium is helpful for those who think too much and deplete their vitality; it imparts a sense of *joie de vivre!*

HOMEOPATHY
The remedy is used for disorders of the urinary tract, including cystitis, stones and gravel.

CULINARY USES
The leaves, flowers and seeds can be eaten raw in salads to give a pungent, peppery flavour. The seeds and flower buds can be pickled and used as capers.

CULTIVATION AND COLLECTION
Sow the seed in early spring. The plant seeds itself freely, so once introduced into the garden it soon becomes naturalised. Nasturtium prefers a light, well-drained soil and a sunny position. Although the plant is commonly used fresh, the leaves can be dried for winter use.

VALERIANA OFFICINALIS

VALERIAN

Family: Valerianaceae (Valerian Family)
Parts Used: essential oil, rhizome, roots

DESCRIPTION AND HABITAT
(See illustration, page 184)
An herbaceous perennial reaching up to 1m tall, with a massive root system and a short rhizome which bears erect, furrowed, usually unbranched stems. Slender branches bear pinnate leaves, divided into six to ten segments. The small, funnel-shaped, white or pinkish flowers are carried in loose clusters at the end of the stem. The whole plant has a rancid or 'sweaty' odour if crushed. Valerian is native to northern Asia and Europe, where it can be found in damp meadows and along streams, banks and ditches.

HISTORY
Valerian takes its name from Latin *valere*, meaning 'to be healthy' – a reference to its medicinal value. In the Middle Ages it was used as a sedative for certain kinds of epilepsy. Despite its foul odour, during the sixteenth century the essential oil was a popular perfume – it must have harmonised with the unwashed bodies of the era! Cats are fascinated by the roots and become almost intoxicated if they nibble them.

PRINCIPAL CONSTITUENTS
Essential oil (including bornyl acetate, isovalerate, valeranone, ionone, eugenyl isovalerate, patchouli alcohol), valepotriates, alkaloids, bitter compounds, tannins, resins.

HERBAL MEDICINE
Valerian is sedative, hypnotic, antispasmodic, hypotensive and carminative. It is one of the most useful remedies for nervous tension, anxiety and insomnia, yet it seems to have an enlivening effect on those suffering from fatigue. The remedy is valuable for intestinal colic, irritable bowel syndrome, period pain, rheumatic pain and migraine. It also has a strengthening action on the heart and can be used for palpitations and high blood pressure.

AROMATHERAPY
The essential oil is obtained by steam distillation of the rhizomes. It is a dark brown liquid with a pungent, 'sweaty', musky aroma. While most people find the aroma unpleasant, there are a few who adore it! It is not much used in aromatherapy because of the smell, though in tiny amounts it may be helpful for insomnia, nervous tension, migraine and indigestion – but only if the aroma is liked. Valerian does not blend well with other essences, although the aroma may be slightly improved if blended with bergamot, cedarwood, lavender, lemon, petitgrain, pine or rosemary. Valerian essence is exceptionally odoriferous, so use sparingly.

FLOWER THERAPY
The flowers are collected in the height of summer and potentised by the Sun Method. Valerian is for those who suffer from insomnia and nervous exhaustion. It is also helpful during convalescence.

HOMEOPATHY
The homeopathic remedy mirrors the herbal uses.

CULTIVATION AND COLLECTION
Seeds are slow to germinate and have only a 50 per cent fertility rate. Valerian is generally cultivated by removing rooted runners from the main rhizome, which should be planted in nutrient-rich, damp soil. The roots and rhizomes of second-year plants are used medicinally. They should be dug up in the autumn and dried in the shade.

CAUTION

Valerian should not be taken in strong doses as it may cause headaches, muscular spasm and palpitations.

VERBENA OFFICINALIS

VERVAIN

Family: Verbenaceae (Vervain Family)
Parts Used: flowering tops, flowers (flower therapy)

DESCRIPTION AND HABITAT

(See illustration, page 184)

A hairy perennial up to 80cm tall, with erect, stiff stems. The opposite, dull green leaves are pinnately divided, often with rounded teeth. The small, slightly two-lipped, pale lilac flowers are arranged in long terminal spikes. Vervain is native to most of Europe including southern England and Wales, much of Asia and North Africa. It can be found growing on waste ground and roadside verges and in meadows.

HISTORY

The common name derives from *verbena*, the Latin term for plants used in religious ceremonies. Vervain was revered for its magical powers and remarkable healing properties. Roman soldiers carried it in their packs as an amulet, and lovers used it in love potions. The Druids held it almost as sacred as mistletoe.

PRINCIPAL CONSTITUENTS

Glycosides, tannins, essential oil, mucilage, saponins, organic acid, mineral compounds, a bitter principle (castine).

HERBAL MEDICINE

Vervain is nervine, tonic, sedative, antispasmodic, diaphoretic, galactagogic, hepatic and vulnerary. Infusions of the plant are beneficial for nervous exhaustion, depression, lethargy, tension headaches, migraine, delayed or irregular periods, feverish conditions, poor digestion, diarrhoea, liver disorders, gallstones, fluid retention and gout. It may also be helpful for ME. The herb is said to promote the flow of breast milk. Externally it can be used as a mouthwash or gargle for infected gums and sore throats, and as a compress for wounds.

FLOWER THERAPY

The flowers are collected during high summer and potentised using the Sun Method. Vervain is for strain and tension felt by those who are overenthusiastic and have fixed ideas (see page 72).

CULTIVATION AND COLLECTION

Vervain can be propagated by cuttings or root division. Alternatively, sow the seed under glass in early spring or outdoors in late spring. The plants require a well-drained, rich soil and a sunny position. Collect the flowering tops before the flowers are fully open in midsummer.

CAUTION

Due to its ability to promote menstruation, the herbal remedy is best avoided during pregnancy.

VIOLA ODORATA

VIOLET, SWEET

Family: Violaceae (Violet Family)
Parts Used: flowers, leaves

DESCRIPTION AND HABITAT
(See illustration, page 184)
A perennial plant rising from a thick, creeping rhizome to a height of 15cm. The heart-shaped leaves are arranged in a basal rosette. The flowers are sweetly scented, usually violet but sometimes white or pink. The plant is native to northern Europe and can be found on moist grassy banks, in hedgerows and in deciduous woodlands. There are numerous cultivated varieties.

HISTORY
Viola, the original Latin name, derives from Greek *ion*, meaning 'violet'. It is associated with a legend concerning Zeus and his lover Io, who was turned into a white heifer; the violet was created in honour of her beauty. From *Viola* has come the common name, through the French *violette*. The specific name, *odorata*, means 'fragrant'. Apart from its medicinal, culinary and perfumery uses, the violet was once a popular ingredient in love potions.

PRINCIPAL CONSTITUENTS
Leaves and flowers: essential oil (including nonadienal, parmone, hexyl alcohol, benzyl alcohol, ionone, viola quercitin), saponins, mucilage, glycoside (violarutin), methyl salicylate, organic acids. The flowers also contain anthocyanin pigments.

HERBAL MEDICINE
Violets are cooling, soothing, expectorant, diuretic, anti-inflammatory, antirheumatic, laxative and soporific. Infusions of the leaves and flowers are helpful for bronchitis, coughs (including whooping cough), colds and flu, rheumatic and arthritic pain, constipation, headaches and migraine. Violet flowers are useful for anxiety and insomnia. Externally, the cooled infusion can be applied in compresses to treat swellings, slow-healing wounds, ulcers and rashes. As a mouthwash or gargle it treats inflamed gums and sore throat.

AROMATHERAPY
The solvent-extracted absolute obtained from the leaves is a dark green, viscous liquid with a strong, green-leaf aroma, quite different from that of the flowers. The genuine *floral* absolute is unobtainable because the synthetic version is comparatively cheap to produce. Violet *leaf* absolute is occasionally used for acne, eczema, rheumatic aches and pains, respiratory ailments, anxiety and nervous tension. It blends well with clary sage, hops, lavender, neroli, rose and ylang ylang. Violet leaf absolute is highly odoriferous, so use sparingly.

FLOWER THERAPY
The flowers are collected in early spring and potentised by the Sun Method. However, the spring sunshine in northern Europe is rarely strong enough to potentise the remedy, so it may be necessary to obtain the Californian (FES) Violet flower essence (see page 265). The remedy is for those who are profoundly shy, reserved, aloof and lonely. It engenders the ability to interact with others whilst protecting individuality.

HOMEOPATHY
The remedy mirrors the herbal uses but is especially suited to those who are tense, nervous and excitable, prone to becoming depressed, mentally congested and tearful.

CULINARY USES
Crystallised violets are used as decoration for cakes and desserts; the fresh flowers lend a delicate flavour to salads.

CULTIVATION AND COLLECTION
Violet is usually propagated by cuttings from the previous season's runners. Alternatively, sow the seed in trays in early spring and allow to germinate under glass. Plant in a half-shady position in moist soil enriched with leaf mould. Leaves and flowers for drying are gathered in the spring.

CAUTION

*Never use violet **root**, which in large doses causes vomiting and diarrhoea.*

ZINGIBER OFFICINALE

GINGER

Family: Zingiberaceae (Ginger Family) **Synonym:** Jamaican Ginger
Parts Used: essential oil, rhizome (root), stem

DESCRIPTION AND HABITAT
(See illustration, page 184)
An erect, reed-like perennial with pungent, thick rhizomes. The flower stem grows directly from the rhizome, producing spikes of fragrant white or yellow blooms. Native to southern Asia, ginger is cultivated commercially in the West Indies and Africa.

HISTORY
Ginger was introduced into Europe by Arab traders before the days of the Roman Empire; the Romans later brought it to Britain. Its healing virtues were praised by the Chinese philosopher Confucius (551–479 BC) and the Greek physician Dioscorides.

PRINCIPAL CONSTITUENTS
Essential oil (including zingiberole, phellandrene, borneol, cineole, citral), starch, mucilage, resin.

HERBAL MEDICINE
Ginger is warming, stimulating, carminative, expectorant and febrifuge. Its main uses are for indigestion, flatulence, nausea, poor circulation, colds and flu. As a gargle, it can relieve sore throats. It is also helpful for nausea, including travel and pregnancy sickness (crystallised stem ginger is convenient).

AROMATHERAPY
The essential oil is captured by steam distillation of the dried rhizomes. The pale amber liquid has a pungent, spicy aroma that lacks the fruity nuances detected in the raw plant. The odour effect is warming and stimulating; a reputed aphrodisiac. Ginger is helpful for arthritis, muscular aches and pains, poor circulation, rheumatism, catarrh, coughs, sore throats, diarrhoea, colic, indigestion, loss of appetite, nausea, colds and flu, infectious illness, mental fatigue and nervous exhaustion. It blends well with cedarwood, citrus essences, coriander, neroli, patchouli, petitgrain, rose, sandalwood and ylang ylang.

HOMEOPATHY
The remedy is used for digestive, respiratory and urinary disorders, also impotence and painful erections.

CULINARY USES
Ginger is used extensively in curries and other oriental dishes. It is also used in baking and for brewing ginger beer. The crystallised stems are eaten as a delicacy or in cakes, biscuits and confectionery.

CULTIVATION AND COLLECTION
Ginger needs a hot, wet tropical climate. For medicinal purposes the rhizomes are cleaned and sun-dried, though fresh ginger is sometimes available from supermarkets.

CAUTION

The essential oil may irritate sensitive skin. Use in the lowest concentrations. Also, if applied to skin shortly before exposure to natural or simulated sunlight it may cause pigmentation.

MINOR DIRECTORY

CONTENTS

The plants in this directory are organised alphabetically by their Latin, or botanical name. For ease of reference, common names for plants are referred to in the index and below.

AESCULUS X CARNEA

CHESTNUT, RED

Family: Hippocastanaceae (Horse Chestnut)
Parts Used: flowering twigs (flower therapy)

DESCRIPTION AND HABITAT
(See illustration, page 185)

A hybrid arising from the common horse chestnut (*A. hippocastanum*) and red buckeye (*A. pavia*), a small horse chestnut native to North America. The rose-pink flowers are borne in clusters of upright panicles. Red chestnut is cultivated all over Europe as a shade tree in avenues, parks and gardens.

PRINCIPAL CONSTITUENTS
Data unavailable, though probably similar to *A. hippocastanum* (see Major Directory).

FLOWER THERAPY
Very occasionally the tree can be found growing wild (as a garden escape). However, young specimens can be obtained from good tree and shrub nurseries. Cultivation is the same as for the common chestnut (see page 161). Gather the flowers, twigs and young leaves in early summer and potentise using the Boiling Method. The remedy is for those who are overconcerned for the health and safety of loved ones (see page 68).

AGRIMONIA EUPATORIA

AGRIMONY

Family: *Rosaceae (Rose Family)*
Parts Used: *flowering stems, flowers (flower therapy), leaves*

DESCRIPTION AND HABITAT
(See illustration, page 185)

An erect perennial herb growing up to 60cm tall. The leaves are pinnate, serrate and downy. The small, star-shaped, yellow flowers are borne on tall, conical spikes and emanate a definite scent of ripe apricots, as do the roots. The closely related *A. odorata* has a more pronounced and camphoraceous aroma. Agrimony is widespread in grassland throughout Europe, though rare in Scotland.

PRINCIPAL CONSTITUENTS
Tannins, bitters, essential oil (including borneol acetate).

HERBAL MEDICINE
Agrimony is astringent, carminative and anti-inflammatory. Infusions are helpful for digestive upset, gastritis and diarrhoea. Externally, the warm infusion can be used as a gargle for sore throat. The cooled infusion can be applied in compresses for skin rashes, cuts and bruises.

FLOWER THERAPY
The flowers are collected in midsummer and potentised using the Sun Method. The remedy is for those who suffer inwardly, hiding their true feelings behind a cloak of joviality (see page 67).

HOMEOPATHY
The homeopathic remedy mirrors the herbal uses.

BOSWELLIA CARTERII

FRANKINCENSE

Family: Burseraceae (Balm Family) **Synonym:** Olibanum
Parts Used: essential oil, gum resin

DESCRIPTION AND HABITAT

A small deciduous tree or shrub which grows wild in north-east Africa and the Red Sea region. Ducts under the bark secrete an oleo gum resin which is extracted by making deep incisions in the trunk. The milky white fluid solidifies into pea-sized amber 'tears'.

PRINCIPAL CONSTITUENTS

Boswellic acid, olibanoresene, bitter principle, water-soluble gum, bassorine, essential oil (including pinene, limonene, thujene, myrcene, phellandrene, terpinene). When the gum resin (not the essential oil) is burned as incense it produces the mood-elevating substance trahydrocannabinole.

AROMATHERAPY

The essential oil is extracted by steam distillation of the frankincense 'tears'. The aroma is warm and balsamic with a hint of lemon and camphor and a warming, head-clearing, calming effect. It blends well with basil, cedarwood, citrus oils, cypress, juniper, neroli, patchouli, rose and sandalwood, and is a popular vaporising oil with a long reputation for facilitating meditation. It helps with skin care (oily and mature), acne, abscesses, scars, wounds, skin ulcers, haemorrhoids, asthma, bronchitis, coughs, catarrh, laryngitis, cystitis, painful menstruation, PMS, nervous tension and stress-related disorders.

CAUTION

Since the oil may promote menstruation, avoid skin applications during the first trimester of pregnancy.

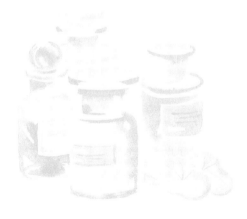

BROMUS RAMOSUS

OAT, WILD

Family: Graminaceae (Grass Family)
Parts Used: flowers (flower therapy)

DESCRIPTION AND HABITAT
(See illustration, page 185)
A tall grass of 1.5m or more. The flower heads are in loose panicles. It is often confused with the cultivated oat (*Avena sativa*), since the latter grows wild as an escape. There is one important distinguishing feature: the wild oat has hairy stems. The grass is native to Europe and can be found on hedge-banks and along the edge of woodland.

PRINCIPAL CONSTITUENTS
Wild Oat is used only as a Bach flower remedy. The cultivated oat, however, is a valuable herbal medicine containing saponins, alkaloids, a sterol, flavonoids, starch, protein, fats, minerals (including silica, iron, calcium, copper, magnesium, zinc) and vitamin B.

HERBAL MEDICINE
The grains of *A. sativa*, and the dry stalks (straw), are used medicinally, most conveniently as a tincture. Oat is primarily nervine, antidepressant, nutritive, demulcent and vulnerary. Infusions of the straw (or the diluted tincture) are prescribed for depression, fatigue, insomnia and convalescence. Externally, fine oatmeal can be used as a cleansing and soothing bath preparation for eczema and other inflamed skin conditions.

FLOWER THERAPY
The flowers are ready when they suddenly open to reveal the brown pollen on the anthers. Gather in late summer and potentise by the Sun Method. The remedy helps those who are seeking their true vocation in life (see page 73).

CALLUNA VULGARIS

HEATHER

Family: Ericaceae (Heather Family) **Synonym:** Ling
Parts Used: flowering stems, flowers (flower therapy)

DESCRIPTION AND HABITAT
(See illustration, page 185)
A short, straggly, evergreen shrub with needle-like leaves. The small, pale pinkish-purple flowers are clustered in dense terminal spikes. When growing *en masse*, the late summer blooms emanates a honey-like fragrance. Heather is widespread throughout Europe on barren acidic soil such as poor grassland, bogs and moors.

PRINCIPAL CONSTITUENTS
Arbutin (hydroquinone-glycoside), hydroquinone, tannins, flavone-glycosides.

HERBAL MEDICINE
Heather has anti-inflammatory, diuretic and mild sedative properties. Infusions of the flowering stems are helpful for rheumatic pain and urinary infections. Externally it is employed as a wash for eczema.

FLOWER THERAPY
The flowering sprays are collected in late summer and potentised using the Sun Method. The remedy is for talkative, self-absorbed people who fear loneliness (see page 69).

CANANGA ODORATA VAR. GENUINA

YLANG YLANG

Family: Anonaceae (Custard Apple Family)
Parts Used: flowers (mainly for the essential oil)

DESCRIPTION AND HABITAT

Ylang ylang (pronounced ee-lang ee-lang) means 'flower of flowers' and is a tropical tree reaching a height of about 30m. The branches, gracefully arched like those of the weeping willow, bear large, oval, shiny leaves and an abundance of intensely fragrant yellow blooms which appear constantly. The tree is native to the Philippines, but is cultivated for its essential oil in Madagascar, Réunion and the Comoros Islands.

PRINCIPAL CONSTITUENTS

Essential oil (including methyl benzoate, methyl salicylate, linalyl acetate, cadinene, caryophyllene, pinene, cresol, eugenol, linalol, geraniol).

HERBAL MEDICINE

Ylang ylang is antidepressant, anti-infectious, antiseptic, hypotensive, nervine, sedative, tonic and a circulatory stimulant. In the Molucca Islands, an ointment is made from ylang ylang flowers in a coconut oil base for cosmetic skin and hair care and for various skin diseases. It is also rubbed into the skin to help fight infections and prevent malaria.

AROMATHERAPY

The essential oil is captured by steam distillation of the flowers. There are four grades or fractions of the oil: ylang ylang extra, and ylang ylang one, two and three. Always use the more expensive 'extra' grade because it has a superior aroma. It is collected from the 'first running' of the distillation process; the plant material is distilled two or three more times to obtain the lower grades. A 'complete' oil, representing all the aforementioned fractions, is also available (though hard to find). But it is sometimes constructed by blending the inferior 1 and 2 grades. The extra grade has an intensely sweet floral aroma reminiscent of azalea flowers. The odour effect is warming and intoxicating; a reputed aphrodisiac. It is helpful for high blood pressure, palpitations, depression, insomnia and nervous tension. Ylang ylang blends well with other floral oils, citrus oils, coriander, ginger, frankincense, geranium and patchouli.

FLOWER THERAPY

The tree cannot be grown in Europe, but the flower essence can be obtained from suppliers of the Californian FES remedies. The blooms are collected during summer and potentised using the Sun Method. The remedy is for emotional upset, stress and tension.

CARPINUS BETULUS

HORNBEAM

Family: Betulaceae (Birch Family)
Parts Used: flowers (flower therapy)

DESCRIPTION AND HABITAT
(See illustration, page 185)
A majestic deciduous tree growing up to 20m tall. The leaves are oval and serrated with numerous strong veins. The trunk has characteristic grey streaks unlike any other tree. The male and female flowers appear on the same tree. The males are yellow catkins; the smaller females emerge from the tips of growing shoots. Hornbeam, native to Asia Minor and Europe, is widely cultivated in Europe and North America for ornament.

PRINCIPAL CONSTITUENTS
Data unavailable.

FLOWER THERAPY
Gather twigs with both male and female catkins in mid-spring and potentise by the Boiling Method. The remedy is for those who lack the strength or enthusiasm to fulfil their daily tasks (see page 70).

CASTANEA SATIVA

CHESTNUT, SWEET

Family: Fagaceae (Beech Family) **Synonym:** Spanish Chestnut
Parts Used: bark, flowers (flower therapy), fruit (chestnuts)

DESCRIPTION AND HABITAT
(See illustration, page 186)
A large tree reaching up to 30m. The bark is at first smooth and olive-green, maturing to greyish brown with vertical spiral ridges. The leaves are alternate, oblong-lanceolate and serrated. Male and female flowers appear on the same tree, the males greenish white in upright catkins, the females bud-like and surrounded by a green, scaly husk. The fruit is a shiny dark brown edible nut: up to three are enclosed in a brownish yellow spiny husk. The tree is native to the deciduous woodlands of southern Europe but cultivated in many other regions.

PRINCIPAL CONSTITUENTS
Leaves, bark, catkins: tannins, flavonoids. Fruit: starch.

HERBAL MEDICINE
Sweet chestnut is primarily astringent. Decoctions of the leaves, bark or male flowers (catkins) are helpful for diar-rhoea and catarrhal coughs. Externally, the remedy is used for bruises and wounds. Roasted sweet chestnuts were formerly regarded as a nutritional food of especial value during convalescence.

FLOWER THERAPY
Male and female flowers, a few leaves and twigs, are gathered in high summer and potentised by the Boiling Method. The remedy is for extreme anguish (see page 72).

HOMEOPATHY
The homeopathic remedy is prepared from the leaves of *C. vesca* and is used for whooping cough and diarrhoea.

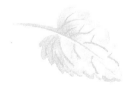

CEDRUS ATLANTICA

CEDARWOOD, ATLAS

Family: Pinaceae (Pine Family) **Parts Used:** essential oil

DESCRIPTION AND HABITAT
(See illustration, page 186)
A hardy, long-lived conifer attaining a height of 36m. The green, cylindrical male and female flowers (cones) appear on the same tree, ripening to dark woody brown. It is native to the Atlas Mountains of Algeria and Morocco, but extensively cultivated for ornament in Europe and North America.

PRINCIPAL CONSTITUENTS
Atlantone, caryophyllene, cedrol, cadinene.

AROMATHERAPY
The essential oil, a dark amber, viscous liquid with a tenacious, sweet, woody aroma, is distilled from the wood, stumps and sawdust. Its odour effect is warming and calming; a reputed aphrodisiac. The oil is antiseptic, circulatory stimulant, antiseborrheic, diuretic, expectorant, fungicidal and sedative. Helpful for oily skin, dandruff, eczema, athlete's foot, arthritis, rheumatism, respiratory disorders, premenstrual distress and nervous tension, and blends well with bergamot, clary sage, frankincense, jasmine, juniper berry, neroli, rose, rosemary and ylang ylang.

> ## CAUTION
> *Several trees yield an essential oil commonly labelled 'Cedarwood', including Juniperus virginiana, whose oil is potentially irritating to sensitive skin and a known abortifacient. Most authorities advise against the use of all cedar oils during pregnancy.*

CENTAURIUM ERYTHRAEA

CENTAURY

Family: Gentianaceae (Gentian Family) **Synonyms:** *C. umbellatum, C. minus*
Parts Used: flowering stems, flowers (flower therapy)

DESCRIPTION AND HABITAT
(See illustration, page 186)
An annual or biennial up to 30cm tall. The lower leaves are narrowly oval, growing in a rosette, with bright rose-pink flowers. Centaury can be found throughout Europe in dry, grassy places such as meadows, clearings and slopes.

PRINCIPAL CONSTITUENTS
Bitter glycosides, alkaloids, tannins, triterpenes, sugars, essential oil (trace).

HERBAL MEDICINE
Centaury, primarily a gastric stimulant, also helps liver and gall bladder problems, rheumatism and gout. Formerly prescribed for melancholy and for calming the nerves. Currently being used by herbalists to boost immunity in cases of ME. Externally, the cooled infusion is an antiseptic for cuts and grazes and heals ulcerated sores.

FLOWER THERAPY
The flowers are gathered during summer and potentised by the Sun Method (but see Caution). The remedy is for those who become the willing slaves of more dominant individuals (see page 67).

> ## CAUTION
> *Centaury is a protected species, so do not collect from the wild. Use only commercial preparations.*

CERATOSTIGMA WILLMOTTIANUM

CERATO

Family: Plumbaginaceae (Plumbago Family) **Parts Used:** flowers (flower therapy)

DESCRIPTION AND HABITAT
(See illustration, page 186)
A low-growing, deciduous shrub with vivid blue, flat-faced flowers in terminal clusters from midsummer to early autumn. The plant is native to the Himalayas and China, where it still grows in the wild.

PRINCIPAL CONSTITUENTS Data unavailable.

HERBAL MEDICINE
Cerato does not feature in modern herbalism. According to Pliny, the leaves and roots are an antidote for lead poisoning.

FLOWER THERAPY
The flower remedy is prepared from cultivated plants grown without the use of artificial fertilisers and poisonous sprays. Young plants can be purchased from tree and shrub nurseries. Plant in late spring and early summer in light, free-draining soil and in full sun. To potentise the remedy, collect the blooms in midsummer and prepare by the Sun Method. Cerato is the remedy for those who cannot trust their own decisions and repeatedly seek the advice of others (see page 67).

CICHORIUM INTYBUS

CHICORY

Family: Compositae/Asteraceae (Daisy Family) **Synonym:** Wild Succory
Parts Used: flowers (flower therapy), leaves (as a salad green), roots

DESCRIPTION AND HABITAT
(See illustration, page 186)
A perennial herb 1.2m tall with a long taproot, branched stem and milky sap. The basal leaves are lanceolate, deeply divided and hairy beneath. The cornflower-blue, dandelion-shaped flowers are arranged in clusters of two or three growing from the upper leaf axils. Chicory grows throughout Europe in fields and hedgerows and on roadsides, especially on lime-rich soils. The related endive (*C. endiva*) is grown as a salad crop.

PRINCIPAL CONSTITUENTS
Dried root: bitter compounds, inulin, tannins, sugars, fixed oil. Leaves: inulin, fructose, resin, cichorin, esculetin.

HERBAL MEDICINE
Chicory has aperitif, stomachic, tonic, hypoglycaemic, mild diuretic and laxative properties. Decoctions of the root are prescribed for liver disorders, gallstones, kidney stones and gout (it promotes the elimination of uric acid). Chicory also lowers blood sugar levels, making it helpful for diabetics. The ground roasted root is often blended with coffee to counteract both the acidic effects of oxalic acid (found in coffee) and the stimulating effects of caffeine.

FLOWER THERAPY
Pick the flowers in late summer and potentise by the Sun Method. They fade very quickly when picked, so cover your palm with a large basal leaf from the parent plant to protect them from the warmth of your hand. The remedy is for those who are possessive and overcritical of others (see page 68).

HOMEOPATHY
The remedy is used for sluggish digestion, constipation and stomach pains, particularly if physical or mental exertion is disliked.

CITRUS AURANTIUM

ORANGE BLOSSOM

Family: Rutaceae (Rue Family) **Synonyms:** *C. vulgaris*, *C. bigaradia*, Bitter Orange, Seville Orange
Parts Used: essential oil, flowers, orange flower water

DESCRIPTION AND HABITAT
(See illustration, page 187)
An evergreen tree with glossy leaves growing up to 10m. The white flowers appear singly or in small groups and are intensely fragrant. They appear even alongside the fruit, which is the bitter Seville orange used for making marmalade. Native to Asia, the tree is cultivated extensively around the Mediterranean.

PRINCIPAL CONSTITUENTS
Flowers: essential oil (including linalol, linalyl acetate, limonene, pinene, nerolidol, geraniol, nerol, indole, citral, jasmone), hesperidine and other flavonoids, bitters.

HERBAL MEDICINE
Orange blossom is antidepressant, antispasmodic, nervine, deodorant, mildly hypnotic, bactericidal, cicatrisant, stomachic and sedative; also a heart and circulatory tonic. Flower infusions are helpful for palpitations, nervous indigestion, anxiety and insomnia. The leaves have similar properties (see Petitgrain). Alternatively, authentic orange flower water (available from specialist suppliers) can be taken internally for the same conditions. The usual dosage is one dessertspoonful three times daily.

AROMATHERAPY
The essential oil (neroli) is captured by steam distillation of the fresh flowers (orange flower water is a by-product). The oil is a pale yellow liquid with a sweet floral scent. The odour effect is uplifting and calming; a reputed aphrodisiac. Neroli is used for skin care (most skin types), palpitations, poor circulation, diarrhoea, PMS, depression and other stress-related ailments. Neroli blends well with citrus essences, floral essences, chamomile (German and Roman), clary sage, coriander and geranium.

CITRUS AURANTIUM VAR. AMARA

PETITGRAIN

Family: Rutaceae (Rue Family) **Synonyms:** *C. vulgaris*, *C. bigaradia*, Bitter Orange, Seville Orange
Parts Used: Leaves (mainly for extraction of essential oil)

DESCRIPTION AND HABITAT
See Orange Blossom.

PRINCIPAL CONSTITUENTS
Leaves: essential oil (including linalyl acetate, geranyl acetate, linalol, nerol, terpineol).

HERBAL MEDICINE
Orange leaves are antiseptic, antispasmodic, deodorant, digestive, nervine, stomachic and tonic. The remedy is little used in herbal medicine, except in France where infusions are prescribed for stress-related ailments such as palpitations, insomnia and mild depression.

AROMATHERAPY
The essential oil (petitgrain) is captured by steam distillation of the fresh leaves and twigs. It is a pale yellow liquid with a dry, almost bitter-sweet aroma, reminiscent of neroli but much less refined. The odour effect is cooling and uplifting. It is helpful for skin and hair care (oily), indigestion, flatulence, insomnia, palpitations, PMS, nervous exhaustion and other stress-related ailments. Neroli blends well with bergamot (and other citrus oils), cedarwood, clary sage, coriander, frankincense, geranium, lavender, neroli and rose.

CITRUS BERGAMIA

BERGAMOT

Family: Rutaceae (Rue Family) **Synonym:** *Citrus aurantium* spp. *bergamia*
Parts Used: fruit (essential oil)

DESCRIPTION AND HABITAT
(See illustration, page 187)
A small evergreen tree with glossy leaves and fragrant, star-shaped flowers which appear continuously throughout the spring and summer, followed by small, orange-like fruit yellow when ripe. Unknown in the wild, it is probably native to tropical Asia. Bergamot is extensively cultivated in southern Italy and grown commercially for its aromatic oil on the Ivory Coast.

PRINCIPAL CONSTITUENTS
The essential oil mainly comprises linalyl acetate, linalol, sequiterpenes, terpenes and furocoumarins (including bergapten). The rectified version, labelled 'Bergamot FCF' (see page 259), is virtually free of furocoumarins.

HERBAL MEDICINE
The oil is antiseptic (pulmonary, genito-urinary), antidepressant, antispasmodic, carminative, deodorant, febrigual, rubefacient, vermifugal and tonic. An Italian folk remedy for reducing fevers (including malaria) and expelling worms, the oil is also used to flavour Earl Grey tea, which is renowned for its uplifting effect.

AROMATHERAPY
The oil is captured by cold expression of the rind of the fruit. It is a pale green liquid with an aroma reminiscent of orange and lemon combined. The rectified oil (see Cautions) is virtually colourless and has a lighter aroma. The odour effect of either is uplifting and refreshing. Helpful for colds and flu, anxiety, depression and premenstrual distress, it blends well with most essences, especially clary sage, coriander, frankincense, geranium, jasmine, juniper berry, lavender, lemon, neroli, orange and petitgrain.

CAUTION

The cold expressed oil can provoke unsightly pigmentation if applied before exposure to natural or simulated sunlight, so for skin it is best to use the rectified version known as bergamot FCF (furocoumarin-free) which is non-phototoxic. Use whole bergamot oil as a mood-enhancing room scent.

CITRUS SINENSIS

ORANGE, SWEET

Family: Rutaceae (Rue Family) **Synonyms:** *C. aurantium* var. *sinensis*, *C. aurantium* var. *dulcis*
Parts Used: essential oil, flowers (flower therapy), fruit, leaves

DESCRIPTION AND HABITAT
(See illustration, page 187)
A glossy-leaved evergreen growing up to 10m, producing abundant fragrant white flowers and the familiar fruit. Since it can take up to a year for the fruit to be formed, there is often blossom and fruit on the tree at the same time. The tree is native to China but cultivated extensively elsewhere.

PRINCIPAL CONSTITUENT
Essential oil (including limonene, citral, citronellal, geraniol, linalol, terpinol) bergapten, auraptenol, organic acids, hesperidine, bitters.

HERBAL MEDICINE
The fruit is little used in modern herbalism, though orange wine is a popular aperitif in France. The French also employ infusions of orange leaves as a remedy for nervous conditions such as palpitations, insomnia and mild depression.

AROMATHERAPY
The best-quality oil is obtained by expression of the rind of the fruit. An inferior grade is distilled from the fruit pulp, a by-product of orange juice manufacture. The expressed oil is yellow/orange with a sweet, refreshing aroma of the fresh fruit. The odour effect is uplifting and cheery. Helpful for palpitations, colds and flu, indigestion, depression and nervous tension. It blends well with other citrus essences, clary sage, coriander (and other spices), frankincense, geranium, lavender, neroli, patchouli, petitgrain, rose and rosemary.

FLOWER THERAPY
Collect the flowers in high summer and potentise by the Sun Method. Orange is for those who feel depressed, hopeless or despairing: the remedy is revitalising, bringing resolution and joy.

CAUTION

Orange oil is potentially phototoxic and should not be applied to skin before exposure to natural or simulated sunlight as it may cause pigmentation. It may also irritate sensitive skin. Always use in the lowest recommended concentrations. The oil deteriorates quickly, so use up within six months of opening the bottle.

CLEMATIS VITALBA

CLEMATIS

Family: Ranunculaceae (Buttercup Family) **Synonyms:** Traveller's Joy, Wild Clematis, Old Man's Beard
Parts Used: flowers (flower therapy)

DESCRIPTION AND HABITAT
(See illustration, page 187)
A deciduous, woody climber with trusses of faintly vanilla-scented, greenish white flowers. The leaves are opposite and pinnate, the leaf stalks long and twisting, enabling the plant to cling as it climbs. In autumn the stamens take on the appearance of an 'old man's beard' formed by the woolly greyish white plumes on the ripe fruits. Wild clematis is native to Europe and North Africa and can be found in woods and hedgerows, especially on chalk and limestone.

PRINCIPAL CONSTITUENTS

The biochemical monologue for C. *vitalba* is not generally available. The flowering stems of the closely related C. *recta* contain glycocides, saponins and other, so far unidentified, substances.

HERBAL MEDICINE

Clematis is rarely used in modern herbalism because of its toxicity. Formerly a preparation of the roots of C. *vitalba* was applied externally to treat 'itch' (pruritis). The flowering stems of C. *recta* were once used for treating venereal disease, gout, rheumatism and bone diseases.

FLOWER THERAPY

Gather flowers by their stalks in late summer and potentise by the Sun Method. The remedy is indicated for a bemused state of mind (see page 68). It is also a component of Rescue Remedy (see page 73).

CAUTION

The fresh leaves of C. recta may cause stubborn eczema and irritate the eyes. If any part of the plant is eaten it may cause severe abdominal pain and diarrhoea. C. vitalba is believed to be less toxic. Clearly, this counters the general view that Bach avoided the use of poisonous plants. Nonetheless, it is only herbal preparations (and pharmaceutical drugs derived from clematis) which are toxic. The flower remedy has been used for over sixty years, and thus proven perfectly benign in its action.

HOMEOPATHY

C. *vitalba* is employed for varicose veins, slow-healing wounds and skin ulcers, especially if the person is also prone to drowsiness and confusion.

ECHINACEA ANGUSTIFOLIA

ECHINACEA

Family: *Compositae/Asteraceae* (Daisy Family) **Synonym:** Purple Cone Flower
Parts Used: rhizome, root

DESCRIPTION AND HABITAT

(See illustration, page 187)
A hairy perennial with unbranched stems and lanceolate leaves, growing up to 60cm. The faintly aromatic, daisy-like florets have purple centres and are distinctly conical. The plant, native to North American prairies as far north as Canada, is cultivated as a garden plant in Britain and elsewhere in Europe.

PRINCIPAL CONSTITUENTS

Essential oil (including humulence and caryophylene), glycoside, echinaceine, phenolics, resin.

HERBAL MEDICINE

The plant is anti-inflammatory, antimicrobial and alterative. An excellent remedy for boosting immunity, it helps those suffering from decreased immunity and allergies resulting from prolonged stress. Particularly efficacious for most bacterial and viral infections, it is currently being used by herbalists for ME. Also helpful for arthritis and gout, and externally it can heal itchy skin conditions such as urticaria and prickly heat. Echinacea is widely available as a tincture prepared from the fresh root.

FAGUS SYLVATICA

BEECH

Family: Fagaceae (Beech Family)
Parts Used: beechmast (nuts), fixed oil (from the mast), flowers (flower therapy), leaves

DESCRIPTION AND HABITAT
(See illustration, page 188)
A forest tree reaching up to 40m. The leaves are ovate and alternate, with male and female flowers on the same tree; the females are a reddish crown of bristly 'mast', the males form a cluster of hanging tassels. The polished red-brown nuts drop to the ground in autumn. Beech is widespread in western, central and southern Europe.

PRINCIPAL CONSTITUENTS
A nutritious fixed oil can be extracted from the nuts; contains essential fatty acids.

HERBAL MEDICINE
No longer commonly used in herbalism. According to Culpeper, the water found in the hollows of decaying beeches will heal scabby skin disorders. The fresh leaves have astringent properties and can be applied to bruises.

FLOWER THERAPY
Gather the shoots and the male and female catkins in early spring, and potentise by the Boiling Method. The remedy is for those who are intolerant of the weaknesses of others (see page 67).

GENTIANELLA AMARELLA

GENTIAN

Family: Gentianaceae (Gentian Family) **Synonyms:** Bitterwort, Autumn Felwort
Parts Used: flowers (flower therapy)

DESCRIPTION AND HABITAT
(See illustration, page 188)
A low-growing herb with bell-shaped, dull purple flowers. The opposite, lanceolate leaves have prominent veins and are generally stalkless. The plant is native to most of Europe, especially in chalk and limestone turf and on dunes.

PRINCIPAL CONSTITUENTS
Bitter principles.

HERBAL MEDICINE
This variety is seldom used: herbalists favour the related G. *lutea*, which is mainly employed for digestive problems.

FLOWER THERAPY
The flowers are collected in late summer and potentised by the Sun Method. The remedy is for those who have a generally pessimistic outlook and are too easily discouraged (see page 69).

CAUTION

Gentian is a protected species so do not collect from the wild. Obtain only commercial preparations of the flower remedy.

HELIANTHEMUM NUMMULARIUM
ROCK ROSE

Family: Cistaceae (Rock Rose Family) **Synonyms:** *H. vulgare, H. chamaecistus*
Parts Used: flowers (flower therapy)

DESCRIPTION AND HABITAT
(See illustration, page 188)
A small, wiry-stemmed perennial with trailing branches, growing to a height of 15–30cm. The leaves are narrow and lanceolate, growing in opposite pairs, green above and downy white beneath. The bright yellow flowers, crumpled like tissue paper, open one or two at a time in sunny weather and fall within a few hours. Rock rose is native to northern Europe and is common in grassy places on chalk and limestone; also on acid soils in Scotland.

PRINCIPAL CONSTITUENTS
Biochemical data is not generally available.

FLOWER THERAPY
The flowers are collected in midsummer and potentised by the Sun Method. Although there are several garden varieties of rock rose, Bach emphasised the importance of using only wild flowers for preparing the essence. The remedy is for acute states of fear, terror or panic (see page 71). Rock rose is also a component of Rescue Remedy (see page 73).

HOTTONIA PALUSTRIS
WATER VIOLET

Family: Primulaceae (Primrose Family)
Parts Used: flowers (flower therapy)

DESCRIPTION AND HABITAT
(See illustration, page 188)
A graceful, floating, aquatic perennial growing up to 90cm. It has feathery leaves on submerged stems which turn up at the tip and emerge from the water before flowering. The primrose-like blooms, mauve with yellow centres, are set in whorls. Water violet is native to northern Europe and can be found growing in ditches and ponds. Unfortunately, the plant is increasingly difficult to find due to extensive drainage of wetlands.

PRINCIPAL CONSTITUENTS
The biochemical data is generally unavailable.

FLOWER THERAPY
The flowers are collected in early summer and potentised by the Sun Method. The remedy is for those who are proud and aloof (see page 72).

ILEX AQUIFOLIUM

HOLLY

Family: Aquifoliaceae (Holly Family)
Parts Used: flowers (flower therapy)

DESCRIPTION AND HABITAT
(See illustration, page 188)
An evergreen tree or shrub with hard, glossy, spiny leaves and bright red berries. The flowers are small, white and four-petalled, tinged with pink and very fragrant: male and female usually grow on different trees, though sometimes a tree may be bisexual. Holly is native to western Asia and Europe.

PRINCIPAL CONSTITUENTS
Leaves: bitter principle (ilicin). Berries: poisonous alkaloids.

HERBAL MEDICINE
Not used in modern herbalism. Extractions of the leaves were formerly administered for catarrh, pleurisy, smallpox, intermittent fevers, rheumatism and jaundice.

FLOWER THERAPY
The flowering leafy twigs are collected in late spring and potentised by the Boiling Method. Holly is for those prone to feelings of envy, jealousy, revenge, suspicion and rage (see page 69).

CAUTION

Holly berries are extremely poisonous. Herbal preparations of the leaves should be avoided by the home user as they are potentially toxic. However, the non-material Bach flower remedy is perfectly benign.

IMPATIENS GLANDULIFERA

IMPATIENS

Family: Balsaminaceae (Balsam Family) **Synonym:** Himalayan Balsam
Parts Used: flowers (flower therapy)

DESCRIPTION AND HABITAT
(See illustration, page 189)
A fast-growing annual up to 2m tall. The smooth, dark green leaves have sharply serrated edges. The large pale mauve to purplish pink flowers are helmet-shaped and emanate an elusive balsamic aroma. The ripe seed pods fascinate children because, at a touch, they shoot open and scatter the seed widely. As its common name implies, the plant is native to the Himalayas, but has become extensively naturalised in Europe. It can be found growing in damp places, especially in ditches and on river banks.

PRINCIPAL CONSTITUENTS
Data unavailable.

FLOWER THERAPY
Bach emphasised the importance of choosing only the pale mauve flowers for making the flower essence. Gather the blooms in late summer and potentise using the Sun Method. The remedy is for those who are impatient and irritable (see page 70). Impatiens is also a component of Rescue Remedy (see page 73).

JASMINUM OFFICINALE

JASMINE

Family: Oleaceae (Olive Family)
Parts Used: flowers, solvent-extracted absolute

DESCRIPTION AND HABITAT
(See illustration, page 189)
A twining, evergreen or semi-evergreen climber with mid-green leaves and an abundance of white, star-shaped blooms whose rich fragrance intensifies after dusk. Jasmine is native to China, northern India and the Middle East, but is cultivated worldwide.

PRINCIPAL CONSTITUENTS
Essential oil (including benzyl acetate, linalol, farnesol, cisjasmone, methyl jasmonate, phenylacetic acid, benzyl alcohol).

HERBAL MEDICINE
Antidepressant, anti-inflammatory, antispasmodic, expectorant, parturient, sedative, uterine tonic. In China, infusions of the flowers are traditionally employed for hepatitis and dysentery. The flowers are also blended with black China tea and taken as an uplifting tisane. A syrup prepared from the flowers was formerly used by British herbalists as a cough medicine. Jasmine infusions alleviate painful periods and facilitate childbirth. Applied as a compress, the flowers arrest the flow of breast milk.

AROMATHERAPY
A solvent-extracted absolute is prepared from the fresh flowers. It is a brown viscous liquid with a richly floral-musky fragrance. The odour effect is warming and intoxicating; a reputed aphrodisiac. It is helpful for muscular aches and pains, catarrh, coughs, painful menstruation, labour pains, PMS, depression and stress-related disorders. Jasmine blends well with other floral oils, cedarwood, clary sage, petitgrain and sandalwood.

FLOWER THERAPY
The flowers are collected in high summer and potentised using the Sun Method. For those seeking a new path in life it can help engender a sense of direction.

CAUTION

Since jasmine exerts a stimulating effect on the uterus, both the absolute and herbal remedy should be avoided during pregnancy.

JUGLANS REGIA

WALNUT

Family: Juglandaceae (Walnut Family)
Parts Used: flowers, leaves, nuts, pericarp (green outer layer of the fruits)

DESCRIPTION AND HABITAT
(See illustration, page 189)
A large deciduous tree with a spreading crown, growing up to 25m. The greyish bark is smooth when young, later fissured. The scented alternate leaves are pinnate with seven to ten leaflets. Male and female flowers grow on the same tree: the males are pendulous catkins, the females bud-like and at the ends of the twigs. The green, rounded fruit contains the familiar crinkled walnut. The tree is native to south-eastern Europe and western Asia, but cultivated elsewhere.

PRINCIPAL CONSTITUENTS
Catkins, leaves, pericarp: tannins, a bitter compound (juglone), flavonoids, organic acids, essential oil (except catkins), hydrojuglone. Nuts: fixed oil, mucilage, albumen, mineral matter, cellulose.

HERBAL MEDICINE
Walnut is primarily astringent, haemostatic, anti-inflammatory and mildly sedative. Decoctions of the leaves, pericarp or catkins are prescribed for eczema, pruritis, rheumatism, gout, night sweats, heavy periods, diarrhoea and dysentery. Externally, the cooled decoction is helpful for vaginal thrush, skin rashes, cold sores, eyelid irritation, cuts and wounds.

FLOWER THERAPY
The flowers are collected in late spring and potentised by the Boiling Method. Walnut is for those who are finding it difficult to adjust to change (see page 72).

HOMEOPATHY
The homeopathic remedy mirrors the herbal uses.

LARIX DECIDUA

LARCH

Family: Pinaceae (Pine Family)
Parts Used: flowers (flower remedy)

DESCRIPTION AND HABITAT
(See illustration, page 189)
A tall deciduous conifer reaching to 40m, with needle-like leaves in bunches, it is the only European conifer to shed its leaves in autumn. The bark is pinkish grey with vertical cracks and scaly ridges. Male and female catkins grow on the same tree: females are red ovoid tufts, males are smaller yellow tufts. Small ovoid cones remain on the branches from previous years. Larch is native to the mountains of central and southern Europe and widely cultivated elsewhere.

PRINCIPAL CONSTITUENTS
Bark: taninic acid, oleo gum resin (including turpentine).

HERBAL MEDICINE
No longer employed. An extract of the oleo gum resin was formerly used as an astringent, stimulant and expectorant. It was deemed particularly efficacious for chronic bronchitis.

FLOWER THERAPY
The male and female catkins, twigs and young leaves are collected in early spring; potentise using the Boiling Method. The remedy is for those who lack confidence (see page 70).

LONICERA CAPRIFOLIUM

HONEYSUCKLE, RED

Family: Caprifoliaceae (Honeysuckle Family)
Parts Used: *L. caprifolium*: flowers (flower therapy)

DESCRIPTION AND HABITAT
(See illustration, page 189)
The richly scented honeysuckle of herbal medicine proper is the yellow-flowered wild *L. periclymenum* variety found growing wild in deciduous woodlands. Red (Italian) honeysuckle is used in Bach flower therapy. The leaves of both are rounded and in opposite pairs. However, the upper leaves of red honeysuckle are unstalked and clasping (the main distinguishing feature). The flowers are borne in terminal clusters of red 'tubes' which are white inside, becoming yellow after pollination.

PRINCIPAL CONSTITUENTS
Biochemical data for *L. caprifolium* is not generally available, although the plant is certainly non-poisonous. The leaves of the closely related *L. periclymenum* contain mucilage, glucoside, salicylic acid and invertin. The flowers produce an essential oil (unavailable commercially).

HERBAL MEDICINE
Infusions of the leaves are helpful for colds, flu, fevers and headaches, and for easing arthritic and rheumatic pain.

Infusions of the flowers can be taken to soothe the nerves. A syrup of the flowers was formerly used as a cough medicine, especially for bronchitis.

HOMEOPATHY
The homeopathic remedy prepared from the leaves of *L. periclymenum* is employed for irritability and aggressive outbursts.

FLOWER THERAPY
If *L. caprifolium* cannot be found growing wild (as a garden escape), prepare the remedy from an organically grown plant. Gather the flowering heads and young leaves in midsummer and potentise by the Boiling Method. Honeysuckle is for those who live too much in the past (see page 69).

MALUS SYLVESTRIS

CRAB APPLE

Family: Rosaceae (Rose Family)
Parts Used: flowers (flower therapy), fruit, leaves

DESCRIPTION AND HABITAT
(See illustration, page 190)
A small deciduous tree reaching 9m. The bark is greyish brown, fissured and cracked, the leaves oval with finely serrated edges. The clusters of fragrant flowers are white, flushed pink, with a yellow stamen. The fruit is a greenish yellow apple, sometimes also flushed pink. The tree, native to northern Europe, is found in woods, hedgerows and scrub. Rarely cultivated, though undoubtedly a parent of orchard apples.

PRINCIPAL CONSTITUENTS
Fruit: water, starch, fructose, organic acids, mineral salts, tannins, vitamin C. Bark: tannins, bitter principle, quercetin (yellow colouring matter).

HERBAL MEDICINE
Decoctions of the bark were formerly used for intermittent fevers, infusions of the flowers and leaves for eye complaints. Crab apple cider in which horseradish has been steeped was found efficacious for dropsy (fluid retention associated with heart disease). The verjuice (a precursor of cider vinegar) was used for chronic diarrhoea. Cider vinegar (taken internally three times daily, diluted 1:4 with water and sweetened with honey) is helpful for arthritic conditions, coughs and colds, and as a gargle for sore throats. Stewed and sweetened with honey, the fruit is good for eczema and other skin problems.

FLOWER THERAPY
Collect flower clusters, a few twigs and leaves in late spring; potentise by the Boiling Method. The remedy is for those who feel 'unclean' or experience self-disgust (see page 68).

CAUTION

The bark is potentially poisonous and must never be used for self-medication.

MIMULUS GUTTATUS

MIMULUS

Family: Scrophulariaceae (Figwort Family) **Synonym:** Monkey Flower
Parts Used: flowers (Flower therapy)

DESCRIPTION AND HABITAT
(See illustration, page 190)
An attractive creeping perennial growing up to 45cm, with broad, toothed, opposite leaves. The bright yellow flowers, with a few red spots on the lower lip, are five-petalled but fuse to form an open mouth. Mimulus was introduced into Britain from North American in the nineteenth century and can sometimes be found growing by shallow streams, especially in Wales.

PRINCIPAL CONSTITUENTS
Biochemical data is generally unavailable. The plant may never have been employed in herbal medicine.

FLOWER THERAPY
The flowers are gathered in high summer and potentised by the Sun Method. Mimulus is for fear, particularly of worldly things like poverty, illness, pain and misfortune (see page 70).

ORNITHOGALUM UMBELLATUM

STAR-OF-BETHLEHEM

Family: Liliaceae (Lily Family)
Parts Used: bulb (culinary use), flowers (flower therapy)

DESCRIPTION AND HABITAT

(See illustration, page 190)

A hairless, unbranched perennial 10–20 cm high with slender, pointed leaves, dark green with a white vein down the centre, growing from the bulb. The brilliant white flowers are borne in umbels, with a green stripe on the back of each of the six petals, opening star-like in the sun. Star-of-Bethlehem is native to Asia, North Africa and Europe on dry grassland. It is usually a garden plant in the British Isles, although it has become naturalised in the south and east of England.

PRINCIPAL CONSTITUENTS

The biochemical data is not generally available. Since Star-of-Bethlehem is related to onion and garlic, it probably contains plenty of sulphur. The edible bulbs were popular in ancient Greek and Roman times. They are still eaten in Middle-Eastern countries, being roasted like chestnuts.

FLOWER THERAPY

The flowering clusters are gathered in late spring and potentised by the Boiling Method. The remedy is used for shock (see pages 71–2). Star-of-Bethlehem is a component of Rescue Remedy (see page 73).

HOMEOPATHY

The remedy is helpful for chronic gastric disorders. It is also used in the treatment of certain cancers of the intestinal tract.

PANAX GINSENG

GINSENG

Family: Araliaceae (Ivy Family) **Synonym:** Oriental Ginseng **Parts Used:** dried root

DESCRIPTION AND HABITAT

(See illustration, page 190)

A smooth perennial herb with large, fleshy, slow-growing roots whose flavour resembles liquorice. Ginseng is native to China, and cultivated there as well as in Korea and Japan.

PRINCIPAL CONSTITUENTS

Starch, hormone-like saponins, essential oils, sterols, sugars, pectin, vitamins (including B1, B2, B12), minerals (including zinc, iron, calcium, magnesium).

HERBAL MEDICINE

Decoctions of the dried root (or a tincture prepared from the fresh root) have an adaptogenic effect and are an excellent remedy for nervous exhaustion. Ginseng also enhances immunity through its ability to stimulate the production of white blood cells. The remedy is excellent for people for people made weak through chronic illness or advanced age.

CAUTION

Not to be confused with its less effective American cousin, Panax quinquefolium. Avoid during acute inflammatory disease such as viral bronchitis, which ginseng's warming and stimulating properties may exacerbate. Also avoid if you have high blood pressure.

POGOSTEMON CABLIN

PATCHOULI

Family: Lamiaceae/Labiatae (Mint Family) *Parts Used:* essential oil, leaves

DESCRIPTION AND HABITAT
A herbaceous perennial growing up to 90cm, with purple-tinged white flowers. The soft, hairy, egg-shaped leaves emanate a peculiar earthy fragrance when rubbed. Native to Malaysia, the plant is cultivated for its oil in other regions such as India, China and South America.

PRINCIPAL CONSTITUENTS
Essential oil (including patchoulol, pogostol, bulnesol, patchoulenol, bulnese, patchoulene).

HERBAL MEDICINE
Patchouli is antidepressant, anti-inflammatory, antiseptic, antiviral, bactericidal, cicatrisant, deodorant, diuretic, febrifugal, fungicidal, nervine, stimulant, stomachic, tonic. The plant is not used in European herbalism, but in China, Japan and Malaysia infusions of the leaves are taken for colds, headaches, nausea, diarrhoea and colic.

AROMATHERAPY
The essential oil, a dark amber, viscous liquid, is obtained by steam distillation of the dried and fermented leaves. The earthy-musky aroma becomes sweeter as the oil ages. Its odour effect is warming and stimulating; a reputed aphrodisiac. It is helpful for skin and hair care (especially oily skin), abscesses, acne, athlete's foot, bed sores, cracked and sore skin, dandruff, weeping eczema, wounds, depression and nervous exhaustion. It is also a good insect repellent. Patchouli blends well with bergamot and other citrus oils, cedarwood, clary sage, geranium, jasmine, lavender, neroli, petitgrain, rose and sandalwood. The oil is highly odoriferous, so use in low concentration.

POPULUS TREMULA

ASPEN

Family: Salicaceae (Willow Family) *Parts Used:* bark, flowers (flower therapy), leaf buds, leaves

DESCRIPTION AND HABITAT
(See illustration, page 190)
A slender deciduous tree reaching up to 30m. The roundish, coarsely serrated leaves flutter and tremble in the slightest breeze, hence its specific name *tremula*. The male and female flowers appear on separate trees: the male catkins are brownish red, the females green. Aspen is native to Europe, North American and Asia.

PRINCIPAL CONSTITUENTS
Phenolic glycosides, salicin, populin, essential oil, bitter compounds.

HERBAL MEDICINE
Preparations of the buds, bark and leaves are diuretic, antiseptic and febrifuge. it is chiefly administered as a decoction for urinary infections, gout and rheumatism. Externally, compresses, bath preparations and ointments are used for haemorrhoids and to treat burns.

FLOWER THERAPY
Collect the male and female catkins, including a few twigs and leaves, in early spring and potentise by the Boiling Method. Aspen is indicated for vague fears of unknown origin, including night terrors and paranoia (see page 67).

HOMEOPATHY
The homeopathic remedy (prepared from the fresh leaves) mirrors the herbal uses.

PRUNUS CERASIFERA

CHERRY PLUM

Family: Rosaceae (Rose Family)
Parts Used: flowering twigs (flower therapy)

DESCRIPTION AND HABITAT
(See illustration, page 191)
A small deciduous tree commonly grown as a hedgerow specimen. The clusters of white blossom appear in early spring. Cherry trees (there are many varieties) are believed to be native of Asia; they were introduced into Europe by the Romans.

PRINCIPAL CONSTITUENTS
This particular species of cherry is not used in herbal medicine, so biochemical data is unavailable.

FLOWER THERAPY
Collect the flowering twigs in early spring, before the leaves appear. The remedy is prepared by the Boiling Method and is used for uncontrolled outbreaks of rage, or a fear of harming oneself or others (see page 68). Cherry Plum is also a component of Rescue Remedy (see page 73).

QUERCUS ROBUR

OAK

Family: Fagaceae (Beech Family) *Synonym:* Pedunculate Oak
Parts Used: acorns, bark, flowers (flower therapy) leaves

DESCRIPTION AND HABITAT
(See illustration, page 191)
A large deciduous tree reaching 30m or more. In ideal conditions the crown can form a perfect dome. The bark is rough and greyish brown, becoming fissured as it ages. The leaves are almost stalkless and deeply lobed. The male flowers are pendulous catkins, the females small red buds at the tip of the twigs. Both appear on the same tree and are followed by the familiar oval nuts (acorns). Oak is native to Europe, south-west Asia, North Africa and eastern Russia.

PRINCIPAL CONSTITUENTS
Tannins, gallic acid, catechins.

HERBAL MEDICINE
The leaves and bark are astringent, antiseptic and anti-inflammatory. Decoctions of the bark or leaves are used for gastroenteritis and diarrhoea. The cooled decoction is used as a compress or bath preparation to treat chilblains, cuts, burns and haemorrhoids, and as a bath preparation or local wash for vaginal thrush.

FLOWER THERAPY
The female flowers are collected in late spring and potentised by the Sun Method. Oak is for those who suffer as a result of relentless effort against all odds and refuse to give in to illness (see also page 70).

HOMEOPATHY
The remedy, prepared from tincture of acorn kernels, is helpful for the recovering alcoholic and for gout and old malarial cases.

SALIX VITELLINA

WILLOW

Family: Salicaceae (Willow Family) **Synonym:** Yellow Willow **Parts Used:** flowers (flower therapy)

DESCRIPTION AND HABITAT
(See illustration, page 191)

A tall, elegant, deciduous tree reaching up to 25m with a deeply fissured bark and slender branches. The alternate leaves are lanceolate and finely toothed, with fine white hairs on the underside. The flowers are long catkins, males (yellow) and females (green) appearing on different trees. The way to distinguish yellow willow (*S. vitellina*) from the closely related white willow (*S. alba*) is by the winter twigs, which are the colour of egg yolk. Willow trees are native to Europe, northern Asia and northern Africa. They are found in damp, low-lying land, often lining the banks of rivers and streams.

PRINCIPAL CONSTITUENTS
The biochemical data for *S. vitellina* is not generally available. The bark of the closely related *S. alba* contains phenolic glycoside, salicin and tannins.

HERBAL MEDICINE
S. alba is tonic, astringent, diaphoretic, antirheumatic and anodyne. Decoctions of the bark were once used for poor digestion, intestinal worms, diarrhoea, rheumatic and arthritic complaints, dysentery, fevers and neuralgia. Externally, the decoction can be added to the bath for rheumatic and arthritic pain, and used in compresses for cuts, skin ulcers and burns.

FLOWER THERAPY
Collect the male or female catkins, including a few twigs and leaves, in mid-spring; potentise by the Boiling Method. It is for those who harbour bitterness and resentment (see page 73).

SANTALUM ALBUM

SANDALWOOD

Family: Santalaceae (Sandal Family) **Synonym:** Mysore Sandalwood
Parts Used: heartwood (mainly for extraction of essential oil)

DESCRIPTION AND HABITAT
(See illustration, page 191)

An evergreen semi-parasitic tree which grows on the roots of other trees during the first seven years of its life, causing the host to die. It takes about thirty years to attain its maximum height of 12–15m. The tree is native to tropical Asia, especially Mysore in India where the highest-quality essential oil is produced.

PRINCIPAL CONSTITUENTS
Essential oil (including santalols, fusanols, borneol, santalone).

HERBAL MEDICINE
Sandalwood is antidepressant, anti-inflammatory, antiseptic (urinary and pulmonary), antispasmodic, astringent, bactericidal, carminative, cicatrisant, diuretic, expectorant, fungicidal, insecticidal, sedative and tonic. In Chinese medicine the essential oil is taken internally for gastrointestinal disorders and skin diseases. In Ayurvedic medicine the oil taken orally is used for chronic diarrhoea, urinary infections and respiratory ailments.

AROMATHERAPY

The essential oil is stream-distilled from the roots and heartwood. It is a yellowish, slightly viscous liquid with a soft, sweet, balsamic aroma of excellent tenacity. The odour effect is soothing and sensual; a reputed aphrodisiac. It is helpful for skin care, acne, eczema, cracked and chapped skin, respiratory ailments, laryngitis, cystitis, nausea, insomnia, PMS, depression and stress-related ailments. Sandalwood blends well with citrus essences, cedarwood, coriander, frankincense, ginger, juniper berry, lavender, patchouli, pine, rose and ylang ylang.

> ### CAUTION
>
> *Not to be confused with West Indian sandalwood or amyris (A. balsamifera), which is a cheap alternative. Amyris has an inferior musky-woody aroma with poor tenacity.*

SCLERANTHUS ANNUS

SCLERANTHUS

Family: Caryophyllaceae (Pink Family) **Synonyms:** Knawel
Parts Used: flowers (flower therapy)

DESCRIPTION AND HABITAT

(See illustration, page 191)
A small, wiry, rather bushy, greyish annual, it grows low on the ground with numerous branched stems. The leaves are small and spiky, clasping the stems in pairs. The plant produces heads of minute petalless green flowers at the end of shoots, though the five-pointed sepals might be mistaken for petals. The plant is native to northern Europe on dry, porous, sandy soil. Although once common on the margins of cornfields, it is now difficult to find due to modern agricultural practices.

PRINCIPAL CONSTITUENTS

The biochemical data is generally unavailable.

FLOWER THERAPY

The flowers are collected in high summer and potentised using the Sun Method. It is for those who vacillate and are unable to decide between two things (see page 71).

SINAPSIS ARVENSIS

MUSTARD

Family: Cruciferae (Cabbage Family) **Synonyms:** Charlock, Field Mustard
Parts Used: flowers (flower therapy), leaves, seed

DESCRIPTION AND HABITAT
(See illustration, page 192)
Mustard or charlock is an erect branched annual attaining a height of 30–60cm. It has roughly oval leaves with opposite lobes at the base, and toothed edges, alternately spaced on the stem. The yellow flowers have four equal-sized petals forming a cross. The fruit is a long capsule with a distinctive beak at the tip. Mustard is native to northern Europe and can be found as a weed on arable land and roadside verges.

PRINCIPAL CONSTITUENTS
Charlock is used in Bach flower therapy rather than herbal medicine proper. However, it is believed to have a similar chemistry to the closely related white mustard (*S. alba*), which contains glycosides, sinapine and fixed oil (mustard oil is high in sulphur).

HERBAL MEDICINE
White mustard has local rubefacient properties, as does charlock to a lesser degree. The ground seeds are used in cold compresses (placed between two pieces of damp cotton fabric) to ease rheumatic pain. Hot mustard compresses, however, may blister the skin. The seeds are laxative and antiseptic.

FLOWER THERAPY
Gather the flowerheads of charlock in early summer and potentise using the Boiling Method. The remedy is for recurrent periods of deep gloom and despair (see page 70).

HOMEOPATHY
The homeopathic remedy is prepared from the seeds of *S. alba* and is prescribed for hayfever and throat inflammation.

ULEX EUROPAEUS

GORSE

Family: Leguminosae (Pea Family) **Parts Used:** flowers (flower therapy)

DESCRIPTION AND HABITAT
(See illustration, page 192)
A viciously spiny, evergreen shrub with abundant golden yellow flowers, like those of the pea family. The blooms emanate a delicious coconut-like (some say almond-like) fragrance. Gorse thrives in dry woodland, thickets and heaths. It is native to western Europe, though extensively naturalised in other parts including western Britain.

PRINCIPAL CONSTITUENTS
Flowers: data unavailable. Seeds: ulexine (a poisonous alkaloid isolated in 1886 and once used for cardiac dropsy).

HERBAL MEDICINE
Not used in modern herbalism. In the past, infusions of the flowers were taken to prevent jaundice. The same remedy was once prescribed for children with scarlet fever.

FLOWER THERAPY
The flowers are collected in summer and potentised by the Sun Method. The remedy is for those who are experiencing great hopelessness and despair (see page 69).

ULMUS PROCERA

ELM, ENGLISH

Family: Ulmaceae (Elm Family) **Parts Used:** flowers (flower therapy)

DESCRIPTION AND HABITAT
(See illustration, page 192)

A deciduous tree reaching up to 30m. The leaves are ovoid, dark green and coarse on the upper surface with a short downy stalk. Small red flowers appear before the leaves in early spring and are borne in tight clusters. Native to most of Europe, the elm was once widespread in town and country, but since the devastation of Dutch elm disease it is being replaced by other species. To protect the few remaining trees, use only commercial preparations.

PRINCIPAL CONSTITUENTS
U. procera, is rarely used in herbal medicine, although it probably shares properties with *U. fulva*, the inner bark of which contains mucilage, bitter compounds and tannin (available in powdered form and known as Slippery Elm).

HERBAL MEDICINE
A decoction of powdered Slippery Elm (from *U. fulva*) has anti-inflammatory and demulcent properties. It is helpful for gastritis, gastric or duodenal ulcers, diarrhoea and colitis. In France, decoctions of the chopped dried inner bark are prescribed for skin complaints such as acne, psoriasis, eczema and pruritus.

FLOWER THERAPY
The flowers and twigs are collected in early spring and potentised by the Boiling Method. The remedy is for those who suddenly experience a sense of inadequacy or overload due to pressing demands (see pages 68–9).

URTICA DIOICA

NETTLE

Family: Urticaceae (Nettle Family) **Synonym:** Stinging Nettle **Parts Used:** flower stems, flowers (flower therapy), leaves

DESCRIPTION AND HABITAT
(See illustration, page 192)

A perennial plant up to 1.5m tall with tough, creeping roots, dull green stems and leaves covered with stinging hairs. Tiny greenish flowers grow in catkin formations in the leaf axils, with males (spreading) and females (pendulous) on separate plants. Found worldwide in temperate regions, it is a common garden weed.

PRINCIPAL CONSTITUENTS
Tannins, histamine, organic acids, vitamin C, provitamin A, mineral salts.

HERBAL MEDICINE
Nettle is astringent, tonic, diuretic, haemostatic, anti-rheumatic, galactogogic and blood-purifying. Infusions are used for urinary, liver and respiratory disorders, high blood pressure, simple anaemia, poor circulation, rheumatism, sciatica and skin disorders, especially childhood eczema.

FLOWER THERAPY
Collect male or female flowers in high summer and potentise by the Sun Method. Nettle is for those who feel apart or have been 'stung' by life, but are unable to express their feelings. The remedy restores the ability to demonstrate righteous anger.

HOMEOPATHY
As for herbal uses, though it may also be used to counter the ill effects of eating shellfish, and for bedwetting, uterine haemorrhage, pruritus and genital herpes.

VIOLA TRICOLOR

HEARTSEASE

Family: Violaceae (Violet Family) **Synonym:** Wild Pansy **Parts Used:** flowers (including flower therapy)

DESCRIPTION AND HABITAT
(See illustration, page 192)
An annual or perennial herb with creeping leafy stems and leaves which are heart-shaped at the base. The leafless flowering stems bear the solitary blooms, which are yellow, white or violet, or a combination. Heartsease is native to Europe on cultivated and waste ground, in mountain pastures and on coastal dunes.

PRINCIPAL CONSTITUENTS
Saponins, essential oil, flavonoids, salicylates, tannins, mucilage.

HERBAL MEDICINE
The plant has diuretic, tonic and anti-inflammatory properties. Internally and externally heartsease is helpful for various skin complaints, including eczema, and for respiratory ailments, feverish conditions and rheumatic pain. The remedy is widely available as a tincture.

HOMEOPATHY
The homeopathic remedy mirrors the herbal uses.

FLOWER THERAPY
The flowers are collected in midsummer and potentised by the Sun Method. As its name suggests, the remedy eases the pain of a broken heart.

VITEX AGNUS CASTUS

CHASTE TREE

Family: Verbenaceae (Verbena Family) **Synonyms:** Chaste Tree, Monk's Pepper
Parts Used: fruit (ripe berries)

DESCRIPTION AND HABITAT
(See illustration, page 192)
A deciduous shrub with small, fragrant, purple flowers borne in clusters on branching panicles. The ripe fruits (reddish black berries) resemble peppercorns. Chaste Tree is native to the shores of the Mediterranean.

PRINCIPAL CONSTITUENTS
Essential oil (unavailable commercially), glycosides, flavonoids, bitter principle (castin).

HERBAL MEDICINE
Chaste tree is primarily a tonic for the female reproductive organs. It is helpful for excessive menstruation, too frequent menstruation, PMS (particularly fluid retention, headache and tender breasts), menopausal hot flushes, vaginal dryness and insufficient breast milk. The remedy also increases a sense of emotional wellbeing. Reputedly anaphrodisiac in men but it can have the opposite effect in women who are experiencing loss of libido. Chaste Tree is widely available as a tincture prepared from the fresh fruit.

HOMEOPATHY
The potentised remedy is employed for male potency disorders, especially in the presence of absentmindedness, nervous depression and fearfulness.

VITIS VINIFERA

VINE

Parts Used: flowers (flower therapy), fruit, leaves, seeds (for their fixed oil)
Family: Vitaceae (Vine Family) **Synonym:** Grapevine

DESCRIPTION AND HABITAT

A deciduous, perennial, trailing climber, growing to 15m or more. The alternate leaves have three to five lobes and are coarsely serrated. The fragrant flowers, small, green and bud-like, are borne in branched clusters emerging from the leaf axils. These are followed by the familiar fruit (grapes). The grapevine is native to Asia, central and southern Europe, Australia, California and Africa.

PRINCIPAL CONSTITUENTS

Fruit: sugars, gum, malic acid, potassium bi-tartrate. Leaves: sugar, glucose, tartaric acid, potassium bi-tartrate, quercetine, quercitrin, tannin, amidon, malic acid, gum, inosite, oxalate of calcium.

HERBAL MEDICINE

The astringent leaves were formerly used internally and externally to staunch bleeding; dried and powdered, they were used for dysentery in cattle. The fruit is diuretic and hepatic, and so helpful for problems of the stomach, liver and kidneys.

AROMATHERAPY

The fixed oil is extracted from the seeds using volatile solvents. Unfortunately, the unrefined oil is unpalatable with an objectionable odour. The refined version is pale green and virtually odourless. A finely textured oil, it can be used as a base for all essential oils.

FLOWER THERAPY

The flowers are gathered in early summer and potentised by the Sun Method. (The Bach flower remedy is prepared from wild vines, such as those growing in Crete.) Vine is for those who tend to be domineering (see page 72).

APPENDICES

FLOWER THERAPY: REPERTORY OF EMOTIONAL/PSYCHOLOGICAL STATES

This section is intended as a quick reference and should be used in conjunction with the Bach flower remedy profiles in Chapter 5. The healing potential of selected flower essences developed in more recent years is described in the Directory of Healing Plants (Chapters 9–11).

When several flower essences seem to be equally appropriate for your particular state of mind (and if pendulum dowsing is not your forte), simply opt for the remedy plant with which you feel a special affinity – a flower or tree that you have seen growing in the wild or in a garden. You may be enamoured of its colour, texture, fragrance and form. Or perhaps you feel drawn to its natural habitat – be it open moorland, meadow, woodland or seashore. In this way you can find the flower that resonates most strongly with the spiritual aspect of your being.

For a list of mail order suppliers, see Useful Addresses on page 264.

> ### KEY
>
> Bach Flower Remedies, Britain (B), Bush Flower Essences, Australia (Aus B), Deva Flower Elixirs, France (Dv), Flower Essence Society, California (FES), Harebell Remedies, Britain (Hb), Master's Flower Essences, Hawaii (Mas), New Perception Flower Essences, New Zealand (NZ). The few flower essences shown in italics have not been profiled in the Directory of Healing Plants, but they are worth exploring

Absent-mindedness: Chestnut Bud, Clematis, Honeysuckle, Mustard, Olive (B), Rosemary, St John's Wort (Hb, FES), White Chestnut, Wild Rose (B)

Accident-proneness: Impatiens (B)

Addiction to substances: Agrimony (B), Angelica, Californian Poppy (FES)

Addiction to experiences: Basil (FES), Chestnut Bud(B)

Adolescence, associated problems: Californian Poppy (FES), Cerato (B), Chamomile (Hb, FES), Crab Apple, Holly, Hops, Larch, Scleranthus, Walnut, Wild Oat, Willow (B)

Ageing, fear of: Honeysuckle (B)

Aggressiveness: Holly, Impatiens, Sunflower (FES), Vine (B)

Aloofness: Rock Water (B), Violet (FES), Water Violet (B)

Ambition, unfulfilled: Walnut, Wild Oat (B)

Ambivalence: Cerato, Scleranthus, Wild Oat (B)

Anger: Chamomile (Hb, FES), Cherry Plum, Holly, Impatiens, Vine (B)

Anger, inability to express righteous: Holly (B), Nettle (Hb)

Anxiety: Agrimony, Aspen, Cerato (B), Chamomile (Hb, FES), Chicory, Cherry Plum, Crab Apple (B), Dandelion (Hb, FES), Elm, Heather, Larch (B), Lavender (Hb, FES), Meadowsweet (Hb), Mimulus, Red Chestnut, Rescue Remedy, Rock Water, Sweet Chestnut (B), Valerian (Dv),

White Chestnut (B), Ylang Ylang (FES). See also Worry

Apathy: Clematis, Gorse (B), Peppermint (FES), Wild Rose (B)

Argumentativeness: Beech (B), Calendula (FES), Chicory, Holly, Impatiens, Vervain, Vine, Willow (B)

Arrogance: Beech (B), Sunflower (FES), Vine (B)

Bitterness: Holly, Willow (B)

Boredom: Hornbeam (B)

Broken-heartedness: Angelica (FES), Chamomile (Hb, FES), Clematis (B), Dandelion (FES, Hb), *Hawthorn*, Heartsease (Hb), Holly, Honeysuckle, Rescue Remedy, Star-of-Bethlehem, Sweet Chestnut, Wild Rose, Willow (B)

Commitment, avoidance of: Evening Primrose (FES)

Communication, to enhance (including public speaking): Calendula (Hb, FES), Larch (B), Sunflower (FES). See also flower essence blend on page 245

Compassion, to engender: Beech (B), Calendula (Hb, FES), Chicory, Heather, Holly (B), Sunflower (FES), Willow (B)

Compulsive lying: Agrimony (B), *Honesty* (Hb).

Concentration, lack of: Chestnut Bud, Clematis, Honeysuckle (B), Peppermint (FES), Rosemary (Hb, FES), White Chestnut (B)

Confidence (to increase): Centaury, Cerato, Elm, Larch, Mimulus, Pine (B), Sunflower (FES)

Control, loss of: Cherry Plum, Rock Rose (B)

Courage, to engender: Larch (B),

Lemon Balm (NZ), Mimulus (B)

Creativity, to release potential: Clematis (B), *Iris* (Dv, FES)

Criticises others: Beech, Chicory, Holly (B), Sunflower (FES), Vine, Willow (B)

Cynicism: Gentian, Holly, Willow (B)

Death and dying (to engender balanced acceptance): Angelica, *Chrysanthemum* (FES), St John's Wort (Hb, FES), Star-of-Bethlehem, Sweet Chestnut, Walnut (B)

Delusions: Angelica (FES), Aspen, Cherry Plum (B), Clematis, Elder, Rescue Remedy (B)

Depression: Chamomile (Hb, FES), Elder (Hb), Gentian (B), Geranium (Hb), Gorse, Larch, Mustard (B), Nasturtium (FES), Oak, Pine (B), St John's Wort (Hb, FES), Wild Rose (B)

Despair: Cherry Plum, Crab Apple, Elm, Gentian, Larch, Oak, Pine, Star-of-Bethlehem, Sweet Chestnut, Willow (B)

Devitalisation: Geranium (Hb), Gorse, Hornbeam (B), Lemon Balm (NZ), Nasturtium (Hb, FES), Olive (B), Rosemary (Dv), St John's Wort (Hb, FES), Wild Rose (B)

Dishonesty: Basil (FES), *Honesty* (Hb)

Disdainfulness: Beech, Crab Apple, Rock Water, Water Violet (B)

Disorientation: Clematis, Honeysuckle, Rescue Remedy (B), Rosemary (Dv), Scleranthus (B)

Domineering temperament: Chicory (B), Sunflower (FES), Vervain, Vine (B)

Duplicity: Agrimony (B), Basil (FES), Cerato, Scleranthus (B), Sunflower (FES). See also Dishonesty

Easily led: Agrimony, Centaury, Cerato, Chestnut Bud, Walnut (B)

Eating, compulsive: Evening Primrose (FES)

Eating Disorders: see flower essence blends on page 245

Egotism: Beech, Chicory, Holly (B), Sunflower (FES), Vine, Water Violet (B)

Empathy: see Compassion

Emotional blackmail (to gain sympathy): Chicory, Willow (B)

Emotional detachment: Rock Water, Sweet Chestnut, Water Violet, Wild Rose (B)

Erratic behaviour: Chamomile (Hb, FES), Impatiens, Scleranthus (B)

Escapism: Agrimony (B), Californian Poppy (FES), Chestnut Bud, Clematis, Honeysuckle (B), Violet (FES), Water Violet, Wild Oat (B)

False persona: Agrimony (B), Californian Poppy, Sunflower (FES). See also Dishonesty

Fanaticism: Californian Poppy (FES), Vervain (B) Vine

Fathering (to engender balanced feelings towards): *Quince*, Sunflower (FES), Vine (B)

Fear: Angelica (FES), Aspen, Cherry Plum (B), Dandelion (Hb, FES), Elder, Holly, Larch (B), Marjoram (Hb), Mimulus, Red Chestnut, Rescue Remedy, Rock Rose (B), St John's Wort (Hb, FES)

Forgetfulness: Chestnut Bud, Clematis, Honeysuckle (B), Rosemary (Dv)

Forgiveness, of others: Beech, Holly, Pine, Willow (B)

Forgiveness, of self: Pine (B)

Freedom, to impart a sense of: Centaury, Cerato, Chestnut Bud (B), Lemon Balm (NZ), Walnut (B)

Frivolity, to impart a sense of: Geranium (Hb)

Frustration: Gentian, Holly, Impatiens, Walnut, Wild Oat (B)

Fussiness: Beech, Cerato, Chicory, Crab Apple, Heather, Rock Water (B)

Greed: Chicory, Heather, Holly (B), *Star Thistle* (FES), Vine (B)

Grief: see Broken-heartedness

Guilt: Pine (B)

Hatred, of others: Holly, Willow (B)

Hatred, of self: Crab Apple (B)

Homesickness: Honeysuckle (B)

Hopelessness: Angelica (FES), Gentian, Gorse, Sweet Chestnut, Wild Rose (B)

Hostility: Cherry Plum, Holly (B)

Hyperactivity: Chamomile (Hb, FES), Impatiens, Vervain (B)

Hypochondria, tendency towards: Heather (B)

Hysteria: Chamomile (Hb, FES), Rescue Remedy, Rock Rose (B), Valerian (Dv)

Idealism: Clematis, Elm, Rock Water, Vervain (B)

Imitative, being: Californian Poppy (FES), Cerato (B)

Impatience: Impatiens (B), Calendula (FES)

Impulsiveness: Impatiens, Vervain (B)

Indecisiveness: Cerato, Larch, Scleranthus, Wild Oat (B)

Infertility, emotionally induced: *She Oak* (Aus B), *Pomegranate* (FES), *Lady's Mantle* (Hb)

Inertia: Chestnut bud, Hornbeam (B), Peppermint (FES)

Inferiority, feeling of: Centaury, Larch, Pine (B)

Insecurity: Aspen (B), Evening Primrose (FES), Mimulus (B), St John's Wort (Hb, FES), Wild Oat (B)

Insomnia: Aspen (B), Chamomile, Lavender (Hb, FES), Rescue Remedy (B), St John's Wort (Hb, FES), Valerian (Dv), White Chestnut (B), Ylang Ylang (FES)

Inspiration, to engender: *Iris* (Dv, FES)

Intolerance: Beech, Impatiens, Rock Water, Vervain, Vine, Willow (B)

Irrational behaviour: Aspen (B)

Irritability: Beech (B), Chamomile (Hb, FES), Chicory, Crab Apple, Impatiens (B), Lavender (Hb, FES), Valerian (Dv), Willow (B)

Jealousy: Holly (B)

Joy, to impart a sense of: Geranium (Hb), Orange (Mas)

Karma, to free oneself from the dictates of others: Centaury, Cerato, Walnut (B)

Karma, to release oneself from repeating the same old mistakes: Chestnut Bud (B)

Laziness: see Inertia

Loneliness: Beech, Chicory, Elm (B), Heartsease (Hb), Heather (B), Holly, Honeysuckle, Impatiens, Mustard, Sweet Chestnut (B), Violet (FES), Water Violet (B)

Love, ability to give and receive: Holly (B), Linden (Dv), Willow (B)

Martyrdom: Centaury, Chicory, Rock Water (B)

Maternal instincts, unfulfilled: Evening Primrose (FES). See also Mothering

Meditation aid: Angelica, Californian Poppy (FES), Impatiens (B), Lavender (Hb, FES), *Lotus* (FES), Rosemary (FES), White Chestnut (B)

Memory, poor: see Forgetfulness

Menopausal distress: Chamomile (Hb, FES), Evening Primrose (FES), *Pomegranate* (FES), *She Oak* (Aus B)

Mental fatigue/congestion: Heather (B), Lemon (Dv, FES), Nasturtium (Hb, FES), Peppermint (Dv), Rescue Remedy, White Chestnut (B)

Mid-life crisis: Walnut, Wild Oat (B)

Miserliness: *Star Thistle* (FES)

Monotonous existence, to help break pattern: Centaury, Gentian (B), *Iris* (FES), Wild Rose (B)

Mood swings: Chamomile (Hb, FES), Mustard, Rescue Remedy, Scleranthus (B)

Mothering, to engender balanced feelings towards: Chicory (B), Linden (Dv), *Pomegranate* (FES)

Motivation, to trigger: Gorse, Hornbeam, Larch, Wild Rose (B)

Nervous breakdown: Cherry Plum, Oak, Rescue Remedy, Vervain (B)

Nervous tension: Aspen (B) Chamomile (Hb, FES), Cherry Plum (B), Dandelion (Hb, FES), Impatiens (B), Lavender (Hb, FES), Mimulus, Rescue Remedy, Valerian (Dv), Vervain (B), Ylang Ylang (FES)

Nervy personality type: Impatiens, Vervain (B)

Nightmares/night terrors: Angelica (FES), Aspen, Cherry Plum, Rescue Remedy, Rock Rose (B), St John's Wort (Hb, FES)

Nostalgia: Honeysuckle (B)

Obsession: Crab Apple, Heather, Red Chestnut, Rock Water, Vervain, White Chestnut (B)

Over-intellectualism: Nasturtium (Hb, FES)

Over-sensitivity: Angelica (FES), Beech (B), Calendula, Chamomile, Lavender (Hb, FES), Red chestnut, Rescue Remedy (B), St John's Wort (Hb, FES), Star-of-Bethlehem, Walnut (B)

Overwhelmed, feeling: Chamomile (Hb, FES), Cherry Plum, Elm, Hornbeam (B), Lavender (Hb, FES), Oak, Rescue Remedy, Sweet Chestnut (B)

Optimism, blind: Chestnut Bud(B)

Overwork: Elm, Impatiens, Oak, Rescue Remedy (B)

Panic: Rescue Remedy, Rock Rose (B)

Paranoia: Aspen (B), Elder (Hb), Holly (B), St John's Wort (Hb, FES)

Perfectionism: Agrimony, Beech, Crab Apple (B), Dandelion (Hb,

FES), Elm, Rock Water, Water Violet (B)

Pessimism: Gentian, Gorse, Larch (B)

Phobias: Aspen, Mimulus, Rescue Remedy (B)

Possessiveness: Chicory, Heather, Red Chestnut (B)

Premenstrual distress: Chamomile (Hb, FES), Evening Primrose (FES), *She Oak* (Aus B)

Pride: Beech (B), *Field Poppy* (Hb), Sunflower (FES), Vine, Water Violet (B)

Procrastination: Cerato, Chamomile (Hb, FES), Scleranthus (B)

Psychism, uncontrolled and resulting in fear: Angelica (FES), Aspen, Clematis, Rescue Remedy (B), St John's Wort (Hb, FES)

Purpose, to engender a sense of: Jasmine (FES), Wild Oat (B)

Reclusive, tendency to be: Mimulus, Rock Water, Water Violet (B)

Rejected, sense of being: Angelica, Evening Primrose (FES), Chicory, Crab Apple, Holly, Honeysuckle, Larch, Pine, Sweet Chestnut, Willow (B)

Resentfulness: Beech, Chicory, Holly, Willow (B)

Sapped by others: Agrimony, Centaury, Clematis, Mimulus (B)

Saps others: Cerato, Chicory, Heather, Holly, Honeysuckle (B)

Seasonal affective disorder (SAD): Mustard (B), St John's Wort (FES)

Self-acceptance, to help engender: Californian Poppy (FES), Chamomile (FES, Hb), *Cornflower* (Hb), Oak (B), Sage (FES, Hb)

Self-aggrandisement: Sunflower (FES), Vine (B)

Self-centredness: Beech, Chicory, Heather (B), Sunflower (FES), Vine, Willow (B)

Self-confidence: see Confidence

Self-deception: Agrimony (B), *Honesty* (Hb)

Self-disgust: Crab Apple (B)

Self-effacement: Centaury, Crab Apple, Pine (B), Sunflower (FES)

Self-esteem, low: Centaury, Cerato, Larch (B), Sunflower (FES)

Selfishness: Chicory, Heather, Holly, Water Violet (B), Willow

Self-neglect: Gorse, Pine, Wild Rose (B)

Self-pity: Chicory, Heather, Willow (B)

Sensory enhancement/awakening: *Iris* (FES), Wild Rose (B)

Sensory overload: Lavender (FES)

Sexual abuse: Crab Apple (B), Evening Primrose (FES)

Sexual desire, loss of: *Fuchsia* (FES), Wild Rose (B)

Sexual insecurity: Basil (FES), Crab Apple (B), Evening Primrose (FES), Larch, Mimulus, Pine (B), Rosemary (FES)

Shame: Agrimony (B), Basil (FES), Crab Apple, Larch, Pine (B)

Shock, effects of past: Star-of-Bethlehem (B)

Shock, immediate: Rescue Remedy, Star-of-Bethlehem (B)

Shyness: Larch, Mimulus (B), Violet (FES), Water Violet (B)

Sleepwalking: Aspen (B)

Stinginess: Chicory, Holly (B), *Star Thistle* (FES), Willow (B)

Stress: Chamomile (Hb, FES), Cherry Plum, Elm, Impatiens (B), Lavender (Hb, FES), Meadowsweet (Hb), Olive, Rescue Remedy, Star-of-Bethlehem (B), Valerian (Dv), Vervain (B), Ylang Ylang (FES)

Subservience: Centaury (B)

Suicidal thoughts: Agrimony, Aspen, Cherry Plum, Mimulus, Rescue Remedy (B)

Superiority, feelings of: Sunflower (FES), Vine, Water Violet (B)

Temper, severe and uncontrolled: Cherry Plum (B)

Terror: Rescue Remedy (B), Rock Rose

Torment, inner: Agrimony (B)

Trauma, past or present: Star-of-Bethlehem (B)

Trivia, over-concerned with: Crab Apple, Heather (B)

Trust, to engender: Angelica (FES), Aspen (B), Basil (FES), Cerato, Cherry Plum (B), *Hawthorn*, Marjoram (Hb), Red Chestnut (B), St John's Wort (Hb, FES)

Unconsciousness: Clematis (B), Rescue Remedy (B) (see page 73)

Ungroundedness: Aspen, Cherry Plum, Clematis, Honeysuckle, Mimulus, Rescue Remedy, Rock Rose (B), Rosemary (Hb, FES), Scleranthus, Star-of-Bethlehem (B), St John's Wort (Hb, FES), Walnut (B). See also flower essence blend on page 245

Unworldliness: Clematis, Honeysuckle (B), Violet (FES), Water Violet (B)

Victim mentality: Centaury, Willow (B)

Violence of actions, thoughts or dreams: Cherry Plum, Holly, Impatiens, Rescue Remedy, Scleranthus, Vine (B)

Vocation, to help find true path in life: Jasmine (FES), Sage (Dv), Wild Oat (B)

Weak will: Agrimony, Centaury, Cerato, Larch, Mimulus, Wild Rose (B)

Wisdom for inner guidance: Calendula, Californian Poppy (FES), Cerato, Chestnut Bud (B), Sage (Dv)

Worry: Agrimony, White Chestnut (B), Ylang Ylang (FES). See also Anxiety

FLOWER ESSENCE BLENDS

Although flower essences are best prescribed according to individual need, here are a few standard formulas which you may find useful. Make up a treatment bottle as usual, adding 2 drops of each flower essence.

EATING DISORDERS

Choose the combination which seems most appropriate to the person's mental state, adding other remedies as necessary. Crab Apple is included in each blend because it is for those who suffer anxiety, self-disgust and compulsive behaviour (especially in relation to various forms of self-cleansing and purging), and have obsessively negative feelings about their own body image.

Important: While flower therapy may suffice in the early stages of an eating disorder, advanced cases will also require professional intervention from a specialist in the field.

Anorexia: Cherry Plum/Crab Apple/Rock Water (B)

Bulimia: Cherry Plum/Crab Apple/Scleranthus (B)

Compulsive Eating: Chicory/Crab Apple (B)

GROUNDING FORMULA

The following combination remedy is especially helpful for therapists who feel disorientated, or in any other way uncomfortable, as a result of having taken on the problems of their clients/patients. It is also beneficial for anyone who feels totally engulfed by the concerns of another and therefore quite unable to be of any assistance. By rising above the situation, greater insight may be gleaned.

Red Chestnut/Rescue Remedy/Walnut (B)

PUBLIC SPEAKING

For dispelling nerves, increasing self-confidence and aiding clarity of thought.

Larch/Mimulus/White Chestnut (B)

Lemon/Sunflower (FES)

STRESS-RELATED INSOMNIA

The following blends soothe a frenzied nervous system and help to quieten mental chatter. The second blend is especially suited to those who may drop off to sleep initially, only to be awakened by disturbing dreams.

Chamomile/Lavender/White Chestnut (FES/B)

Rescue Remedy/St John's Wort/White Chestnut (FES/B)

DR AUBREY WESTLAKE'S RADIATION REMEDY

We live in a world subject to increasing levels of radiation emanating from high-voltage power lines, radio, television, computer terminals, X-rays, hi-tech medical scanning devices and many other sources. It is believed that over-exposure to radiation in its many guises may be responsible for a wide range of health problems, including fatigue, nervous tension, headache, insomnia, diminished libido, low fertility and, in extreme cases, certain forms of cancer.

The following flower essence composite was devised by the late Dr Aubrey Westlake, a British physician who spent many years researching into vibrational methods of healing. He believed that the mixture would generally alleviate the negative effects of radiation upon the subtle body or electro-magnetic field. The remedy is certainly worth considering if you spend many hours each day in front of a computer screen, if you are constantly exposed to high-voltage electrical equipment, or if you have to undergo medical treatment involving radiological devices.

Radiation Remedy consists of seven Bach flower essences: Cherry Plum, Gentian, Rock Rose, Star-of-Bethlehem, Vine, Walnut and Wild Oat. (It would also seem appropriate to add Crab Apple, the cleanser.) To prepare the remedy, put 1g of finely ground sea salt in a 50ml dark glass medicine bottle, then fill the bottle almost to the top with spring water. Shake well to disperse the salt crystals. Add 2 drops of each flower essence to the bottle and shake again. Take 4 drops directly on the tongue 3–4 times daily. Continue for as long as required.

QUICK GUIDE TO HERBS AND OILS FOR SPECIFIC AILMENTS

Holistic treatment strategies for many of the ailments can be found in Chapter 8. For advice on preparing and using herbs and essential oils, see Chapter 6.

ACNE

Essential Oils: cedarwood (Virginian or Atlas), chamomile (German and Roman), frankincense, garlic (capsules), geranium, juniper berry, lavender, patchouli, rose otto, rosemary, tea tree.

Herbs: calendula, dandelion, echinacea, elm, heartsease, lemon, nasturtium, nettle, rose petal, sage, violet (sweet).

ALCOHOL WITHDRAWAL SYMPTOMS

Also helpful for those recovering from other addictive substances

Essential Oils: as for *Anxiety and Stress.*

Herbs: angelica, evening primrose oil (capsules). See also herbs for *Anxiety and Stress.*

ALLERGIES

Essential Oils: first carry out a skin test (page 88): chamomile (German and Roman), lavender, melissa (true), rose otto.

Herbs: chamomile, echinacea, evening primrose oil (capsules), ginseng, lemon balm, rose petal.

ANAEMIA

Herbs: angelica, centaury, nasturtium, nettle.

ANXIETY AND STRESS

Essential Oils: angelica, basil (but see Cautions, page 193), bergamot (and other citrus oils), chamomile (German and Roman), clary sage, frankincense, jasmine, hops, juniper berry, lavender, marjoram (sweet), melissa (true), neroli, patchouli, petitgrain, rose, sandalwood, valerian, ylang ylang.

Herbs: basil, calendula, Californian poppy, chamomile, evening primrose (leaves and stems), honeysuckle, hops, jasmine flowers, lavender, lemon (leaves), lemon balm, linden blossom, oat, orange blossom, rose petal, St John's wort, valerian, violet (sweet).

APPETITE, LOSS OF after illness

Essential Oils: The aromas of almost all essential oils stimulate the appetite (if found pleasing), though the following are especially recommended: angelica, bergamot, coriander, ginger, lemon, orange, peppermint, rosemary.

Herbs: most aromatics, especially culinary herbs and spices like basil, chicory, coriander, ginger, peppermint and marjoram (sweet). Also agrimony, angelica, centaury, hops.

ARTHRITIS AND RHEUMATISM

Essential Oils: angelica, cedarwood (Virginian and Atlas), chamomile (German and Roman), coriander, eucalyptus, ginger, juniper berry, lavender, marjoram (sweet), pine, rosemary.

Herbs: apple (cider vinegar), aspen, centaury, chamomile, chicory, dandelion, evening primrose oil (capsules), elder (flowers and berries), feverfew, ginger, heartsease, juniper berry, lemon, lilac (infused oil, see page 96), marjoram (sweet), meadowsweet, mustard, nettle, olive (fixed olive externally), pine needle, rosemary, sage, St John's wort, valerian, violet (sweet), willow.

ASTHMA

Essential Oils: eucalyptus, frankincense, garlic (capsules), lavender, melissa (true), marjoram (sweet), peppermint, pine, rose otto, rosemary, tea tree.

Herbs: angelica, chamomile, echninacea, eucalyptus (leaves), evening primrose (leaves and stems), feverfew, lavender, linden blossom, marjoram (sweet), lemon balm, peppermint, pine needle, rosemary.

ATHLETE'S FOOT
Essential Oils: cedarwood (Atlas), eucalyptus, lavender, patchouli, pine, tea tree.
Herbs: calendula, echinacea, eucalyptus (leaves).

BED SORES
Essential Oils: chamomile (German), patchouli.
Herbs: calendula, St John's wort.

BLOOD PRESSURE (high)
Essential Oils: chamomile (German and Roman), clary sage, garlic (capsules), lavender, lemon, melissa (true), valerian, ylang ylang.
Herbs: Californian poppy, evening primrose oil (capsules), lemon, lemon balm, linden blossom, nettle, olive (leaves), valerian.

BLOOD PRESSURE (low)
Essential Oils: angelica, coriander, geranium, ginger, lemon, marjoram (sweet), neroli, pine, rose otto, rosemary.
Herbs: angelica, coriander (seed), dandelion (root), ginger, ginseng, lemon, marjoram (sweet), orange flowers, rosemary.

BLOOD SUGAR (high)
Herbs: chicory, eucalyptus (leaves), olive (leaves), walnut (leaves).

BOILS AND ABSCESSES
Essential Oils: bergamot FCF, chamomile (German and Roman, though preferably the former), clary sage, eucalyptus, garlic (capsules), lavender, lemon, tea tree.
Herbs: calendula, dandelion (root), echinacea, heartsease, lemon, nettle, violet (sweet).

BRONCHITIS
Essential Oils: angelica, cedarwood (Atlas and Virginian), eucalyptus, frankincense, garlic (capsules), lavender, lemon, marjoram (sweet), orange, peppermint, pine, rose otto, rosemary, sandalwood, tea tree.
Herbs: angelica, basil, echinacea, ginger, heartsease, honeysuckle, lemon, marjoram (sweet), nasturtium, pine needle, sage, vervain, violet (sweet).

BRUISES
See *Sprains and Bruises*.

BURNS AND SCALDS (minor)
Essential Oils: chamomile (German and Roman), eucalyptus, frankincense, geranium, lavender, tea tree.
Herbs: calendula, elder (leaves), oak (bark), St John's wort, witch-hazel (distilled water).

CATARRH
Essential Oils: angelica, basil (but see Cautions, page 193), cedarwood (Atlas or Virginian), eucalyptus, frankincense, ginger, juniper berry, lavender, lemon marjoram (sweet), orange, peppermint, pine, rose otto, rosemary, sandalwood, tea tree.
Herbs: angelica, basil, chamomile, elder (flower), feverfew, heartsease, juniper berry, lemon balm, linden blossom, marjoram (sweet), nasturtium (seeds), peppermint, pine needle, rosemary, sage, violet (sweet).

CHILBLAINS
Essential Oils: chamomile (German and Roman), lavender, lemon, marjoram (sweet).
Herbs: calendula, ginger, lemon balm, nettle, oak (bark, leaves), peppermint.

CHILDBIRTH (to facilitate labour)
Essential Oils: clary sage, jasmine, lavender.
Herbs: clary sage, jasmine (flowers).

CIRCULATION, SLUGGISH
Essential Oils: angelica, bergamot FCF, coriander, eucalyptus, garlic (capsules), geranium, ginger, lavender, lemon, marjoram (sweet), melissa (true), neroli, orange, peppermint, rose otto, rosemary.
Herbs: angelica, basil, dandelion (root), horse chestnut, lavender, lemon balm, mustard, nasturtium, nettle, peppermint, pine, rosemary, sage, vervain.

COLDS AND FLU
Essential Oils: angelica, basil (but see Cautions on page 193), bergamot FCF, cedarwood (Atlas and Virginian), coriander, eucalyptus, ginger, lavender, lemon, marjoram, orange, peppermint, petitgrain, pine, tea tree.
Herbs: chamomile, elder (berries, flower), ginger, honeysuckle, lemon, lemon balm, linden blossom, marjoram (sweet), mustard, peppermint, pine needle, rose (petal, hips), meadowsweet, sage, violet (sweet).

COLD SORES
Essential Oils: bergamot FCF, chamomile (preferably German), eucalyptus, melissa (true), tea tree.
Herbs: calendula, chamomile, echinacea, lavender, lemon balm, St John's wort, walnut (leaves).

COLIC
Essential Oils: angelica, chamomile (German and Roman), coriander, ginger, hops, marjoram (sweet), melissa (true), peppermint, valerian.
Herbs: angelica, Californian poppy,

chamomile, coriander, evening primrose (leaves and stems), hops, valerian.

COLITIS
Essential Oils: agrimony, cranesbill (listed under Geranium in the Directory of Healing Plants), meadowsweet, oak (bark), slippery elm (listed under Elm in the Directory of Healing Plants).

CONSTIPATION
Essential Oils: marjoram (sweet), orange, rose otto, rosemary.
Herbs: apple (stewed), basil, centaury, chamomile, chicory, dandelion (root), elder (berry), marjoram (sweet), mustard (seeds), nasturtium (seeds), olive (extra virgin grade oil), rose (leaves), sunflower (roots), violet (sweet).

COUGHS
Essential Oils: angelica, cedarwood, clary sage, eucalyptus, frankincense, garlic (capsules, but see page 132), ginger, jasmine, marjoram (sweet), pine, rose otto, rosemary, sandalwood, tea tree.
Herbs: apple (cider vinegar and honey), basil, chestnut (sweet), clary sage, dandelion (flowers), elder (berry), honeysuckle (flowers), jasmine (flowers), marjoram (sweet), peppermint, pine needle, rose (petals), sage, vervain, violet (sweet).

CUTS AND GRAZES
Essential Oils: chamomile (German and Roman), eucalyptus, frankincense, geranium, lavender, lemon, pine, tea tree.
Herbs: agrimony, calendula, centaury, horse chestnut, lavender, St John's wort, walnut (leaves), witch-hazel (distilled water).

CRACKED SKIN
Essential Oils: patchouli, sandalwood.
Herbs: calendula.

CYSTITIS
Essential Oils: bergamot FCF, cedarwood (Atlas), chamomile (German and Roman), eucalyptus, frankincense, juniper berry, lavender, pine, sandalwood, tea tree.
Herbs: angelica, aspen (buds, bark, leaves), chamomile, dandelion (root), eucalyptus (leaves), heather, meadowsweet, nasturtium (seeds), pine needle.

DANDRUFF
Essential Oils: cedarwood (Atlas), eucalyptus, lavender, patchouli, rosemary, tea tree.
Herbs: eucalyptus (leaves), lavender, nasturtium (leaves, seeds), rosemary.

DEPRESSION (including Post Natal Depression)
Essential Oils: basil (but see Caution, page 193), bergamot (and other citrus oils), clary sage, coriander, frankincense, geranium, jasmine, juniper berry, lavender, neroli, patchouli, petitgrain, rose, rosemary, sandalwood, ylang ylang.
Herbs: basil, feverfew, ginseng, honeysuckle, lavender, lemon balm, linden blossom, orange (flowers, leaves), lemon (leaves), nasturtium, oat, rosemary, St John's wort, vervain.

DERMATITIS
See *Eczema*.

DIARRHOEA
Essential Oils: chamomile (German and Roman), garlic (capsules), ginger, marjoram, neroli, peppermint, sandalwood.
Herbs: agrimony, angelica, evening primrose (leaves and stems), ginger,

meadowsweet, oak, peppermint, rose (hips, petals), sage, slippery elm (listed under Elm in the Directory of Healing Plants), St John's wort.

DYSENTERY
Essential Oils: external applications of essential oils are virtually ineffective.
Herbs: cranesbill (listed under Geranium in the Directory of Healing Plants), walnut, willow.

EARACHE
Essential Oils: chamomile (German and Roman), lavender, peppermint, rosemary.
Herbs: see *Coughs and Colds and Flu*.

ECZEMA
Essential Oils: cedarwood (Atlas), chamomile (German and Roman), geranium, juniper berry, lavender, melissa (true), patchouli, rose otto, sandalwood. But carry out a skin test first (see page 88).
Herbs: calendula, chamomile, echinacea, elm (bark), heartsease, heather, nettle, oat, rose petal, violet (sweet), walnut (leaves).

EYE INFECTIONS
Essential Oils: none. Use only genuine distilled rosewater as an eyewash.
Herbs: agrimony, calendula, chamomile, echinacea, elder (flower), rose petal, sage, walnut (leaves).

FATIGUE AND NERVOUS EXHAUSTION
Essential Oils: angelica, bergamot FCF (and other citrus oils), coriander, geranium, ginger, jasmine, juniper berry, lavender, marjoram (sweet), melissa (true), peppermint, pine, rose otto, rosemary.
Herbs: agrimony, angelica, basil,

echinacea, ginger, ginseng, lemon balm, marjoram (sweet), oat, pine needle, rose (hip), rosemary, sage, vervain.

FEVERS

Essential Oils: angelica, bergamot FCF, clary sage, eucalyptus, juniper berry, lemon, patchouli, peppermint, tea tree.

Herbs: clary sage, ginger, heartsease, honeysuckle, horse chestnut, lemon (rind), nasturtium (seeds), olive (leaves), sage, sunflower (flowers, leaves), vervain, willow.

FLATULENCE

Essential Oils: chamomile (Roman), coriander, ginger, marjoram (sweet), peppermint, rosemary.

Herbs: angelica, basil, chamomile, ginger, juniper berry, lemon balm, marjoram (sweet), peppermint, rosemary.

FIBROSITIS

Essential Oils: ginger, pine, rosemary.

Herbs: St John's wort (infused oil).

FLUID RETENTION

Essential Oils: external applications of essential oils are not especially effective. Massage (particularly the form known as lymphatic drainage massage) greatly improves the condition, with or without essential oils.

Herbs: dandelion (root), juniper berry, meadowsweet, pine needle, rosemary, St John's wort, vervain.

GASTRITIS

Essential Oils: chamomile (German and Roman).

Herbs: chamomile, cranesbill (listed under Geranium in the Directory of Healing Plants), meadowsweet,

slippery elm (listed under Elm in the Directory of Healing Plants).

GINGIVITIS

Essential Oils: bergamot FCF, eucalyptus, geranium, lemon, tea tree.

Herbs: agrimony, calendula, echinacea, rose (leaves), sage, vervain.

HAEMORRHOIDS

Essential Oils: frankincense, geranium.

Herbs: calendula, cranesbill (listed under Geranium in the Directory of Healing Plants), horse chestnut, oak, St John's wort.

HAIR (to promote healthy growth)

Essential Oils: cedarwood (Atlas), juniper berry, patchouli, rosemary, ylang ylang.

Herbs: nasturtium, rosemary.

HALITOSIS (offensive breath)

Essential Oils: bergamot FCF, lavender, peppermint.

Herbs: peppermint.

HAYFEVER

Essential Oils: chamomile (preferably German), eucalyptus, garlic (capsules), melissa (true), peppermint, pine, rose otto.

Herbs: chamomile, elderflower, feverfew, lavender, lemon balm, peppermint, pine needle, rose petal.

HEADACHE

Essential Oils: chamomile (German and Roman), clary sage, hops, lavender, marjoram (sweet), melissa (true), peppermint, rose, rosemary, valerian.

Herbs: basil, Californian poppy, clary sage, feverfew, honeysuckle, hops, lavender, linden blossom,

meadowsweet, peppermint, rosemary, sage, valerian, vervain, violet (sweet).

HEADLICE

Essential Oils: eucalyptus, garlic (capsules), geranium, lavender, pine, rosemary, tea tree.

INDIGESTION AND HEARTBURN

Essential Oils: angelica, chamomile (German and Roman), clary sage, coriander, ginger, lavender, marjoram (sweet), melissa (true), neroli, peppermint, petitgrain. Heartburn: chamomile (preferably German).

Herbs: agrimony, angelica, basil, calendula, centaury, chamomile, chicory, coriander, dandelion (root), evening primrose (leaves and stems), ginger, lavender, lemon balm, linden blossom, marjoram (sweet), orange (flowers, leaves), sage, slippery elm (listed under Elm in the Directory of Healing Plants), valerian, vervain. Heartburn: meadowsweet, slippery elm.

INCONTINENCE (urinary)

Herbs: agrimony, St John's wort.

INFECTION AND LOW IMMUNITY (to boost immune system)

Essential Oils: garlic (capsules).

Herbs: echinacea, ginger, ginseng, nasturtium (seeds), sage.

INSECT BITES AND STINGS

Essential Oils: chamomile (German and Roman), eucalyptus, lavender, tea tree.

Herbs: Calendula, chamomile, lavender, peppermint, sage, St John's wort, witch-hazel (distilled).

INSECT REPELLENTS

Essential Oils: cedarwood,

eucalyptus, garlic (capsules), lavender, patchouli, peppermint, rosemary, tea tree.
Herbs: lavender, peppermint, rosemary, sage.

INSOMNIA

Essential Oils: chamomile (Roman), clary sage, hops, lavender, marjoram (sweet), melissa, neroli, petitgrain, rose, sandalwood, valerian, ylang ylang.
Herbs: basil, Californian poppy, chamomile, feverfew, honeysuckle, hops, lavender, lemon balm, linden blossom, oat, orange (flowers, leaves), rose petal, valerian, violet (sweet).

IRRITABLE BOWEL SYNDROME

Essential Oils: chamomile (German and Roman), hops, lavender, marjoram (sweet), melissa (true), neroli, peppermint (capsules), rose otto.
Herbs: agrimony, chamomile, hops, lemon balm, marjoram (sweet), peppermint, slippery elm (listed under Elm in the Directory of Healing Plants), valerian.

JETLAG

Essential Oils: chamomile (German and Roman), clary sage, frankincense, geranium, juniper berry, lavender, melissa (true), neroli, petitgrain, pine, rose, rosemary, sandalwood, valerian, ylang ylang.
Herbs: Californian poppy, hops, rosemary, sage, valerian, vervain.

LIBIDO (to enhance or restore)

Essential Oils: angelica, cedarwood (Atlas and Virginian), clary sage, coriander, ginger, jasmine, neroli, patchouli, rose, rosemary, sandalwood, ylang ylang (all are reputed aphrodisiacs).

Herbs: angelica, chaste tree (has the opposite effect in men), clary sage, coriander, ginger, jasmine (flowers), orange blossom, rose petal, rosemary.

LIBIDO (to lessen)

Essential Oils: hops (usually only in men), marjoram (sweet), valerian (all are reputed anaphrodisiacs).
Herbs: chaste tree (usually only in men), hops (usually only in men), marjoram, valerian.

MENSTRUAL PROBLEMS (loss of periods, scanty or irregular periods)

Essential Oils: angelica, basil (but see Cautions, page 193), clary sage, hops, juniper berry, marjoram (sweet), rose otto.
Herbs: angelica, basil, calendula, chaste tree, feverfew, hops, juniper berry, marjoram (sweet), rose petal, sage, vervain.

MENSTRUAL PROBLEMS (painful periods)

Essential Oils: angelica, chamomile (German and Roman), clary sage, frankincense, hops, juniper berry, lavender, marjoram (sweet), melissa (true), rose otto, rosemary, valerian.
Herbs: angelica, calendula, chamomile, chaste tree, clary sage, hops, jasmine flowers, lemon balm, marjoram (sweet), rose petal, rosemary, St John's wort, valerian.

MENSTRUAL PROBLEMS (heavy periods)

Essential Oils: chamomile (German and Roman), geranium, jasmine, lemon, rose otto.
Herbs: agrimony, cranesbill (listed under Geranium in the Directory of Healing Plants), jasmine (flowers), lemon (rind), oak (bark), rose petal, sage, sweet chestnut (leaves), walnut (leaves).

MENOPAUSAL SYMPTOMS

Essential Oils: clary sage, frankincense, geranium, hops, jasmine, melissa (true), rose otto (see also essential oils for *Anxiety and Stress*).
Herbs: calendula, chaste tree, cranesbill (listed under Geranium in the Directory of Healing Plants), evening primrose (oil capsules), ginseng, hops, lemon balm, oat, rose petal, St John's wort, walnut.

MENTAL FATIGUE

Essential Oils: angelica, basil, geranium, lavender, lemon melissa (true), peppermint, pine, rose, rosemary.
Herbs: angelica, basil, lemon balm, peppermint, rose petal, rosemary.

MIGRAINE

Essential Oils: angelica, chamomile (German and Roman), clary sage, coriander, lavender, marjoram (sweet), melissa (true), peppermint, rose otto, rosemary, valerian.
Herbs: angelica, basil, chamomile, elderflower, feverfew, ginseng, hops, lavender, linden blossom, marjoram (sweet), peppermint, rosemary, valerian, vervain, violet (sweet).

MILK FLOW (to decrease)

Essential Oils: jasmine, peppermint.
Herbs: jasmine (flowers), sage.

MILK FLOW (to promote)

Essential Oils: basil (but see Cautions on page 193), hops. Also lemongrass, sweet fennel (not profiled in the Directory of Healing Plants).
Herbs: basil, chaste tree, hops, nettle, vervain.

MOUTH ULCERS

Essential Oils: chamomile (preferably German), lemon,

peppermint, tea tree.
Herbs: calendula, oak (bark), sage.

MULTIPLE SCLEROSIS (MS)
Essential Oils: rosemary. See also
Anxiety and Stress, *Depression*, *Fatigue*.
Herbs: evening primrose (oil
capsules), St John's wort oil (infused
oil for massage).

MUSCULAR ACHES AND PAINS
Essential Oils: basil (but see
Cautions on page 193), chamomile
(German and Roman), clary sage,
coriander, eucalyptus, ginger,
jasmine, juniper berry, lavender,
lemon, marjoram (sweet),
peppermint, pine, rosemary.
Herbs: Californian poppy,
peppermint, pine needle, St John's
wort (infused oil for massage). See
also herbs for *Anxiety and Stress*.

NAPPY RASH
Essential Oils: none. Essential oils
may further irritate a baby's sensitive
skin.
Herbs: calendula, St John's wort
(ointment).

NAUSEA
Essential Oils: angelica, chamomile
(preferably Roman), coriander,
ginger, lavender, melissa (true),
peppermint, sandalwood.
Herbs: angelica, basil, chamomile,
coriander, ginger, meadowsweet,
peppermint. See also *Pregnancy
Sickness*, *Travel/Motion Sickness*.

NEURALGIA
Essential Oils: geranium,
peppermint, pine.
Herbs: Californian poppy,
chamomile, St John's wort, valerian,
willow.

NIPPLES (SORE CRACKED)
Essential Oils: chamomile
(preferably German), rose otto.
Herbs: calendula, St John's wort.

PALPITATIONS
Essential Oils: chamomile (German
and Roman), lavender, melissa
(true), neroli, orange, petitgrain,
rose, ylang ylang.
Herbs: Californian poppy,
chamomile, lemon (leaves), lemon
balm, linden blossom, orange
(flowers, leaves), rose petal, valerian.

PHLEBITIS (inflammation of the veins)
Herbs: Horse chestnut.

PREGNANCY SICKNESS ('EARLY MORNING SICKNESS')
Essential Oils: ginger, lavender,
peppermint (vaporiser or dry
inhalation only).
Herbs: chamomile, ginger
(crystallised stem), meadowsweet,
peppermint.

PREMENSTRUAL SYNDROME
Essential Oils: bergamot (and other
citrus oils), chamomile (German and
Roman), frankincense, geranium,
hops, juniper berry, lavender,
marjoram (sweet), melissa (true),
neroli, rose, sandalwood, ylang ylang.
Herbs: calendula, chamomile, chaste
tree, dandelion (root), evening
primrose (oil capsules), ginseng,
hops, lemon balm, oat, orange
(flowers, leaves), rose petal, St John's
wort, vervain.

POST-VIRAL FATIGUE SYNDROME (ME)
Essential Oils: garlic (capsules). See
also oils for *Anxiety and Stress*,
Depression, *Fatigue*.

Herbs: centaury, echinacea, St John's
wort, vervain.

PRICKLY HEAT
Essential Oils: chamomile
(preferably German), lavender.
Herbs: calendula, echinacea.

PRURITIS (ITCHING)
Essential Oils: cedarwood (Atlas),
chamomile (preferably German),
juniper berry, lavender.
Herbs: calendula, olive oil (extra
virgin), St John's wort (infused oil),
walnut (leaves).

PSORIASIS
Essential Oils: bergamot FCF,
chamomile (German and Roman),
lavender.
Herbs: chamomile, dandelion (root),
elm (bark), heartsease, hops, linden
blossom, nettle, oat, valerian.

RASHES
Essential Oils: chamomile
(preferably German), lavender,
patchouli, sandalwood.
Herbs: calendula, evening primrose
oil, violet (sweet).

RINGWORM
Essential Oils: eucalyptus, geranium,
lavender, lemon, patchouli,
peppermint, pine, tea tree.
Herbs: calendula, echinacea, horse
chestnut.

SCABIES
Essential Oils: bergamot FCF, garlic
(capsules), patchouli, peppermint,
pine, rosemary, sandalwood.

SCARS AND STRETCHMARKS (promotes proper healing of skin; essentially a preventative treatment)
Essential Oils: frankincense, laven-
der, neroli, patchouli, sandalwood.

Herbs: calendula (infused oil), olive oil (extra virgin).

SEASONAL AFFECTIVE DISORDER (SAD)
Essential Oils: see *Depression, Fatigue.*
Herbs: St John's wort.

SINUSITIS
Essential Oils: eucalyptus, garlic (capsules), lavender, lemon, peppermint, pine, tea tree.
Herbs: agrimony, echinacea, elder(flower), feverfew, lavender, peppermint, pine needle, rosemary.

SPOTS (PIMPLES)
Essential Oils: lavender, tea tree.
Herbs: calendula (tincture).

SPRAINS AND BRUISES
Essential Oils: chamomile (German and Roman), eucalyptus, geranium, lavender, marjoram (sweet), pine, rosemary.
Herbs: agrimony, beech (leaves), calendula, elder (leaves), feverfew, peppermint, St John's wort, sweet chestnut (leaves), witch-hazel (distilled).

STRAIN, MUSCULAR
Essential Oils: see *Sprains and Bruises.*
Herbs: calendula (infused oil), St John's wort (infused oil).

SUNBURN
Essential Oils: chamomile (German and Roman), geranium, lavender, rosemary, tea tree.
Herbs: calendula, horse chestnut, St John's wort.

THROAT PROBLEMS (hoarseness)
Essential Oils: clary sage, sandalwood.
Herbs: sage.

THROAT PROBLEMS (laryngitis)
Essential Oils: clary sage, eucalyptus, frankincense, lavender, lemon, sandalwood.
Herbs: agrimony, echinacea, eucalyptus (leaves), elder (leaves), lavender, oak (bark), sage.

THROAT PROBLEMS (sore throat, throat infection)
Essential Oils: garlic (capsules), bergamot FCF, clary sage, eucalyptus, frankincense, geranium, ginger, lavender, lemon, peppermint, pine, sandalwood, tea tree.
Herbs: agrimony, basil, echinacea, ginger, lemon, oak, pine needle, sage, violet (sweet).

THROAT PROBLEMS (tonsillitis)
Essential Oils: bergamot FCF, clary sage, geranium, garlic (capsules)
Herbs: echninacea, sage.

THRUSH, VAGINAL
Essential Oils: garlic (capsules by mouth), lavender, tea tree.
Herbs: agrimony, calendula, echinacea, lavender, oak (bark), rosemary, sage, walnut (leaves).

TRAVEL/MOTION SICKNESS
Essential Oils: as for *Nausea.*
Herbs: ginger (crystallised stem).

ULCER, GASTRIC
Essential Oils: peppermint. See also *Anxiety and Stress.*
Herbs: calendula, chamomile, meadowsweet, peppermint, slippery elm.

ULCER, MOUTH
See *Mouth Ulcers.*

ULCER, SKIN
Essential Oils: geranium.
Herbs: calendula, echinacea.

ULCER, VARICOSE
Herbs: Calendula, horse chestnut.

URTICARIA (HIVES)
Essential Oils: chamomile (preferably German).
Herbs: echninacea, elm (leaves).

VARICOSE VEINS
Essential Oils: frankincense, garlic (capsules taken internally), geranium, lavender, lemon, rose.
Herbs: calendula, cranesbill (listed under Geranium in the Directory of Healing Plants), horse chestnut, nettle, rosehip, St John's wort.

WARTS AND VERRUCAE
Essential Oils: lemon, tea tree.
Herbs: dandelion (latex pressed from stem).

WOUNDS
Essential Oils: bergamot FCF, chamomile (German and Roman), eucalyptus, frankincense, juniper berry, lavender, patchouli, rosemary, tea tree.
Herbs: calendula, elder (leaves), feverfew, olive (leaves), rose (leaves), rosemary, St John's wort, sweet chestnut (leaves), vervain, violet (sweet), walnut (leaves).

WORMS, INTESTINAL
Essential Oils: garlic (capsules).
Herbs: lemon (crushed pips), willow (bark).

GLOSSARY OF BOTANICAL TERMS

Achene: a small, dry, nut-like, one-seeded fruit that does not split open when ripe to release the seed.

Alternate (of leaves): arranged successively on opposite sides of the stem.

Annual: a plant that completes its life cycle within one year.

Aromatic: a plant with a distinctive, usually pleasing, aroma; applied to parts other than the flowers.

Axil: the upper angle between a leaf and the stem on which it grows.

Basal (of leaves): at the base of the stem.

Berry: a soft, fleshy, or pulpy fruit, usually many-seeded.

Biennial: a plant that completes its life cycle within two years, developing in the first year and flowering and fruiting in the second.

Bud: an immature shoot, leaf or flower; also a partially opened leaf or flower.

Bulb: an underground storage organ with fleshy leaves, the whole enclosing next year's bud.

Capsule: a dry fruit with one or more seeds, which when ripe splits open by pores or slits.

Catkin: a dense spike of small male or female flowers, usually long and tassel-like.

Compound (of leaves): composed of two or more similar parts.

Cone: the flower, and usually the fruit, of a cone-bearing tree, consisting of numerous overlapping, spirally arranged scales.

Coniferous: a cone-bearing tree.

Deciduous: applied to a tree or shrub that sheds it leaves in the autumn.

Escape: an introduced or cultivated plant that has escaped from gardens and become naturalised in an area.

Evergreen: a tree or shrub that bears leaves all year, continually shedding and replacing them.

Female flower: a flower with a *pistil* but no *stamens*.

Floret: small individual flower of a dense *inflorescence*.

Fruit: the ripe seeds and their surrounding structures, which can be fleshy or dry.

Genus: a biological classification made up of closely related but distinct species and given a common name. The genus is denoted by the first word in the botanical name.

Herb/herbaceous: any non-woody, soft and leafy plant. The word 'herb' also means any plant used in medicine and cooking.

Hybrid: a plant resulting from a cross between different species.

Inflorescence: the flowering part of the plant.

Lanceolate (of leaves): narrow, with the base broadest, tapering at the tip like a lance or spear.

Latex: milky fluid exuded from some plants when injured.

Leaflet: a subdivision of a compound leaf.

Linear (of leaves): long and narrow, almost parallel-sided (e.g. a blade of grass).

Lobed (of leaves): divided towards the central vein of the leaf, but not into separate leaflets, each division rounded at the apex (e.g. oak leaves).

Male flower: a flower with *stamens* but no *pistil*.

Nut: a non-splitting, one-seeded fruit with a hard, woody outer covering.

Oleo gum resin: an odoriferous exudation from trees and plants, consisting of essential oil, gum and resin (e.g. frankincense).

Oleoresin: a natural odoriferous exudation from trees and plants, consisting of essential oil and resinous material (e.g. myrrh). Also, a prepared resin from which the essential oil has been captured (i.e. *resinoid*).

Opposite (of leaves): growing in pairs at the same level on opposite sides of the stem.

Ovate/ovoid (of leaves): broadest below the middle (like a hen's egg).

Palmate (of compound leaves): lobed or divided in hand-like fashion, usually five- or seven-lobed.

Panicle: a branching flower cluster.

Perennial: a plant that lives for more than two years and usually flowers each year; herbaceous perennials grow from the rootstock each year, dying down to ground level for the winter.

Pinnate (of compound leaves): leaflets are arranged on either side of a central stalk.

Pistil: the female organ of a flower comprising ovary (the 'seedbox'), stigma (the sticky or feathery tip of the pistil which receives the pollen) and style (the part that connects the ovary and stigma).

Resin: an exudation from certain trees which becomes solid or semi-solid on exposure to air (e.g. mastic).

Resinoid: a viscous, highly odoriferous substance (e.g. benzoin), extracted from resinous plant material by means of hydrocarbon solvents. Resinoids are also called *oleoresins*.

Rhizome: a creeping, usually horizontal, underground storage stem which sends up leafy shoots each season.

Rosette: a flattened, circular cluster of leaves, usually at the base of the stem.

Serrate (of leaves): saw-toothed at the edge.

Simple (of leaves): not divided into leaflets.

Stamen: the male organ of a flower comprising anther (which contains pollen grains) and filament (the stalk below the anther).

Taproot: the main root, which grows vertically downwards with smaller lateral roots (e.g. carrot).

Terminal: at the end of a stem or branch.

Umbel: a flat-topped *inflorescence*.

Whorl: three or more flowers or leaves arranged in a ring.

GLOSSARY OF MEDICAL TERMS

Abortifacient: causes abortion.

Acute illness: of rapid onset, intense severity and brief duration (see also *Chronic illness*).

Adaptogenic: restores the body's ability to heal itself.

Alterative: formerly known as a 'blood cleanser'. Gradually restores the proper function of the body and increases health and vitality.

Anaemia: a deficiency in the number of red blood cells or in the quantity of oxygen-carrying haemoglobin in these cells.

Anaesthetic: reduces or eliminates sensation.

Analgesic (also anodyne): pain-relieving.

Anaphrodisiac: reduces sexual desire.

Androgen: a male sex *hormone* (e.g. testosterone) synthesised both in the testes and by cells in the cortex of the adrenals on top of the kidneys. Primarily responsible for male body-hair distribution and muscle development. Androgens are produced in the female body (by the adrenals), albeit in smaller quantities. Testosterone, e.g., is thought to influence the libido in both sexes.

Antibacterial: destroys bacteria.

Antibiotic: destroys or inhibits the growth of micro-organisms, especially bacteria.

Antidepressant: helps alleviate depression.

Antidote: a substance that counteracts a poison.

Antihaemorrhagic: prevents or arrests profuse internal or external bleeding.

Anti-infectious: prevents the spread of infection.

Anti-inflammatory: counteracts inflammation.

Antipyretic: see Febrifugal.

Antirheumatic: relieves rheumatism.

Antiseborrheic: controls the production of sebum, the oily secretion of skin.

Antiseptic: destroys micro-organisms.

Antispasmodic: prevents or eases spasms or cramp.

Antithrombotic: prevents or interferes with the formation of a blood clot (thrombus).

Antiviral: inhibits the proliferation of viruses.

Aperitif: stimulates the appetite.

Aphrodisiac: increases or stimulates sexual desire.

Astringent: causes contraction of the tissues and thus reduces secretions and discharges.

Carminative: stimulates the digestive system and relaxes the stomach, thereby preventing flatulence.

Cholagogic: stimulates the secretion and release of bile from the gall bladder into the duodenum.

Choloretic: stimulates the production of bile in the liver.

Chronic illness: of long duration, involving very slow changes. It does not usually resolve itself without some kind of healing intervention. See also *Acute illness*.

Cicatrisant: promotes healing by increasing the regeneration of skin cells and the formation of scar tissue.

Conjunctivitis: inflammation of the mucous membrane (conjunctiva) lining the inside of the eyelids.

Cytophylactic: increases the production of white blood cells (which help defend the body against infection).

Demulcent: soothes and protects irritated or inflamed internal tissue.

Deodorant: masks or removes unpleasant odours.

Diaphoretic (sudorific): increases or induces perspiration.

Digestive: aids the digestion of food.

Diuretic: increases the flow and excretion of urine.

Dropsy: swelling of a part of the body due to a build-up of fluid in the tissues; an obsolete term for oedema.

Emmenagogic: stimulates and/or normalises menstruation.

Emollient: soothes and softens the skin.

Endometriosis: a condition in which the tissue which forms the lining of the womb (the endometrium) grows outside the uterine cavity in other areas of the pelvis, often causing painful and/or heavy periods, sometimes infertility.

Endorphin (also encephalin, beta endorphin, casomorphin and dynorphin): a morphine-like family of molecules produced in the body cells, especially in parts of the brain and spinal cord. They block pain and elevate mood. Feelings of relaxation and/or joy raise the level of these 'happiness chemicals' which also stimulate our immune defences.

Expectorant: aids the removal of excess mucus (sputum) from the respiratory tract.

Febrifugal: reduces or combats fever.

Fibrositis: a general term for an aching condition of the muscles (also called muscular rheumatism).

Fungicidal: destroys fungi or inhibits their growth.

Galactagogic: increases the secretion of milk.

Gastric: pertaining to the stomach.

Genito-urinary: pertaining to the reproductive organs and urinary tract.

Haemostatic: arrests bleeding.

Hormone: according to the classical definition, a chemical secreted in the blood which acts on cells elsewhere in the body. However, the revised definition is a chemical secreted by body cells (including brain cells) which diffuses into the body fluids to act on other cells both near and distant (see also *Neurotransmitters*).

Hypoglycaemic: lowers blood sugar levels.

Hypnotic (soporific): promotes sleep.

Hypertensive: raises low blood pressure.

Hypotensive: lowers high blood pressure.

Laxative: promotes evacuation of the bowels.

ME: myalgic encephalomyelitis, also known as post-viral syndrome or chronic fatigue syndrome. Since a causative virus has never been found, many believe that it is not a condition as such, but a set of symptoms which can be produced by more than one causative factor. In all cases there is marked immune deficiency, resulting in depression, perpetual tiredness, debility and increased susceptibility to infectious illness.

Mucilaginous: substances with a gelatinous consistency, usually having demulcent and emollient properties.

Mucous membrane (mucosa): the moist membrane lining many body cavities and passages, including the respiratory and digestive tracts.

Mucus: a slimy protective secretion of the mucous membrane.

Narcotic: induces stupor and insensibility and relieves pain.

Nervine (also nervine tonic): tones and strengthens the nervous system.

Neurotransmitters (also neuro-hormones): Until recently, horomones were defined as substances which deliver their message to glands and neurotransmitters to nerves, but definitions are evolving. Neurotransmitters are now classified as brain hormones.

Neuralgia: a stabbing pain along the course of one or more nerves.

Oedema: fluid retention.

Oestrogen: a female hormone synthesised both in the ovaries and by cells in the cortex of the adrenal glands on top of the kidneys. Its role is to initiate the body's preparation for possible fertilisation and pregnancy. The hormone is also produced in lesser amounts (by the adrenals) in the male body, but its role is unclear.

Parturient: promotes and eases labour in childbirth.

Pheromone: a volatile hormone-like secretion, the subtle odour of which evokes a response in another member of the same species – often, but not exclusively, sexual.

Phlebitis: inflammation of the wall of a vein, commonly associated with thrombosis (clotting) within the vein.

Phytohormone (also phytosteroid): a plant substance with a similar chemical composition to certain hormones secreted by the human organism.

Precursor: a nutrient or biochemical required for the manufacture of a particular substance within the body (e.g. carrots contain the precursor substance carotene, which is converted in the body to vitamin A).

Progesterone: one of the female hormones synthesised both in the ovaries and in the cortex of the adrenal glands on top of the kidneys. Its function is to sustain the endometrium (the inner secretory lining of the womb) and to protect the fertilised ovum (egg) until about the third month of pregnancy.

Pulmonary: pertaining to the lungs.

Purgative: causes bowel evacuation, but more quickly and forcefully than a laxative.

Rubefacient: when rubbed into the skin, causes the superficial blood vessels (capillaries) to dilate, resulting in reddening of the skin.

Sciatica: a form of *neuralgia* causing intense pain along the sciatic nerve which extends from the buttocks to the foot.

Sedative: calms the nervous system and reduces stress.

Soporific: see *Hypnotic*.

Steroid: a biochemical compound derived from cholesterol – includes the sex hormones oestrogen, progesterone and testosterone.

Stimulant: increases physiological activity, especially of an organ.

Stomachic: stimulates digestive secretions in the stomach and improves appetite.

Testosterone: see *Androgen*.

Tonic: strengthens and enlivens either specific organs or the whole body.

Urticaria (hives): an allergic skin eruption not unlike that caused by nettles.

Uterine: pertaining to the uterus; a substance that strengthens and tones the uterus.

Vulnerary: aids the healing of wounds and cuts.

GENERAL GLOSSARY

Absolute: a highly concentrated aromatic material, usually captured by alcohol from the waxy *concrete*. The alcohol is then removed by means of vacuum distillation, leaving behind the viscous or semi-viscous absolute.

Allopathy: a method of treating disease by the use of drugs which induce in the body effects different (usually opposite) from those of the ailment, e.g. a laxative for constipation.

Aromatherapy: the therapeutic use of essential oils, with or without massage.

Aromatherapy oil: essential oil diluted in a vegetable base oil.

Concrete: a highly odoriferous, solid, waxy substance extracted from aromatic plant material by means of hydrocarbon-type solvents. The extraction process may continue in order to obtain an *absolute*.

Constitution: a person's overall state of health, including inherited tendencies.

Crude vegetable drug: plant material that has not undergone any material elaboration or separation into constituents.

Decoction: a herbal remedy extracted from fibrous plant material, such as roots, bark and seeds, by simmering in water.

Distillation: the process of evaporating a liquid and condensing its vapour, the classic method for obtaining essential oils.

Essential fatty acids: organic acids, including linoleic and linolenic acids, required by the body for health.

Essential oil (also aromatic oil, essence, ethereal oil, volatile oil): the odoriferous, volatile (i.e. evaporates in the open air) component of an aromatic plant, usually captured by steam distillation or *expression*.

Expression: a method employed for capturing the essential oils of citrus fruits. The oil in the outer skin is obtained by machines using centrifugal force.

FCF (furocoumarin-free); furocourmarins are sweet-smelling *phototoxic* substances found in a number of aromatic plants. Bergamot FCF, for example, has been *rectified* in order to remove the furocourmarin bergaptene.

Fixed oil: ordinary vegetable oil such as olive or corn which, unlike an essential oil, does not evaporate when left in the open air.

Flower essences: totally benign, unperfumed water/alcohol extractions of certain flowers. They are believed to emanate the vital healing force or vibratory pattern of the flowers from which they derive. Not to be confused with highly odoriferous essential oils (also known as essences) used in aromatherapy and perfumery.

Flower therapy: the use of flower essences to remedy imbalances within the psycho-spiritual aspect of our being.

Fractionated oil: an essential oil or vegetable oil which has had a fraction of its chemical components removed.

Herbal medicine (also herbalism, phytotherapy): the therapeutic use of crude vegetable drugs.

Holistic treatment (also constitutional treatment): the aim is to treat the whole person, body, mind and spirit, not just the presenting symptoms. It takes into account inherited tendencies, personal history, past medical treatment, individual attitude to the life experience and environmental factors. Treatment is geared to strengthening natural immunity and enhancing a general level of wellbeing.

Homeopathy (also homoeopathy): the treatment of disease by minute doses of drugs that in a healthy person would produce symptoms of the disease.

Infused oil (also herbal oil, macerated oil): plant material is placed in vegetable oil and gently heated until the aroma has permeated the oil. It is then strained and used as a massage oil for muscular aches and pains, or as a healing agent for skin complaints.

Oxidation: a process by which a substance is chemically combined with oxygen and its original structure is altered or destroyed.

Pharmacognosy: the science of drugs, especially relating to products in their natural or crude state.

Pharmacology: the science of the action of drugs on physiological processes.

Phototoxic: a substance which increases the skin's sensitivity to natural or simulated sunlight, sometimes resulting in unsightly pigmentation.

Phytotherapy: see *Herbal medicine*.

Psychoneuroimmunology (PNI): the science of the effects of thought and emotion upon the functioning of the body's immune defences.

Rectified oil: an essential oil which has been redistilled to remove impurities or a fraction of its chemical composition.

Synergy: agents working harmoniously together; the effect of the whole is greater than the sum of its separate parts.

Synthetic drug: the building of a chemical compound by the union of various chemical components, sometimes to mimic the actions of a natural drug ('nature identical'), or to produce a compound which cannot be found in nature. But so-called nature identical drugs always contain 'shadow' chemicals (an inevitable consequence of laboratory synthesis) which are not found in the crude drug.

Tincture: a herbal remedy or perfumery material obtained by macerating plant material in alcohol and water.

Xenoestrogens (also xenobiotics): the name given to environmental pollutants derived from petrochemicals, capable of disrupting biological processes.

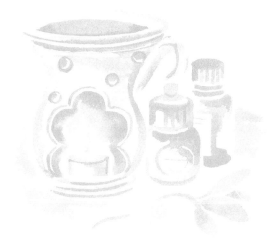

BIBLIOGRAPHY

BARNARD, J., *Collected Writings of Edward Bach*, Flower Remedy Programme, 1987

BARNARD, J., AND BARNARD, M., *The Healing Herbs of Edward Bach*, Ashgrove Press, 1995

BOERICKE, W., *Homoeopathic Material Medica*, Homoeopathic Book Services, 1995

BONAR, A., *Gardening for Fragrance*, Ward Lock, 1990

BONAR, A., *Herbs – A Complete Guide to Their Cultivation and Use*, Tiger Books, 1996

BECKETT, K., AND BECKETT, G., *Planting Native Trees and Shrubs*, Jarrold, 1976

BRUNTON, N., *Homeopathy*, Optima, 1989

BUNNY, S. (ed.), *The Illustrated Book of Herbs*, Octopus, 1984

CAINER, J., AND RIDER, C., *The Psychic Explorer*, Piatkus, 1986

CASTRO, A., *The Complete Homeopathy Handbook*, Macmillan, 1990

COLEMAN, V., *Life without Tranquillisers*, Piatkus, 1985

COLES, W., *The Art of Simpling*, 1657

COLLINGS, J., *Life Forces*, New English Library, 1985

COOMBES, A.J., *A–Z of Plant Names*, Hamlyn, 1994

CULPEPER, N., *Culpeper's Complete Herbal*, Bloomsbury Books, 1992

DUFF, G., *Natural Fragrances*, Sidgwick & Jackson, 1989

EVERARD, B., *Wild Flowers of the World*, Rainbow Books, 1970

FENTON, S., *Moon Signs*, Thorsons, 1987

FISHER, R.B., *A Dictionary of Body Chemistry*, Paladin, 1983

FREETHY, R., *Woodlands of Great Britain*, Bell & Hyman, 1986

GATTEFOSSÉ, R. (ed. Robert Tisserand), *Gattefossé's Aromatherapy*, C.W. Daniel, 1993

GENDERS, R., *The Scented Wild Flowers of Great Britain*, Collins, 1971

GENDERS, R., *Herbs for Health and Beauty*, Robert Hale, 1975

GERBER, R., *Vibrational Medicine*, Bear & Co. (USA), 1988

GOLDER, C., *Moon Signs for Lovers*, Piatkus, 1992

GOODRICK-CLARKE, N. *Paracelsus – Essential Readings*, Crucible, 1990

GREENISH, H.G., *The Text Book of Pharmacognosy*, Churchill, 1933

GREGORY, P.L. (ed.), *The Oxford Companion to the Mind*, Oxford University Press, 1982

GRIEVES, M., *A Modern Herbal*, Penguin, 1982

GRIGGS, B., *The Green Pharmacy*, Jill Norman & Hobhouse, 1981

GROSS, R.D., *Psychology*, Hodder & Stoughton, 1987

HARVEY, C., AND COCHRANE, A., *The Encyclopaedia of Flower Remedies*, Thorsons, 1995

HAY, R. (ed.), *Reader's Digest Encyclopaedia of Garden Plants*, Reader's Digest, 1978

HILLIER, E., *Hillier's Manual of Trees and Shrubs*, David & Charles, 1989

HOFFMANN, D., *Welsh Herbal Medicine*, Abercastle Publications, 1978

HOFFMANN, D., *The New Holistic Herbal*, Element, 1991

HOPE, M., *The Psychology of Healing*, Element, 1989

HOWARD, M., *Traditional Folk Remedies*, Century, 1987

INGLIS, B., *Natural Medicine*, Collins, 1979

JOHNSON, A.T., AND SMITH, H.A., *Plant Names Simplified*, Collingridge, 1931

KAPLAN-WILLIAMS, S., *The Elements of Dreamwork*, Element, 1990

KENTON, L., *Passage to Power*, Vermilion, 1996

KIMINSKI, P., AND KATZ, R., *Flower Essence Repertory*, Flower Essence Society (USA), 1992

LAWLESS, J., *The Encyclopaedia of Essential Oils*, Element, 1992

MABEY, R. (ed.), *The Complete New Herbal*, Penguin, 1988

MAURY, M., *Marguerite Maury's Guide to Aromatherapy*, C.W. Daniel, 1989

McCLINTOCK, D., AND FITTER, R.S.R., *The Pocket Guide to Wildflowers*, Collins, 1975

McINTYRE, A., *The Complete Floral Healer*, Gaia, 1996

McINTYRE, M., *Herbal Medicine for Everyone*, Arcana (Penguin), 1988

MARKHAM, U., *Women Under Pressure*, Element, 1990

MESSEGUE, M., *Health Secrets of Plants and Herbs*, Pan, 1979

MILNER, J.E., *The Tree Book*, Acacia Publications, 1992

MINTER, S., *The Healing Garden*, Headline, 1993

NICHOLS, R., *The Book of Druidry*, Aquarian, 1990

PALAISEUL, J., *Grandmother's Secrets*, Penguin, 1973

PHILLIPS, R., *Trees in Britain, Europe and North America*, Pan, 1981

PODLECH, D., *Herbs and Healing Plants*, Collins, 1996

RYMAN, D., *Aromatherapy – The Encyclopedia of Plants and Oils and How They Can Help You*, Piatkus, 1991

SCHEFFER, M., *Bach Flower Therapy*, Thorsons, 1986

SCOTT, J., *Natural Medicine for Children*, Unwin Hyman, 1990

STRETHLOW, W., AND HERTZA, G., *Hildegard of Bingen's Medicine*, Bear & Co. (USA), 1988

SUTTON, D., *Larousse Pocket Guide – Wild Flowers of Britain and Northern Europe*, Larousse, 1995

VALNET, J., *The Practice of Aromatherapy*, C.W. Daniel, 1982

VAN TOLLER, S. AND DODD, G.H. (eds), *The Psychology and Biology of Fragrance*, Chapman & Hall, 1991

WATTS, G., *Pleasing the Patient*, Faber & Faber, 1992

WEEKS, N., *The Medical Discoveries of Edward Bach*, C.W. Daniel, 1973

WEEKS, N., AND BULLEN, V., *The Bach Flower Remedies – Illustrations and Preparations*, C.W. Daniel, 1994

WEINER, M., *Maximum Immunity*, Gateway, 1986

WESTLAKE, A.T., *The Pattern of Health*, Element, 1985

WILDWOOD, C., *Create Your Own Perfumes*, Piatkus, 1994

WILDWOOD, C., *Flower Remedies*, Element, 1995

WILDWOOD, C., *The Bloomsbury Encyclopedia of Aromatherapy*, Bloomsbury, 1996

WILDWOOD, C., *The Complete Guide to Reducing Stress*, Piatkus, 1997

WINTER, R., *The Smell Book*, Lippincott (USA), 1976

WOODWARD, M. (ed.), *Gerard's Herbal*, Senate, 1994

SUGGESTED READING

AROMATHERAPY AND HOLISTIC HEALING

WILDWOOD, C., *The Bloomsbury Encyclopedia of Aromatherapy*, Bloomsbury, 1996

WILDWOOD, C., *The Complete Guide to Reducing Stress*, Piatkus, 1997

HERBAL MEDICINE

HOFFMANN, D., *The New Holistic Herbal*, Element, 1991

MABEY, R. (ed.), *The Complete New Herbal*, Penguin, 1988

FLOWER THERAPY

HARVEY, C., AND COCHRANE, A., *The Encyclopaedia of Flower Remedies*, Thorsons, 1995

WILDWOOD, C., *Flower Remedies*, Element, 1995

ORGANIC HERB GARDENING AND WILD FLOWER CULTIVATION

BAINES, C., *How to Make A Wildlife Garden*, Elm Tree Books, 1985

BONAR, A., *Herbs – A Complete Guide to Their Cultivation and Use*, Tiger Books, 1996

HAMILTON, G., *Successful Organic Gardening*, Dorling Kindersley, 1989

MCINTYRE, A., *The Apothecary's Garden*, Piatkus, 1997

USEFUL ADDRESSES

UNITED KINGDOM

AROMATHERAPY

For a list of accredited suppliers of essential oils contact:

The Secretary,
The Essential Oil Trade Association
61 Clinton Lane
Kenilworth
Warwickshire
CV8 1AS
Tel: 01926 55980

If you would prefer to use certified organic essential oils, please contact:

Chrissie Wildwood
Florial UK
Tel: 01497 847002

To obtain rose oil captured by the new Phytonics process (as described on page 38) contact:

Dr Peter Wilde
91 Front Street
Sowerby
Thirsk
YO7 1JP

For lists of accredited aromatherapists and training courses:

International Federation of Aromatherapists
Stamford House
2–4 Chiswick High Road
London W4 1TH

The Register of Qualified Aromatherapists
PO Box 6941
London N8 9HF
Tel: 0181 341 2958

International Society of Professional Aromatherapists
41 Leicester Road
Hinckley
Leicestershire
LE10 1LW
Tel: 01455 633231

For lists of accredited aromatherapy training courses and general information:

The Aromatherapy Organisations Council
3 Latymer Close
Braybrooke
Market Harborough
Leicestershire
LE10 1LW
Tel: 01858 434242

For up-to-the-minute information, you may wish to subscribe to the longest-running aromatherapy magazine which is read in over fifty countries:

Aromatherapy Quarterly
5 Ranelagh Avenue
London SW13 0BY
Tel/fax: 0181 392 1691

HERBAL MEDICINE

The following three companies are mail order suppliers of high-quality herbs and tinctures. Malcolm Simmonds also supplies hormone-free herbal formulas for women's problems.

Malcolm Simmonds Herbal Suppliers
3 Burton Villas
Hove
West Sussex
BN3 6FN
Tel: 01273 202 401

The following company has a wide selection of organically grown herbs:

Hambleden Herbs
Court Farm
Milverton
Somerset
TA4 1NF
Tel: 01823 401205

The following company has a wide selection of herbs, tinctures, essential oils, infused oils and other related products. Many of their herbs and some of their essential oils are certified organic.

Neal's Yard Remedies
2 Neal's Yard
Covent Garden
London WC2H 9DP
Tel: 0171 379 7222

For lists of registered medical herbalists and information about training courses:

The National Institute of Medical Herbalists
56 Longbrook Street
Exeter
Devon
EX4 6AH
Tel: 01392 426022

FLOWER THERAPY

Mail order suppliers of Bach flower remedies:

Nelsons Homeopathic Pharmacy
73 Duke Street
Grosvenor Square
London W1M 8DR
Tel: 0171 629 3118

Bach flower remedies are also available from Boots the chemist, most health food stores and many independent pharmacies.

For lists of registered Bach flower remedy practitioners and information about training programmes, please write enclosing a stamped addressed envelope to:

Dr Edward Bach Centre
Mount Vernon
Sotwell
Wallingford
Oxfordshire
OX10 0PZ
Tel: 01491 834678

Flower remedies and training courses: the organisation below has no connection with the Bach Centre in Oxfordshire, but their exceptionally vibrant flower remedies are prepared in accordance with the traditional methods advocated by Dr Bach. The remedies can also be found in many health food stores and pharmacies.

Healing Herbs – The Flower Remedy Programme
PO Box 65
Hereford
HR2 0UW
Tel: 01873 890218

For a comprehensive catalogue of flower essences from around the world, including those explored in this book, contact:

Flower and Gem Remedy Association
Suite 1
Castle Farm
Clifton Road
Deddington
Oxfordshire
OX15 0TP
Tel: 01869 337349

For a two-year professional training course in flower therapy, employing flower essences from all around the world:

Clare Harvey
Middle Piccadilly Natural Healing Centre
Holwell
Nr Sherborne
Dorset
DT9 5LW
Tel: 01963 23468/23774

HOMEOPATHY

Mail order suppliers of homeopathic remedies and organic herbal preparations:

Weleda (UK) Ltd
Heanor Road
Ilkeston
Derbyshire
DE7 8DR
Tel: 0115 944 8200

For lists of registered homeopathic practitioners, please write enclosing a large stamped addressed envelope to:

The Society of Homoeopaths
2 Artizan Road
Northampton
NN1 4HU
Tel: 01604 21400

The organisation below also offers an information pack on how to obtain homeopathic treatment on the NHS.

The Homoeopathic Society
Hahnemann House
2 Powis Place
London WC1N 3HT
Tel: 0171 837 9469

NUTRITIONAL THERAPY

For general information and consultations.

The Institute for Optimum Nutrition
34 Wadham Road
London SW15 2LR
Tel: 0181 871 2949

The organisation below also offers home study courses and a Nutrition Consultant's Diploma course.

Higher Nature Ltd
The Nutrition Centre
Burwash Common
East Sussex
TN19 7LX
Tel: 01495 883 880

The organisation below offers low-cost nutritional consultation by post and telephone for women who suffer from PMS or menopausal difficulties.

Women's Nutritional Advisory Service
PO Box 268
Lewes
East Sussex
BN7 2QN
Tel: 01273 487 366

FULL-SPECTRUM LIGHTING

Unit 1
Riverside Business Centre
Victoria Street
High Wycombe
Bucks
HP11 2LT

MUSIC FOR RELAXATION

New World Music Ltd
Becks Green
St. Andrews
Nr. Beccles
Suffolk NR34 8NB
Tel: 01986 781682
Fax: 01986 781645

UNITED STATES

AROMATHERAPY AND HERBAL MEDICINE

For essential oils, aromatherapy products and information:

Aroma Vera Inc.
PO Box 3609
Culver City
California 90231
Tel: 310-280-0395

For essential oils, infused oils, herbs and other botanic preparations, many of which are certified organic:

Neal's Yard USA
284 Connecticut Street
San Francisco
California 94107

For lists of accredited aromatherapists and training schools, please write enclosing a stamped addressed envelope to:

American Society for Phytotherapy and Aromatherapy
PO Box 3679
South Pasadena
California 91031

National Association for Holistic Aromatherapy
PO Box 17622
Boulder
Colorado 80308

For lists of fully accredited medical herbalists and information about training programmes:

American Botanical Council and Herb Research Foundation
PO Box 201660
Austin
Texas 78720

Californian School of Herbal Studies
9309 HWY 116
Forestville
California 95436

For up-to-the-minute information on aromatherapy, you may wish to subscribe to the following leading magazine:

Aromatherapy Quarterly
PO Box 421
Inverness
California 94937-0421
Tel/fax: 1 (415) 663 9519

FLOWER THERAPY

For flower essences and information about professional training: The organisation below supplies the FES Quintessentials flower essences. It is also the North American distributor for the Healing Herbs line of flower remedies (see UK listing), prepared using the traditional methods advocated by Dr Edward Bach.

Flower Essence Services
PO Box 1769
Nevada City
California 95959
Tel: 916-265-9163

Suppliers of other American flower essences mentioned in this book:

Master's Flower Essences
14618 Tyler Foot Road
Nevada City
California 95959
Tel: 916-292-3345

AUSTRALIA

AROMATHERAPY

For essential oils and aromatherapy courses:

Essential Therapeutics
58 Easey Street
Collingwood
Victoria 3066

House of Pan
PTY Ltd
PO Box 187
Montrose
Victoria 3765

In Essence Aromatherapy
3 Abbot Street
Fairfield
Victoria 3078

For lists of accredited aromatherapists and information about training courses, please write enclosing a stamped addressed envelope to:

International Federation of Aromatherapists
1st Floor
390 Burwood Road
Hawthorn
Victoria 3122

HERBAL MEDICINE

For herbs and essential oils:

Mediherb Pty Ltd
124 McEvoy Street
Warwick
Queensland

Nonesuch Botanicals Pty Ltd
PO Box 68
Mt Evelyn
Victoria 3796

FLOWER THERAPY

For Bach flower remedies:

Martin & Pleasance Wholesale Pty Ltd
PO Box 4
Collingwood
Victoria 3066

Suppliers of the Bush Flower Essences and information about training:

Bush Flower Essences
8a Oaks Avenue
Dee Why
NSW 2099
Tel: 02 972 1033

GENERAL INDEX

INDEX OF HEALING PLANTS

Page numbers in bold denote plant illustrations